THE MOST EFFECTIVE
WAYS TO Live
LONGER

REVISED EDITION

THE MOST EFFECTIVE WAYS TO Live LONGER

REVISED EDITION

THE SURPRISING, UNBIASED TRUTH ABOUT WHAT YOU SHOULD DO TO PREVENT DISEASE, FEEL GREAT, AND HAVE OPTIMUM HEALTH AND LONGEVITY

Jonny Bowden, Ph.D., C.N.S.

with Beth Traylor, M.D., FAAFP

FAIR WINDS

The secret to a long life, from Frank Buckles, 110, the longest surviving veteran of World War I: "When you start to die, don't."

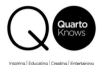

Brimming with creative inspiration, how-to projects, and useful information to enrich your everyday life, Quarto Knows is a favorite destination for those pursuing their interests and passions. Visit our site and dig deeper with our books into your area of interest: Quarto Creates, Quarto Cooks, Quarto Homes, Quarto Lives, Quarto Drives, Quarto Explores, Quarto Gifts, or Quarto Kids.

First Published in 2010 by Fair Winds Press, an imprint of The Quarto Group, 100 Cummings Center, Suite 265-D, Beverly, MA 01915, USA.
T (978) 282-9590 F (978) 283-2742 QuartoKnows.com

Fair Winds Press titles are also available at discount for retail, wholesale, promotional, and bulk purchase. For details, contact the Special Sales Manager by email at specialsales@quarto.com or by mail at The Quarto Group, Attn: Special Sales Manager, 100 Cummings Center, Suite 265-D, Beverly, MA 01915, USA.

23 22 21 20 19   1 2 3 4 5

ISBN: 978-1-59233-862-7

Digital edition published in 2019
eISBN: 978-1-63159-650-6

Originally found under the following Library of Congress Cataloging-in-Publication Data
Bowden, Jonny.
  The most effective ways to live longer: the surprising, unbiased truth about what you should do to prevent disease, feel great, and have optimum health and longevity / Jonny Bowden.
     p. cm.
Includes bibliographical references and index.
ISBN-13: 978-1-59233-340-0
ISBN-10: 1-59233-340-0
1. Dietary supplements. 2. Longevity. 3. Health. I. Title.
RM258.5.B695 2010
613.2—dc22
2009031146

Design: The Quarto Group
Cover Image: Shutterstock
Page Layout: Megan Jones Design
Photography and illustration: istock, fotolia, and Shutterstock except illustrations on pages 94–95 by Robert Brandt and images on pages 141–143 by Jack Deutsch
Printed in China

The information in this book is for educational purposes only. It is not intended to replace the advice of a physician or medical practitioner. Please see your health care provider before beginning any new health program.

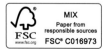

For Logan Elliot Gilman

Born November 1, 2018, the day this manuscript was being submitted, a few days before my 72nd birthday.

Here's my wish for you:

When you reach 72, may you feel as healthy, lucky in life, madly in love, and looking forward to the future as I do right now.

I love you, Logan!

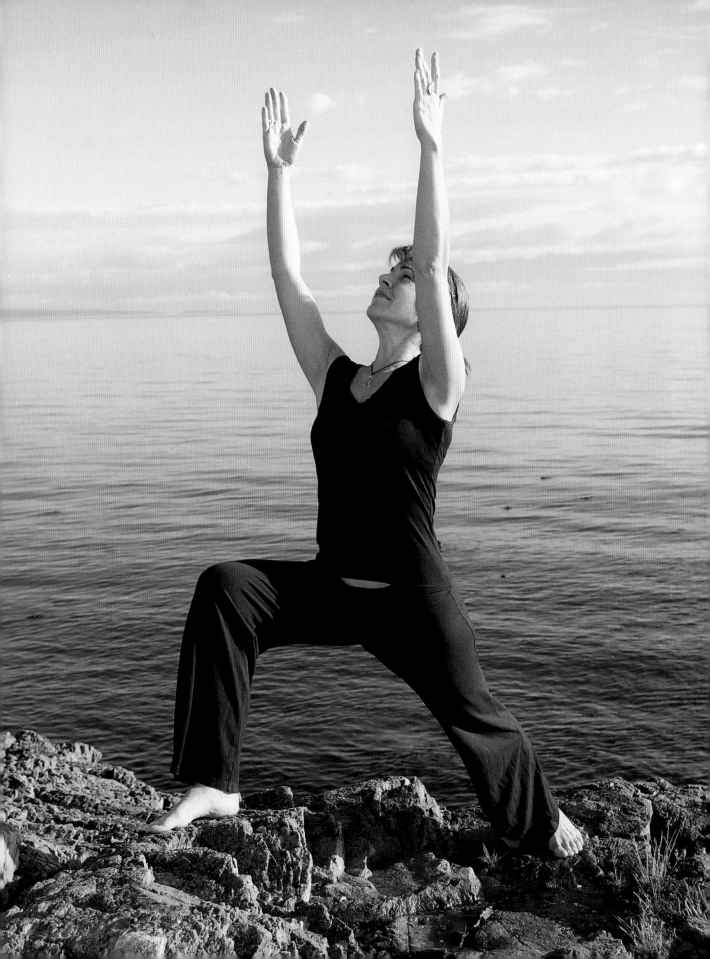

Contents

INTRO

Read This First!

So here's the thing that's true of most of my books: They were meant to be used, not read.

Let me explain.

With the possible exception of *The Great Cholesterol Myth*, none of my books needs to be read sequentially, and this one is no exception. I designed them all to be dipped into, sampled, used as a reference, and studied when needed. If you're browsing through *The 150 Healthiest Foods on Earth* and you're interested in finding out about jicama, there's no need to read about avocados first, you can just jump to the relevant page.

This method has one big advantage and one (small) disadvantage.

The big advantage is that you can read what you're interested in and it will be complete in and of itself. If your immediate challenge is your immune system, jump right to chapter 10, and if you're immediate challenge is heart disease, go to chapter 7.

The disadvantage is that there is, of necessity, some repetition. For example, omega-3 fats (fish oil) are incredibly important for the brain, the heart, the bones, and the muscles. They're also vital for quenching inflammation—one of what we call "the four Horsemen of aging." So you'll read about omega-3s in many different places in the book. In my opinion, this is a small price to pay for having the information you need for any given situation available to you right there without having to read a bunch of stuff you're not interested in.

And for those of you who *do* like to read through a book from chapter one through the end, I've tried to make the information sufficiently varied so that you'll keep learning something new. And if you're already an expert on any topic that's mentioned multiple times in the book, well then, just skip that section!

Upon entering medical school, every new student hears a variation of the statement, "Fifty percent of what we are about to teach you in the next four years is wrong—the problem is, we don't know what 50 percent that is." The same might be said for any book that purports to sum up what we "know" about any field (except maybe physics). Much of it is going to turn out to be wrong. We just don't know what.

We're pretty sure the same is true with this book.

I wrote the original version of this book alone back in 2008. When I was asked to do a revised and updated edition, I suggested to the publishers that the new version have a medical doctor as a co-author. The person I most wanted for a writing partner on this particular project was Dr. Beth Traylor. Dr. Traylor—in addition to being an expert on age-management medicine—happens to be my personal physician and has been for more than a decade. She's my go-to source for anything having to do with anti-aging. And fortunately for both me and you, she is indeed the co-author on the volume you are now holding.

Together, we've gone over all the stuff that was originally included, removed anything that is no longer relevant, and added much new material to bring the book totally up to date. But we were both pleasantly surprised to find how much of the original was true today and has been confirmed by even more research since the original publication. The finding that saturated fat is not a cause of heart disease is a great example.

It's still as true as it was back in 2008 that five basic lifestyle interventions can prevent about 80 percent of heart disease, but we now know that there are a couple of other interventions that may work just as well. You'll hear about all seven of them many times in this book. You'll also learn what the latest research shows about what we call

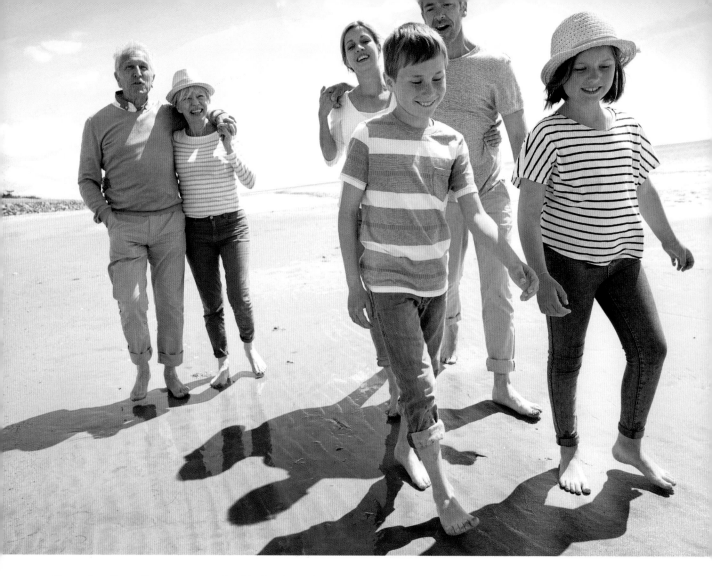

"the eight pillars of longevity—gut health, food, supplements, detoxification, exercise, sleep, stress reduction, and social relationships—and what you can do to maximize each of them. And, of course, you'll learn what the dreaded "Four Horsemen of Aging" are and how to tame them. (Spoiler alert—the "Four Horsemen of Aging" [inflammation, oxidation, stress, and sugar] are the same four promoters of heart disease we identified in *The Great Cholesterol Myth*. In fact, those same "Four Horsemen of Aging" promote, amplify, or make worse just about every degenerative disease ever seen on the planet, including heart disease, Alzheimer's, cancer, obesity, and diabetes.)

And one more thing. To make this book as user-friendly as possible, we've included a kind of "quick start guide" at the end of the book. While we're hoping you'll read this book in its entirety, we didn't want to make it a prerequisite for improving your health. So the "CliffsNotes" section is for those of you who just want to get started. If that's you, feel free to jump right to chapter 12 (page 206) and begin implementing the suggestions. If and when you want to know why we recommend, just go back and read the relevant theory and research earlier in the book.

Finally, a word about our recommendations throughout this book—and it's a word no one in the scientific community likes to use: guesswork.

The truth of the matter is that while we have terrific science on a lot of things at the molecular level, at some point, you just have to make educated guesses. It's extremely rare that we get a good, randomized, double blinded study on a combination of specific supplements at specific doses. Any good experienced health professional or health consumer is going to have to essentially guess what makes sense to use with what. If I have good evidence that compound A is anti-inflammatory and compound B is anti-inflammatory, it might be an untested leap of faith to assume that using them in combination is a good thing, but it's a darn good guess and sometimes that's all we have.

Speaking of recommendations, we've made a lot of them. But they're not meant to be taken as some kind of orthodoxy. They're meant to be starting points. You may not decide it's worth it to take all the supplements we recommend for the brain, for example, especially when you've got a bunch of things you want to take for the heart. That's fine. Look to see what overlaps. Do some research on your own. Try some things and discard others—see what works for you (and what doesn't seem to).

My motto for all things in life is based on the acronym AIM: Assess, Investigate, and Modify.[1] Assess what you're doing and how it's working for you. Investigate what modifications you could make to make it more effective (or simpler). Then, if necessary, modify what you're doing.

Rinse and repeat for life.

Stay engaged, participate, remain curious and open, discover what's really important to you, and then do more

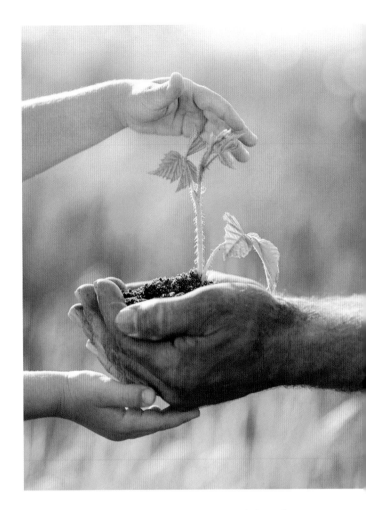

of it. You're only as old as you feel you are, and if you do even 50 percent of what we recommend in this book, you should feel a lot less "old" after you finish this book than you did before you started reading.

Enjoy the journey.

—Dr. Jonny Bowden/Los Angeles, California/2018

---

1   Thank you, Dr. Jade Teta

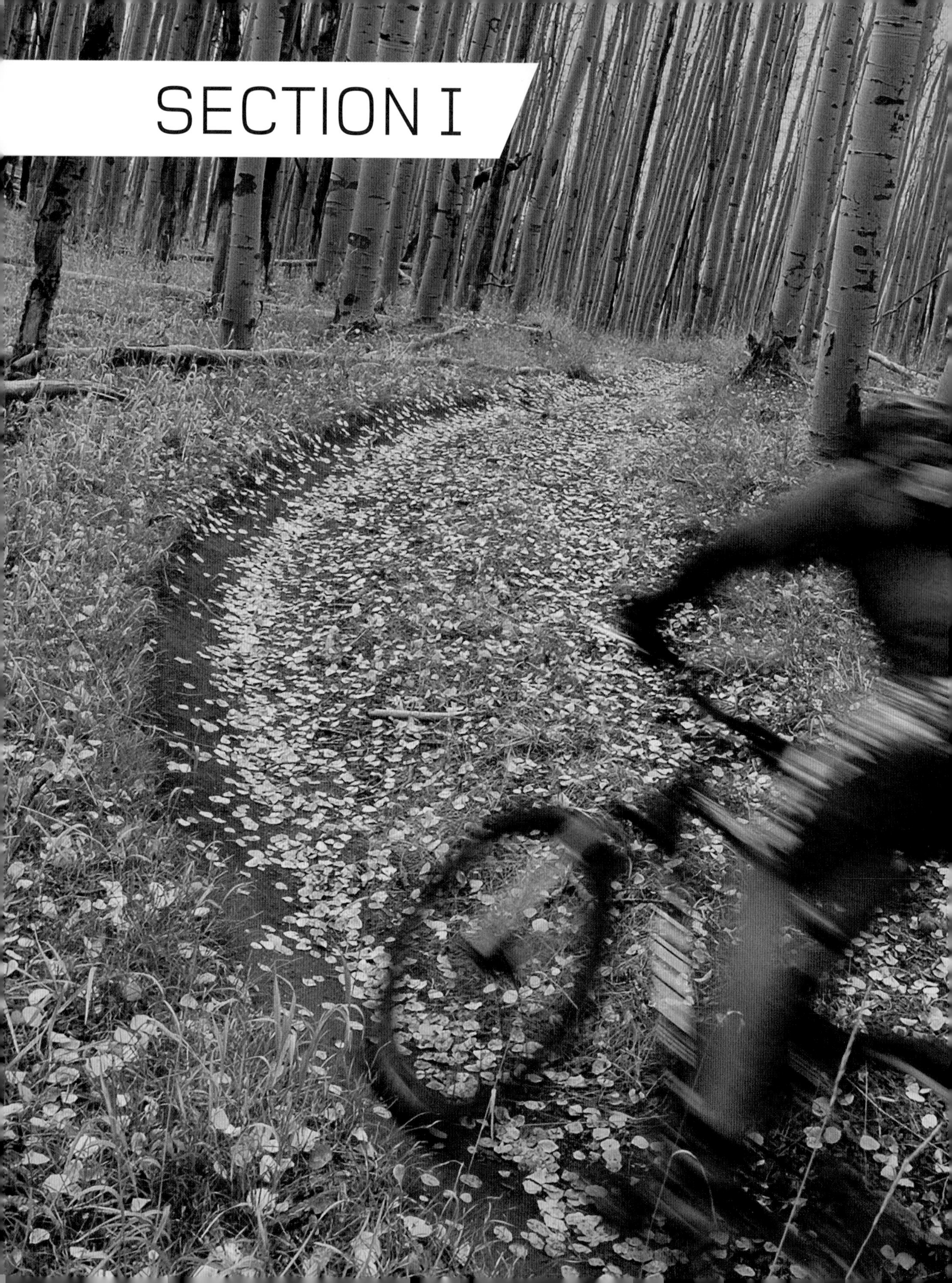

Rein in the Four Horsemen of Aging

....

Don Wildman is a personal trainer who lives in Malibu, California. Which is kind of like saying, "Babe Ruth is a baseball player from New York."

Wildman has completed the Ironman triathlon nine times; the Aspen, Colorado, downhill ski race; a three-thousand-mile bike race called the "Race Across America"; and the Los Angeles and New York City marathons. In his spare time, he snowboards the Alaskan backcountry and competes in sailing events—he's in the record books for winning all three of the Chicago Yacht Club's Mackinac races in a single season.

At his private gym in Paradise Cove, California, he leads a legendary workout known as "The Circuit," which features more than 3,000— yes, *thousand*—repetitions of weight lifting mixed with abdominal and balancing exercises. Participants cycle through twenty multipart exercises six times. There's only one rule: You can't stop until it's done. Not surprisingly, few people can do it, so classes are small. Those who do manage to finish it can barely drive home afterward—Wildman usually spends the rest of the day mountain biking.

By the way, he's an avid snow boarder and surfer and is considered a world-class sailor.

Oh, one more thing. Don Wildman is, as of this writing, seventy-eight years old.

ACTIVE AND AGING

Maybe you don't aspire to be exactly like Don, and truth be told, few of us could, even if we wanted to. But Don Wildman is one of the thousands of people who are changing the way we look at aging. They're showing us what's possible. And they're demonstrating, time and again, that aging doesn't have to be what it looked like back in your grandmother's day.

There are shepherds in their seventies who right now climb punishing hills each day in Sardinia and glow with good health. There are folks in Okinawa who tend vegetable gardens and hoe fields well into their nineties. Explorer and writer Dan Buettner recently met a lovely hundred-year-old woman named Panchita in the Nicoya peninsula off Costa Rica, who spends her days cooking, splitting logs, and clearing brush with a machete. He wrote about her and her eighty-year-old son Tommy, who bicycles to see her every day, in his book, *The Blue Zones.* Closer to home, Thomas Perls, M.D., director of the New England Centenarian Study, told *Time* magazine about a man who was repairing roofs in his nineties (he lived to be 103 years old).

There are countless other examples. At ninety-six, Bill Finch was a champion badminton player and the world record holder for the 1,500-meter (1,640 yd) run among ninety-five- to ninety-nine-year-olds. Astonishingly, they have enough athletes in that age group to create an entire competitive class of runners. He continued dating well into his mid-nineties. And when the first edition of this book was going to press, the mountain climbing world was all in a dither as professional climbers all over the globe vied for the privilege of accompanying legendary mountain climber Fred Beckey, who, at age eighty-five, was about to depart for uncharted territories in Northern Spain.

More recently, the fashion world was all adither when a shirtless model named Wang Deshun walked the runway during fashion week in Bejing. Deshun, who is 80, has a body most 25-year-old men would kill for, causing news outlets to run stories with the title, "80-year old model reshapes China's views on aging."

WHAT AGING WELL LOOKS LIKE

So maybe you don't aspire to be an elite runner at ninety, or the world's fittest man at seventy-eight, or conquering mountains at eighty-five. But I'm betting you wouldn't be reading this book if you weren't interested in living long and living vigorously. Think about it: Would you like to

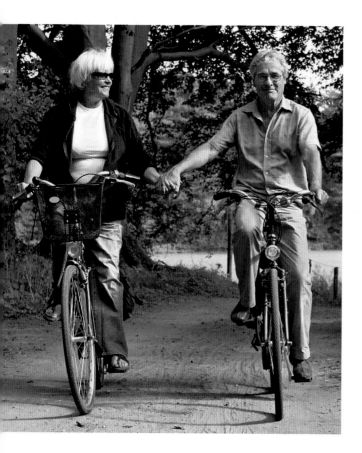

wake up in the morning with energy and enthusiasm, with all your faculties intact, able to take care of yourself physically, and free of any major aches, pains, and disabilities? Would you like to live well into your nineties feeling basically happy, content, fulfilled, and healthy?

Let me guess: The answer is "yes."

And here's the thing: It's totally possible.

There's been a major paradigm shift in the study of aging and longevity. By observing societies that have unusual numbers of centenarians, we've been able to discover patterns associated with long life and good health. By experimenting in the lab, we've been able to discover the genes that have an impact on life and health (see sirtuin genes chapter 5) and what you can do to "turn those genes on" (more on that later). Scientists now have a pretty good idea of what behaviors are linked to longevity and why. And there's a ton of research showing just what people actually die of and what factors influence those deaths.

Take, for example, the ten top causes of death in the United States. Heart disease, cancer, and stroke top the list, and those three diseases—out of the more than 100,000 diseases listed in the World Health Organization's *International Statistical Classification of Diseases and Related Health Problems*—account for a whopping 60 percent of the deaths in the United States! Genetics are a factor in about 10 percent of your risk for heart disease, while lifestyle choices contribute to the other 90 percent! The two single biggest culprits when it comes to causing cancer are diet and tobacco, according to a 1981 landmark study in the *Journal of the National Cancer Institute*—and that's as true today as it was then. One 1996 study from the Harvard School of Public Health attributed a full 30 percent of cancer deaths specifically to diet (the same percentage attributed to smoking)! Ten years later, a study

in *JAMA* found essentially the same thing: 28.6 percent of all cancer deaths attributable to smoking. And data from the National Cancer Institute suggests that the percentage of cancer cases in which diet and lifestyle play major roles ranges from 35 percent to an unbelievable 60 percent!

Then there's diabetes, which comes in at number six on the top ten list. And diabetes—and its relative, metabolic syndrome (or prediabetes)—puts you at enormous risk for heart disease. As many as 80 percent of diabetics die from vascular problems like stroke or heart disease. As you'll learn in this book, diabetes is *almost 100 percent preventable, or reversible*, if you make the right lifestyle choices. Which, by the way, are not all that difficult.

We've been conditioned to believe our fate is determined by our genes or by factors outside of our control. And we've also been taught—subtly and overtly—that there's a pill for everything that ails us. The result is that collectively, we've spent a lot less time worrying about the factors we can't control and not paying enough attention to the ones that we can. Ironically, the factors we can control turn out to make the most difference.

Your health is mostly in your hands, and that may seem scary at first but I hope you'll come to see it as empowering.

In a 2016 paper entitled "Genetic Factors Are Not the Major Causes of Chronic Diseases," Stephen Rappaport, Ph.D.—a Professor of Environmental Health Sciences at Berkeley School of Public Health and the Director of the Berkeley Center for Exposure Biology—argued that a whopping 84 percent of the risk of chronic disease is not genetic at all. Rather, he argues, it's environmental and behavioral.

Rappaport—and other researchers—refer to the cumulative environmental and behavioral "exposures" over the course of a life—as the "exposome." The exposome is to the environment what the geonome is to genetics—only it's way more important. It's every single thing *other than genetics* that influences your health. The exposome is basically everything that happens to you in your lifetime, beginning at conception.

Just to be clear on definitions, an "exposure" isn't sitting next to someone on an airplane who has the flu. An "exposure" is anything at all from environment, diet, lifestyle, stressful occupations, exercise, stress, alcohol, tobacco, mercury exposure, nutritional supplements, prescription drugs, dancing the mambo, you name it—everything, Researchers who study the exposome want to understand how each of these "influencers" (i.e., diet, exercise, lifestyle) interact with our own characteristics such as physiology, metabolism, and genetics.

Why is this so important? Well, it's hard to sum it up better than the paragraph below from the CDC's website, "Exposome and Exposomics," entitled, Why Should We Study the Exposome?

If genetics only turns out to account for 10 percent of diseases, we better start learning what accounts for the other 90 percent. And researchers have been pouring over epidemiological data for decades looking for the answer.

One of the promises of the human genome project was that it could revolutionize our understanding of the underlying causes of disease and aid in the development of preventions and cures for more diseases. **Unfortunately, genetics has been found to account for only about 10% of diseases,** and the remaining causes appear to be from environmental causes. So to understand the causes and eventually the prevention of disease, environmental causes need to be studied.

EPIDEMIOLOGY: THE REDHEADED STEPSISTER OF SCIENCE

It's important to understand that epidemiological studies are observational, not interventional. They don't give half the people in the study a drug and half a placebo and then see how they're doing after six months—that's an experimental (clinical) study. Epidemiological studies are about *watching* people, not doing things to them. Researchers look at data on thousands of individuals over many years—what they eat, if they smoke, how and when they exercise, etc. Then, they compare the individuals who got sick and/or died during the course of the follow-up with those who are still alive and healthy. In these kinds of studies, researchers are searching for any differences in behavior patterns that might shed light on why some folks do relatively well and some folks wind up dead.

A caution, though, before we proceed. Epidemiological evidence may show that two things are found together in the environment—for example, raindrops and umbrellas—but it does *not* prove that one *caused* the other. Still, when two variables (rainbows and umbrellas, or vegetable eating and healthy arteries) show up at the same time, in multiple observational studies, over and over and over again, it's a good bet that there's a connection of some kind worth exploring.

There have been a number of large studies that collected massive amounts of data on a large amount of participants over multiple years, sometimes for decades. As you can imagine, this has been a goldmine for discovering associations of all kinds (i.e., lack of vitamin D and rickets). And I'll cut to the chase: In study after study after study, five behaviors have consistently and reliably shown a clear and positive association with good health and long life.

1. Not smoking
2. Exercising[1]
3. Maintaining a "healthy" weight[2]
4. Eating a healthy diet[3]
5. Consuming alcohol in moderation *or* not at all.[4]

In addition to those five core behaviors, a couple of additional behaviors have also been connected with longer and healthier lives. One is sleeping 7 to 9 hours a night, a subject we'll get into more later on. The other is having strong supportive relationships.

This last one can't be overemphasized. The people living in the Blue Zones—five areas around the globe that have been found to have the highest concentrations of healthy centenarians—don't all eat the same food or exercise the same way or share the same religion. But all have one thing in common: strong social networks with active engagement. It's one of the best and most consistent predictors of longevity. Ironically, though strong social networks probably make the most difference, it's a factor we tend to focus on the least when we're talking about improving our health.

Which kind of reminds me of tennis. (Feel free to swap out your own favorite sport, I guarantee it'll apply . . . .)

I can't help noticing how much health is like tennis. Tennis players like me get caught up spending a ton of energy on things like the right racket—the right string pattern, tension, material, size, and weight. The whole tennis

---

1 Exercise is defined as about half-hour a day of heart-raising activity.

2 Overweight is defined as a BMI over 25.

3 Eating a healthy diet can mean a lot of things to a lot of people but most researchers include high amounts of omega-3s, low amounts of sugar, zero amount of trans fat and hefty intakes of fiber, vegetables, fruits, beans, and the other usual suspects as part of the definition.

4 Moderate drinking means up to one drink a day for women and two drinks a day for men, while "not at all" means, well, not at all. (If you're not currently drinking, in other words, don't start to get the "benefits" of moderate alcohol intake—you already have them.)

industry exists because we all believe that these things are going to make a huge importance to our game and give us an edge over everyone else. And don't get me wrong— these things do make a difference . . . a little.

But in terms of really making a difference in your game, that stuff doesn't hold a candle to the basics—having a strong stroke, a good serve, and quick footwork. That's a whole lot more work than just shelling out 200 bucks for the latest Babalot racket.

I'm sure it's as true in any sport as it is in tennis, just as it's true in health and in life. Basics are basics, and they're always what makes the most difference.

The payoff for attending to the basics, just in terms of extra healthy years, is absolutely amazing. The Nurses Health Study, which has been going on since 1976 and involves more than 84,000 women, found that the same five attainable strategies we've been talking about—not smoking, moderate (or no) consumption of alcohol, exercise, a healthy diet, and a healthy weight—resulted in an astonishing 83 percent reduction in risk for major coronary events (including those that typically result in death).

And there's no need to stop there. While the seven behavioral strategies just mentioned are a great place to start if you want to add years to your life, doing some of the "hacks" we discuss in this book—like supplements, and hormone replacement, and anti-inflammatory foods— can add more life and passion to your years.

You can significantly increase the odds of living a really long time just by following those seven strategies. But how about being in your seventies and practically jumping out of bed each day because you can't wait to get to the tennis court for a couple hours before starting a day you're really excited about? With great gratitude, I can say that is an accurate description of my life in my seventies, and I hope it will continue to be an accurate description for a very long time.

So my goal is to not *just* keep you around a long time, but to keep you around being vital, vigorous, and sexy. (Yes, you read that right. You can—and should—be sexy at any age.)

The take-away is simple: Your future is in large measure determined by your own choices. Your life is in *your* hands. And while not everybody who makes all the right choices will live to be one hundred in great health, there's an awful lot you can do to increase the odds that you'll be one of the growing number of folks who will.

Living well, living long, and living with a high degree of function up to the very (peaceful) end is the goal of everyone reading this book—and it's completely doable.

Which brings us to a concept I call "the functionality curve."

THE FUNCTIONALITY CURVE

If you drew a graph showing age on one axis and function on the other (function meaning everything from how well your heart performs to your ability to have passionate sex), you'd see a depressing slope in which function decreases as age increases. It would look like Figure A, at right.

Notice how the slope goes down?

Well, it doesn't have to. "The goal of anti-aging medicine is to rectangularize the functionality curve," says Ron Rothenberg, M.D., author of *Forever Ageless*. "That is, to maintain all functions—heart, brain, muscle, lungs, etc.— at a high level to the end and then fall apart quickly all at once."

A "rectangularized" functionality curve might look like Figure B.

"Isn't that what everyone wants?" asks Rothenberg.

Let me guess: The answer is a resounding "yes."

"For most of us, death will be preceded by a decline in function and we would all like that period of decline to be as brief as possible," write David Jones, M.D., Jeffrey Bland, Ph.D., and Shelia Quinn in an article on healthy aging.

In labs all over the country, scientists labor tirelessly to discover the secrets of unlocking longevity genes. Examples are David Sinclair, Ph.D., a professor of genetics at Harvard University and co-Director of the Paul F. Glenn Center for the Biology of Aging, whose research on calorie restriction and life extension led to the discovery of resveratrol, and Charles Brenner, Ph.D., a professor of biochemistry and internal medicine at the University of Iowa, who discovered a new form of vitamin B3 (nicotinamide riboside) that has significant anti-aging potential.

Cynthia Kenyon, director of the Hillblom Center for the Biology of Aging at the University of California, San Francisco, has found a way to lengthen the life span of worms from a normal 18 days to 144 days—an increase of 800 percent! Dr. Charles Brenner—a professor of biochemistry at the University of Iowa and a director of the Obesity Initiative at the University of Iowa—discovered a unique form of vitamin B3 called nicotinamide riboside which is causing a huge stir in the anti-aging community because it is the first substance shown to raise NAD levels in humans. (Why that matters we'll go into later, but trust me, it does.) There's a lot of hope that these amazing discoveries will eventually translate into useful products or strategies for humans.

But let's get back to basics. An enormous amount of research has shown that healthful lifestyle activities are associated with less disability, less loss of function, and

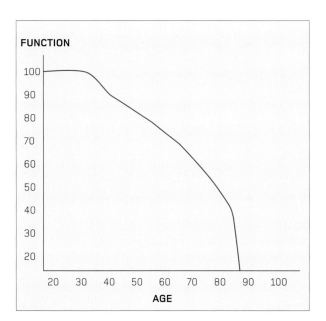

Figure A: Function over age

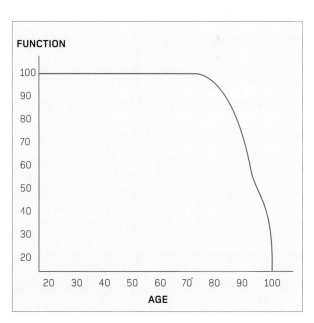

Figure B: Function over age, rectangularized

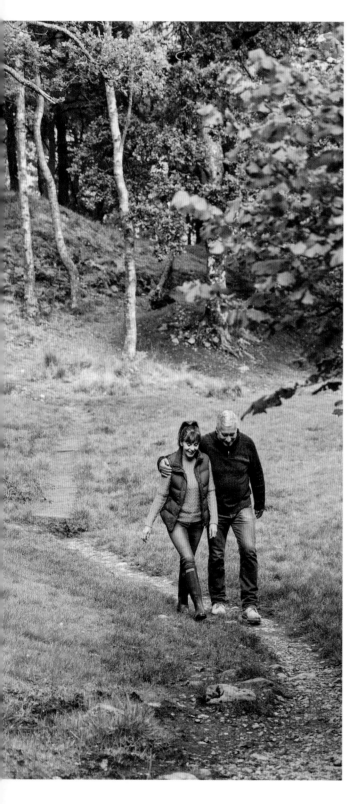

fewer chronic illnesses during the life span. This is empowering news that should make everyone happy. There are things you can do *right now* on a daily basis that will make all the difference in how *long* you live and how *well* you live.

One study on more than 1,700 University of Pennsylvania alumni followed for more than thirty years showed that just three factors accounted for major differences in the length of disability at the end of life and for the severity of that disability. In other words, by manipulating just three factors you could go a long way toward "rectangularizing" the functionality curve. Those three factors are (1) smoking, (2) weight, and (3) patterns of exercise. Starting to sound familiar? Those are three of the seven key strategies we've been talking about that are associated with a longer life in study after study after study.

For example: research at Harvard corroborated the importance of the same three factors and added a couple more, including "a stable marriage," which could easily be seen as a sub-category of "strong supportive relationships" discussed above.

Refining, fleshing out, and adding to that list of things you can actually do to "rectangularize" the curve is the subject of this book.

The take-home point is this: What you do *matters*. Very much. "Research is making it increasingly clear that there are many behaviors (diet, exercise, stress reduction) and treatments (antioxidants, essential fatty acids, minerals, certain amino acids, the B vitamins, and much more) that can counteract the functional decline that leaves us vulnerable to disease and disability as we age," writes Jones.

WHAT IS AGING ANYWAY?

If you think computers are complex, welcome to the world of aging. There are so many interconnected parts in that collection of 100 trillion cells we call our bodies that the number of possible places where things can break down is almost infinite.

And it doesn't end there. There's also the powerful influence of another whole ecological system of microbes that live on and in your body, a vast system that scientists call the *microbiome*. The influence of the microbiome on our health is an exploding area of research.

In many ways, the Internet is a good model for the body. As anyone who spends any time online knows, connections can get lost, systems can crash, servers can go down, viruses and spyware can lurk, and because of the *interconnectedness* of everything, something that happens in one part of the system can have deep consequences in another. Although your body isn't as large as the Internet, it's certainly as complex. (The interconnectedness model is the philosophical basis of functional medicine—more on that in just a minute.)

Your computer can crash because of things that go wrong inside your actual desktop, sure; but malfunctions can *also* happen because of outside influences (think virus and spyware or electrical surges). On the simplest level, your computer won't work if there's an electrical outage in your neighborhood; it needs a steady supply of current just to get up and running. Similarly, we humans need a steady supply of outside energy to keep functioning at our best. At the most basic level, we need food, especially the right kind of food (which you'll read a lot about in this book).

On a more global level, we need social contacts and connections. Without them, we literally wither away and die no matter how good our "hardware" performs.

(Remember that strong social networks are one of the most reliable predictors of old age.)

Although there are many theories of aging and though scientists continue to debate the many metabolic pathways, organs, and genes that are undoubtedly involved, there are four specific processes that are unquestionably linked to the breakdown of systems within the body and that contribute to aging and to virtually every degenerative disease known. When these processes wreak havoc on the eyes, you have dimming vision. When they work their mischief on the brain, you have memory loss. When they turn their collective attention to the circulatory system, you have heart disease. Understanding that these four processes have

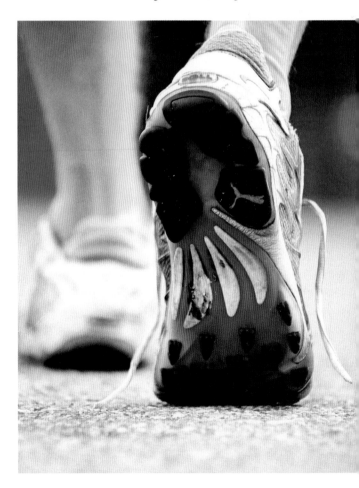

a hand in virtually every disease of aging can help us really get to the core of the issue and yield a much more productive approach than concentrating on the symptoms.

I'll give you an example.

I was recently interviewed by one of the biggest Internet portals in the world for an article on anti-aging. The reporter asked me typical questions that are on the mind of so many of us: "What can I do to protect my brain?" "Are there specific nutrients I can take or foods I can eat that will help protect my aging eyes?" and "What can I do/take/eat to keep my heart healthy?"

These are reasonable questions and ones to which we'd all like some answers.

After all, heart disease and Alzheimer's are both in the top ten list of things that kill us, so who wouldn't want to protect the organs that are affected by them? But what disturbed me was that the questions were being framed as if the events that happen in the eyes or the brain or the heart are fundamentally *different* and require *different* interventions. Although there are undoubtedly issues that are specific to each body system—and we'll discuss those in section ll—the bigger issue is *what all these age-related breakdowns have in common!*

Enter: Functional Medicine.

WHAT IS FUNCTIONAL MEDICINE, AND WHY SHOULD I CARE?

Functional medicine is to conventional medicine what a computer is to a typewriter. This book is being written from a functional medicine perspective, so it's important to understand what it means. One of the best explanations of what functional medicine is about comes from my friend Chris Kresser, M.S., L.Ac., who teaches functional medicine to doctors. "If you've got a pebble in your shoe that's

causing pain, and you go to a conventional doctor, you're going to get a prescription for a pain killer," Chris told me when I interviewed him recently. "If you go to a functional medicine doc, he's going to look for the cause of that pain. Eventually, he's going to ask you to take off your shoe, look inside, see the pebble, and remove it." (Talk about fast-acting painkillers without side effects!)

In other words, conventional medicine treats symptoms; functional medicine treats the underlying cause.

According to Mark Hyman, M.D.—one of the best-known practitioners of functional medicine in the country—functional medicine is the future of medicine, except it's available now. Functional medicine, in Hyman's words, "seeks to identify and address the root causes of disease, and views the body as one integrated system, not a collection of independent organs divided up by medical specialties. It treats the whole system, not just the system."

That's the real fundamental difference between conventional and functional medicine. Functional medicine looks not just at the individual parts of the body—the GI tract, the brain, the heart, the hormones—but at how they interact together and influence one another. The functional medicine doc is interested in how the parts work together—how the pebble gets into the shoe which presses against the toe which results in pain. Functional medicine docs would never just measure your thyroid with a single test, any more than they would treat the painful toe without looking for a pebble. Traditional medicine measures thyroid (usually with a single test), finds it to be low, and offers a script for thyroid meds. Functional medicine docs know that 95 percent of low thyroid is actually caused by the autoimmune disease Hashimoto's, which requires quite a different treatment plan than merely doling out Synthroid. They also know that your adrenal glands have a profound affect on the thyroid, something conventional docs rarely even look at. (Remember the philosophy: the *interconnectedness* of everything.)

When it comes to common patient concerns like losing weight, functional medicine docs know that it's almost never *just* a matter of calories and exercise, the prescription conventional medicine has been peddling, ineffectively, for decades. Functional medicine docs and nutritionists may look at calories and exercise, but they'll just be two points of data. Functional practitioners treating weight issues will look at hormones like cortisol and insulin which often go unmeasured or unnoticed in conventional treatment for weight loss. They may look at leptin, an appetite-regulating hormone. They will investigate food intolerances, inflammation, and leaky gut. It's a way more comprehensive and modern way of looking at the human body and at human health.

A functional medicine perspective is really the only one you want when it comes to what's now known as age-management medicine. Aging is such a complex, multi-determined phenomena, that to look at it only in terms of individual symptoms (aches, pains, low libido) is just ludicrous, even though that's exactly what most conventionally trained docs do.

Functional medicine looks at the patient, not the disease. It treats the person, not the lab test. Functional medicine docs are by nature medical detectives. They will ask about every aspect of your life because they are acutely aware of how all the elements in your life interact and affect each other.

So here's the first take-home point from this book: Find a doctor who's trained in functional medicine. Doctors who are trained in this kind of medicine come from all kinds of backgrounds, from internal medicine to cardiology. Then, they take additional training to get certified in this specialty. If you're dealing with a chronic condition (and that includes some of the symptoms of aging), an M.D., D.O., or N.D. trained in functional medicine is the best choice.

And make no mistake—it's chronic diseases that are killing us. Seven out of the top 10 causes of death were chronic diseases, and two of them—heart disease and cancer—accounted for almost 46 percent of all deaths. As of 2012, about half of all adults in America—roughly 117 million folks—had one or more chronic diseases with one in four having multiple chronic diseases. Of the nation's approximately $3 trillion dollar annual health care expenditures, 86 percent is spent on chronic diseases. And chronic diseases—including aging—is where conventional medicine fails us miserably.

Don't get me wrong—conventional medicine is unparalleled for dealing with emergencies. If I'm ever in a car accident, I want to be taken to Cedars Sinai post-haste—forget the herbalists and acupuncturists and integrative medicine gurus. Here in America, we've got the superheroes of triage. Conventional, traditional, pharmaceutical medicine gets an "A plus" when it comes to life-or-death situations.

Unfortunately, it gets an "F" for keeping us from getting sick in the first place. And if you want to live longer (and healthier), the first rule is not to get sick and the second is that if you *do* get sick, get well quickly.

Which brings us to the big question of the day: Why do we get sick anyway? What breaks our bodies down? It's time to introduce the Four Horsemen of Aging.

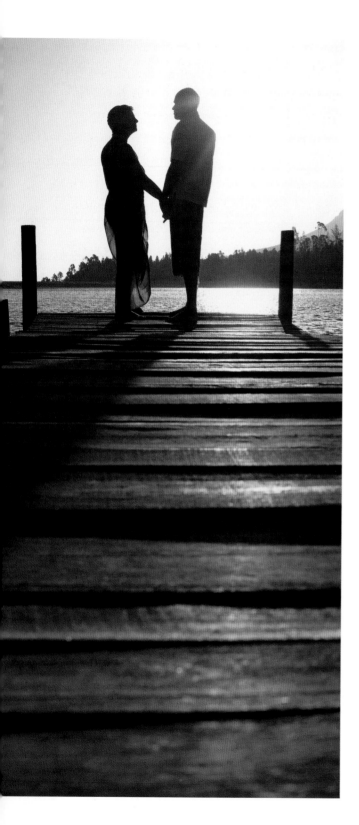

THE FOUR HORSEMEN OF AGING

I've nicknamed the four dangerous processes that age
our bodies "The Four Horsemen of Aging." Wherever
something breaks down in the body—be it the brain,
muscles, circulatory or immune system, you name it—
you don't have to dig too deeply to find the handiwork
of one or more of the Four Horsemen. These Four
Horsemen *together* are probably responsible for the *bulk*
of what happens to our bodies when they break down.

Oh, and by the way: In the time between the first edition of this book and the one you're now reading, I wrote a
book on heart disease with the famous integrative cardiologist, Stephen Sinatra, M.D. The book was called *The Great
Cholesterol Myth*, and in it, we identified four things that
promote heart disease and that we believe are far more
important than cholesterol. Those four promoters of heart
disease were identical to The Four Horsemen of Aging.
We could easily have called them The Four Horsemen
of Heart Disease. And guess what—you could also call
these same four factors The Four Horsemen of Obesity.
Or The Four Horsemen of Diabetes.

These four bad actors ultimately age you at the cellular
level. They damage the cells, particularly structures called
the mitochondria, which are the energy factories inside the
cell responsible for making ATP (adenosine triphosphate),
which is the currency of cellular energy, a molecule used
for every human activity from detoxification to blinking
your eyes to dancing the mambo. Injured *mitochondria*
mean the cells can't do their basic operations as well
and everything—from energy, to vitality, to fat burning,
to detoxification—suffers.

Furthermore, these four bad actors are all made worse by a diet high in sugars, starches, and grains.

By now you're probably saying, "Okay already, what exactly *are* these horsemen he keeps talking about anyway?" Or, more to the point, "Why should I care?" And here's the answer: Anything bad that's happening in your body—from the beginnings of disease to the loss of memory to the weakening of your muscles to the accumulation of body fat—is being driven by the engine of these four processes.

The names of these processes may not yet be familiar to you, but guaranteed, they are behind the scenes of every disease of aging ever experienced by the human species.

So without further ado, allow me to introduce them to you:

1. Oxidative damage
2. Inflammation
3. Glycation (Sugar)
4. Stress

Many of the strategies I talk about in this book pertain to preventing or combating the damaging effects of these four processes. The four of them, collectively, can damage cells and DNA, wear down organs and systems, deeply damage the vascular pathways that deliver blood and oxygen to your entire body, and even shrink the size of your brain. They're involved in heart disease, cancer, diabetes, obesity, Alzheimer's, and cognitive decline, not to mention a host of "less serious" diseases that can vastly diminish the quality of your well-being.

Even though these four processes often overlap and work together to cause serious damage to both your physical health and your mental well-being, let's break them down into manageable chunks and tackle them one by one. In a short time, it will be apparent how each contributes to the damage the other does and how the same weapons—whole foods, nutrients, stress reduction, exercise, detoxification, relationship improvement, and the many other things we'll be discussing in this book—actually do double duty, effectively battling more than one of the four processes that effectively shorten your life.

So let's get started.

CHAPTER 1

Fight the First Horseman of Aging: Free Radicals

If you've ever seen rust on metal, you're familiar with oxidation (also known as oxidative damage), even if you didn't know the technical name for it. You're also familiar with oxidation if you've ever left apple slices out on a picnic table where they were exposed to the air. They turned brown, didn't they? *That's* oxidative damage. Oxidative damage to metal looks like rust. Oxidative damage to your skin looks like ... well, aging skin.

Preventing—or combating—oxidative damage (also known as oxidative stress or oxidation for short) is one of the major anti-aging strategies under your control, and you're more likely to do it if you understand why it's so important.

For those of you who don't remember high school chemistry (or would understandably prefer to forget it), electrons travel in pairs and orbit around atoms. Every so often, one of those electrons gets "loose" and pandemonium ensues. The molecule with the unpaired electron—known as a free radical—starts running around like a headless chicken trying to find its head. Free radicals are like college sophomores on spring break—temporarily free from the constraints of dormitory living, they basically go nuts and will "mate" with anyone! Free radicals "hit on" existing, stable pairs of electrons thousands of times a day, trying to find an electron they can pair-bond with and meanwhile, inflicting enormous damage upon your cells, your cell membranes, and even your DNA.

Once one of the paired electrons breaks off, the molecule or atom where it *used* to reside is now running around with an unpaired single electron. The presence of that "unpaired" electron turns our formerly stable molecule into what is known as a free radical—the raging bull of molecules. It's not a happy camper.

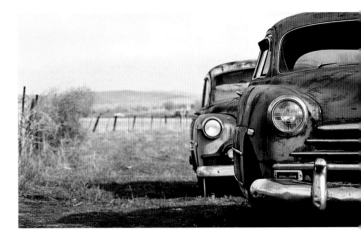

The irony, of course, is that when it *does* finally steal an electron away from a stable molecule, that molecule becomes unstable itself and turns into a free radical (because it's now left with an unpaired electron). And the process begins again. The whole process is kind of like having a vampire on the loose: Each time a new victim gets bitten, it turns into a vampire and the whole sequence repeats. Anti-aging expert Ron Rothenberg, M.D., has a clever name for the sequence: He calls it "Cellular World War III."

Every time these free radicals "hit" on your cells looking for a mate for their unpaired electron, they damage the cells. This cumulative damage is a huge part of aging. "If the DNA is damaged when the cell divides to make new cells, the copies will be wrong and whatever function that cell performs will not be done correctly," Rothenberg says.

If "aging" is another name for "breakdown," then you can see immediately why free radicals age us. Cells break down, organ systems don't function as well, DNA becomes damaged, DNA replication—an incredibly complex and delicate, enzyme-dependent process—doesn't happen efficiently, and DNA can become mutated. When this kind of damage, accumulates in the body, it contributes to all sorts of disorders typical of aging. For example, when it accumulates in the heart or vascular system, you have heart disease. When it accumulates in the skin, you have aging skin.

There's not a disease of aging in which free radical damage is not an important component. That's why fighting free radical damage is such a running theme throughout this book and why you'll be hearing the term "antioxidants" in virtually every chapter.

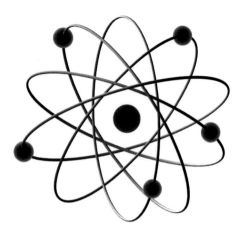

The cellular and DNA damage that result from free radicals contributes to just about every disease you can think of.

Antioxidants refers to a class of substances, including certain vitamins, minerals, and many plant chemicals, that help neutralize oxygen free radicals, soaking them up like little sponges, thus limiting the damage they can do to your body. The reason cut apple slices don't turn brown so quickly when you squirt lemon juice on them is because lemon juice contains a fair amount of vitamin C, a powerful antioxidant.

THE FREE RADICAL THEORY OF AGING

The role of free radicals in aging has been recognized at least since the 1950s, when an innovative scientist (and 1995 Nobel Prize nominee) named Denham Harman, M.D., Ph.D., proposed the free radical theory of aging. Harman believed that as go the cells, so goes the body; if our cells age, our whole body ages (which makes perfect sense because we are, after all, made up of nothing but cells). Harman saw aging as the cellular accumulation of free radical damage over time—that our bodies are essentially "rusting from within."

Years later, the free radical theory of aging was expanded to include not just aging, but degenerative diseases in general. We now know that oxidative damage plays a major role in every degenerative disease of aging, from Alzheimer's and cancer to heart disease and diabetes and even immune dysfunction.

AVOID ENVIRONMENTAL FREE RADICALS BY GOING ORGANIC

There are several sources of free radicals, including the environment: tobacco smoke, air pollution, pesticides, herbicides, and contaminants in our water. All of these form free radicals—which we then take into our body by breathing, drinking, and eating—that contribute to the aging process and the diseases that kill us. This is what we mean when we talk of a "toxic environment" (and this is why I consider detoxification one of the "Seven Pillars of Longevity"—more on this later).

People who are constantly assaulted by these environmental free radicals—and who don't have good defenses against them—tend to age badly. The free radicals come into our body and attack our cells. They destroy genetic material, damage and mutate DNA, burden the immune system, and virtually destroy a cell's identity. The damage is enormous, and it's a huge part of what ages us.

Some of the obvious sources of free radicals—tobacco smoke, pesticides, and certain chemicals—are also sources of cancer-causing chemicals called *carcinogens*. The combination is lethal to anyone wanting to live in optimal health for nine or more decades. Smoking, for example, creates free radicals that damage the lungs and just for good measure, exposes us to carcinogenic chemicals. Tobacco smoke is literally a turbocharged free radical factory on steroids.

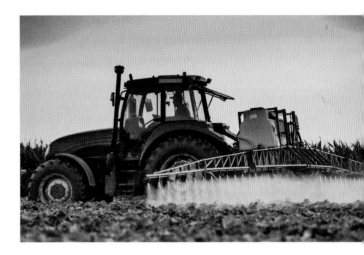

Then, there are the pesticides sprayed on crops. "Pesticides kill the pest by *creating* free radicals," says Hari Sharma, M.D., a fellow of the Royal College of Physicians and Surgeons and a consultant to the National Institutes of Health. "If you consume them, you will be damaged by those free radicals, also." At least fifty-three carcinogenic (cancer-causing) pesticides are applied in large amounts to the major food crops, according to a study by the U.S. Food and Drug Administration. In the first edition of this book, I mentioned a 2005 study that found 73 percent of fresh vegetables and fruits contained pesticide residues, as did 61 percent of processed fruits and vegetables, 22 percent of soybeans, 75 percent of wheat, a whopping 99 percent of milk and cream, and 16 percent of bottled water.

Alarming right? But since then, it's gotten worse. Data released by the U.S. Department of Agriculture in 2016 shows that the percentage has risen. In the latest study, 85 percent of the 10,187 samples tested had pesticide residues. No wonder that when the Centers for Disease Control and Prevention tested for 116 pesticides and other artificial chemicals in the blood and urine of 2,500 volunteers they found detectable levels of 89 chemicals, including pesticides, phthalates, herbicides, pest repellants,

Buy Organic—But Buy Wisely

Choosing organic foods is especially important with foods that are known to have a high level of contamination. Since organic foods are a lot more expensive, I personally use the EWG dirty dozen list to prioritize what to buy organically. (For example: I worry much less about avocados and pineapples than I do about strawberries, one of the most sprayed crops ever.)

I always add three items to my "must buy organic" list, to add to whatever 12 foods happen to make the EWG "dirty" list.

→ Meat

→ Milk

→ Coffee

Meat and milk are frequently laced with antibiotics, steroids, and growth hormone, and coffee is a widely sprayed crop. These unwelcome additions—including, by the way, the notoriously controversial herbicide RoundUp—are the primary reason for recommending organic foods as part of an anti-aging lifestyle. Although studies have been mixed about whether the nutritional content of organic food is any greater than that of conventionally grown food, the primary reason for eating organic food is not because they're necessarily more nutritious. It's to avoid the intake of the chemicals used in nonorganic farming.

and disinfectants. The Environmental Working Group—a nonprofit, consumer advocacy group, has been testing fruits and vegetables in the American food supply for many years, and each year publishes a list of what they call the "dirty dozen"—fruits and vegetables assessed to be the most contaminated of all. The list is updated every year, along with a complementary list called "the clean 15"—those fruits and vegetables that tested to have the lowest levels of contaminants and chemicals. You can find (and download) the "Dirty Dozen" list from the EWG website: www.ewg.org. "The effects of these chemicals may be difficult to separate from normally mildly debilitating aspects of the aging process," says professor Harvey Blatt of the Institute of Earth Sciences at Hebrew University of Jerusalem.

AGING FREE RADICALS FROM OUR OWN BODIES

The environment isn't the only source of these toxic free radicals. Our bodies are a virtual free radical *factory*. Now why in the world would you produce free radicals in your body, you might ask, especially because these are such dangerous and health-robbing compounds?

Good question, and the answer is simple: All free radicals aren't bad.

Our immune system, for example, produces free radicals to help protect us from harmful microorganisms and fight infections. The very process of creating energy—respiratory metabolism, or in simpler terms, *breathing*—creates free radicals. Free radicals can help activate enzymes and produce hormones. The problem arises when the *amount* of free radicals in our body is excessive and out of control. Then, the damage significantly outweighs the benefits.

Although free radicals can search for that extra electron anywhere, they cause the most damage when they are derived from oxygen. Yup, oxygen—the stuff you breathe and without which you couldn't live for more than a few moments. But oxygen has a dark side. Oxygen free radicals are actually one of the most damaging kinds on the planet. When oxygen molecules are the ones that give up their electrons, we're in big trouble. It's like those wild unpaired electrons decided to pick on the biggest, toughest guy in the schoolyard—and mayhem ensues. Free radicals derived from oxygen are known collectively as *reactive oxygen species*, and they are a virtual aging factory.

Oxygen-derived radicals are a normal part of aerobic metabolism, so they're constantly being formed. In fact, anywhere there's oxygen, there are oxygen free radicals. Doing some aerobic exercise? You're making oxygen free radicals! Just breathing? Oxygen free radicals! White blood cells are especially talented at producing oxygen free radicals, which they then use as a defense against invading microbes. But all those toxins from the environment that we spoke about earlier also have oxidizing effects on cells and produce tons of oxygen free radicals. So does radiation, which actually produces the most damage in tissues that

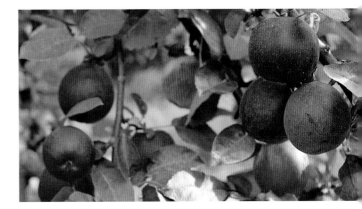

have a heavy concentration of oxygen (we call these heavily oxidized tissues).

Another way free radicals age us is through their effect on DNA. You may remember from high school biology that your DNA is kind of like your own individual genetic instruction manual. It's found in every cell, and it's like a set of master blueprints that tell every *other* cell what to do. When free radicals attack the DNA in your cells, they screw up their ability to replicate properly and pass on their instructions. This kind of DNA damage eventually shortens your DNA strands and triggers a process called *apoptosis*, or "programmed cell death." It's as if you were passing on a repair manual that constantly got dropped in the dirt, burned at the edges, or dropped in the water and finally became so worn that anyone trying to use it couldn't read the words anymore and had to guess what was written on the page. A mechanic relying on a manual like that couldn't be counted on to do a good job with your car, and DNA that's been damaged like that doesn't do a good job of repairing and rebuilding your cells, tissues, and organs. The result? What we know as aging!

But wait, there's more!

ANTI-AGING ACTION PLAN:

Protect Your Cells with the Best Fats

I recommend that you consume healthy oils every day to strengthen cells so they can fight off free radicals. In addition to fish oil, use oils such as walnut oil, flaxseed oil, extra-virgin olive oil, or almond oil as part of salad dressings. For cooking, macadamia oil, avocado oil, ghee, Malaysian palm oil, and coconut oil are particularly good. Remember that oils have to be used at the correct temperature. Some of the most valuable and healthful oils—like flaxseed oil—are not at all good for high heat cooking. They just have to be used for things like salad dressings or extremely low heat sautéing. The more refined oils stand up to heat better, but they also produce the most toxic compounds. Take home point: Use the best oils you can find and cook with them at the right temperature. Contrary to conventional wisdom, extra-virgin olive oil (EVOO) is also a suitable oil for cooking at temperatures up to 392°F (200°C).

Oils

→ **Flaxseed oil:** I don't recommend this oil for cooking, though some folks would argue it's okay for very low heat. Its smoke point is 225°F (107°C).

→ **Extra-virgin olive oil:** Olives are an incredibly rich source of plant compounds called polyphenols (see Olive Leaf Extract, page 167). I use EVOO as drizzles and on salads to maximize consumption of the incredible anti-inflammatory nutrients. (And I'll confess to taking a swig out of Cobram Estates extra-virgin olive oil—the best-tasting olive oil I've ever had.) Interestingly, research shows that the higher an oil is in polyphenols, the more stable it remains when heated.

→ **Grapeseed oil:** I'm not quite sure why grapeseed oil is such a fan fave among health-conscious consumers. It does have a high-ish smoke point of 420°F (215°C), but its omega-6 to omega-3 ratio is 676:1. And—if you'll excuse the pun—we're already *over*-saturated with omega-6s in our diet.

→ **Walnut oil (unrefined):** Like all oils, if you refine walnut oil, the smoke point goes up from 320°F (160°C) to 400°F (204°C), with a not-bad-at-all omega-6 to omega-3 ratio of 5.1:1.

→ **Almond oil:** This has a nice smoke point of 420°F (215°C), but it only contains omega-6.

→ **Macadamia nut oil:** Like avocado and olive oil, it's mostly made up of healthy, anti-inflammatory monounsaturated fat. The smoke point is 390°F (199°C)—higher than extra virgin olive oil but lower than avocado oil.

→ **Coconut oil:** Unrefined coconut oil—like Barlean's organic virgin coconut oil—is one of my favorite foods, but the smoke point is only 350°F (177°C), so watch the heat. Barlean's makes a slightly more refined culinary coconut oil that brings the smoke point up to a respectable 450°F (232°C).

- → **Avocado oil:** One of the greatest oils for cooking, it has a really high smoke point of 520°F (271°C) and about 70 percent healthy anti-inflammatory monounsaturated fats.

- → **Malaysian palm oil:** I love this oil. Its reddish color is due to the rich content of nutrients like tocotrienols and carotenoids. It has a nice high smoke point of 450°F (232°C), albeit lower if it's more unrefined. And for those concerned about the palm oil industry in some countries harming animal habitats, that is *not* the case in Malaysia, where 50 percent of forests are protected and palm is harvested in a sustainable way.

- → **Grass-fed butter:** Grass-fed butter is the only kind I recommend. Its smoke point is 350°F (177°C).

- → **Ghee:** Clarified butter, a.k.a. ghee, is considered a health food in India. It's basically "clarified" by removing all of the dairy proteins and sugars. It also has a nice high smoke point of 485°F (252°C).

- → **Lard:** Yup, lard. It's making a comeback both in chef circles and Paleo circles, but with a caveat: It absolutely must be lard from pasteured pork, which is raised both humanely and in a far healthier manner. Remember: I am not talking about Crisco or any kind of vegetable shortening. The smoke point of lard is 370°F (188°C).

In case you're wondering where soy oil and canola oil are, I can only say that I haven't been a fan or either one for a long time. I know there's controversy about them and I know the cases to be made for both sides of those controversies—I've listened to them for well over a decade. Nonetheless, these two oils remain banned from my kitchen.

High-Fat Anti-Aging Foods

- → **All nuts:** ½–1 ounce (15 to 28 g), up to five times a week, is great!
- → **Avocado:** Use in salads or guacamole.
- → **Cold-water fish, such as wild Alaskan salmon, tuna, mackerel, and sardines:** Eat at least twice a week, more if you can!
- → **Yogurt:** A good "daily" food. Avoid the no-fat kind for two reasons. One, it contains too much sugar. Two is because recent research has shown that people who had the most dairy fat in their diet had about a 50 percent reduction in their risk for diabetes.

Do Not Fear Saturated Fats from Whole Foods

- → Free-range eggs
- → Grass-fed butter
- → Grass-fed meat
- → Ghee
- → Malaysian red palm oil
- → Coconut and coconut oil
- → Raw, organic milk

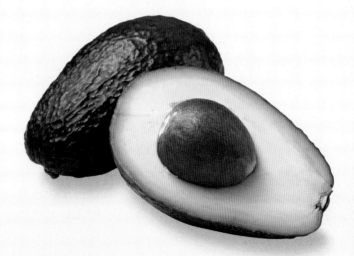

EAT THE RIGHT FATS FOR FLEXIBILITY

One of the best-known toxic effects of oxygen free radicals is the damage to cellular membranes. Nothing will age you faster than an assault on your cell membranes, even though it takes place under the radar and even though you can't see it (except with a microscope). Why? *Because the membranes are critical to cell health*—they're what hold the cell together. Cell membranes have to be flexible enough to allow information to pass in and out, but stiff enough so that they don't collapse. They're delicate structures. (One of the reasons trans fats are so harmful is that they damage the cell membrane.)

Lipid peroxidation is the technical name for the damage to cell membranes caused by oxygen free radicals. It has a number of effects, none of them good. It can make the membranes stiffer. It can decrease the activity of enzymes that are bound in the membranes. It can alter the activity of membrane receptors. Ultimately, on the cellular level, lipid peroxidation ages you from the inside out.

To me, one of the most God-awful missteps made by conventional medicine and conventional public health policy has been to focus on cholesterol lowering as an anti-aging strategy when in fact the big risk factors for disease are oxidative damage and inflammation. Cholesterol itself doesn't do any damage in the body at all—until it's *oxidized*. When cholesterol just sits there minding its own business, it is perfectly harmless. Only when it gets attacked by oxygen free radicals does it become a problem.

If we could prevent the oxidation of cholesterol by fighting off free radical damage, as well as preventing or reversing the inflammation that nearly always accompanies this oxidative damage, we'd be sitting pretty. Oxidized cholesterol is indeed a health risk, but blaming cholesterol is like blaming the St. Bernard for the avalanche.

The Great Cholesterol Myth

Speaking of fat and cholesterol, let's take a moment to examine one of the central tenants of conventional health wisdom—the notion that saturated fat and cholesterol are terrible for us and should be avoided at all costs. You'll be reading a ton of stuff in this book that contradicts that conventional wisdom—which as it turns out, is very far from wise—so let's confront the elephant in the room right now so you don't have to spend the rest of the book wondering, *"Why on earth are these guys recommending so many high-fat foods? Aren't they worried about cholesterol?"*

Well, actually, no. They're not. And here's why.

Whenever celebrities die of heart related issues—George Michael, Carrie Fisher, and Alan Thicke being examples from the last decade—it raises our collective awareness about heart disease, the number one cause of death in the United States. Awareness is always a good thing, but it's even better when accompanied by action. Unfortunately, mainstream medicine's *prescription* for action—lowering cholesterol—is way past its expiration date.

As I stated on *The Dr. Oz Show*, "Trying to lower heart disease by lowering cholesterol is like trying to lower calories by taking the lettuce off your whopper."

About half the people admitted to hospitals for coronary artery disease have perfectly normal cholesterol. Tim Russert, the popular moderator of *Meet the Press*, died of a massive heart attack on a treadmill, his cholesterol perfectly under control. His LDL was 68 and his total cholesterol was a jaw-dropping 105, figures that would make any conventional doctor very happy.

But if I had those numbers, I'd be seriously scared.

Low cholesterol is associated with a baker's dozen of bad outcomes, including increased risk for cancer, stroke, and . . . counterintuitively . . . heart disease itself. It's even associated with a significantly increased risk of suicide.

Cholesterol is a vitally important molecule for the brain, for the immune system, and for the creation of sex hormones and vitamin D. And our obsessive fixation on lowering it has actually caused us to lose sight of the meaningful steps we can take to lower our risk for *heart disease*. If you take away nothing else from this, remember that *lowering heart disease* and *lowering cholesterol* are very far from the same thing.

This is not the place to go into the fascinating history of how we got the whole cholesterol thing wrong (while, until very recently, giving sugar—a far more dangerous substance—a free pass). There are excellent books on the subject for anyone interested in how we got here—Nina Teicholz's *The Big Fat Surprise*, Malcolm Kendrick's *The Great Cholesterol Con*, Gary Taubes' *The Case Against Sugar*, and the aforementioned *The Great Cholesterol Myth* by myself and cardiologist Stephen Sinatra. For now, let's talk about what to do next.

In our book, we identified four factors that promote heart disease, not coincidentally these are the exact same four factors that promote many other degenerative diseases as well, the four factors that we're calling *The Four Horsemen of Aging*: stress, sugar, inflammation, and oxidative damage. Rather than spending another minute worrying about cholesterol, I'd much rather see us focus on lowering inflammatory markers like homocysteine, IL-6, and small particle LDL-b, reducing triglycerides and blood pressure, reducing oxidative damage to our cells and organs with antioxidant-rich foods, managing our stress, and eating less sugar. *That's* a plan for reducing heart disease. Cholesterol has almost nothing to do with it.

We've already talked about the five basic lifestyle interventions that can reduce heart attacks by up to 80 percent. And throughout this book, we'll be talking about ways to reduce that risk even more. (See page 100.)

Meanwhile, here are a few more things that increase your odds of dodging the heart disease bullet.

Omega-3. Wild salmon and fish oil supplements contain two powerful omega-3s which have been found to lower triglycerides and blood pressure. Omega-3s are also one of the most anti-inflammatory molecules on the planet, and virtually everyone can benefit from more. Buy the best you can afford. (You'll be reading much more on omega-3s throughout the book.)

Breathing. Four or five minutes with your eyes closed, sitting quietly or lying down, breathing deeply (5 counts in, hold for 5, exhale for 5) will do wonders for your stress levels, blood pressure, and state of mind. Of course, if you can meditate, that's even better!

Magnesium. Almost no one gets enough of this important nutrient which relaxes both the mind and the arteries and helps regulate blood sugar to boot.

Sleep. Not getting enough sleep—or getting poor quality sleep—is a huge stressor to the body, raising cortisol levels and generally causing metabolic dysfunction. Keep the room dark and cool and don't sleep with the TV on!

Sitting breaks. Recent research has shown that sitting for long periods causes metabolic havoc, even for people who exercise. Take a few-minute break every hour or so, even if you just walk down the hallway and back.

Relationships. One of the best predictors of long life, according to research done in the so-called Blue Zones, was connectedness, purpose, and relationships. And I'm talking real people, real interactions. None of the people in the Blue Zones had a Facebook account.

Undoubtedly, there are more actions you could take. Getting on a good supplement program which includes probiotics, vitamin D, vitamin K, resveratrol, and curcumin. Eating an anti-inflammatory diet with lots of plant foods in it, especially nuts, berries, apples, and greens. Eating only clean, grass-fed meat. Ditching processed foods fast, and fast foods faster. Taking a slow, relaxed 15-minute walk five times a week. Spending some time in the sun and around greenery. Drinking pomegranate juice, green tea, and lots of water. And following the principle of HALT—don't get too hungry, angry, lonely, or tired.

All good stuff, all in good time. Meanwhile, the steps outlined above are a terrific place to start for just about everybody.

Get those down first. The rest is details.

FREE THE RADICALS FROM YOUR BODY

By now, it should be pretty apparent that there's no aging without free radical damage, and there's no way to fight the effects of aging without a strong army to fight off that damage. If your body didn't have any built-in defenses against the constant assault of free radicals, you probably wouldn't be here reading this book. In fact, you'd be quite dead.

Fortunately, nature hardwired into our DNA the ability to make chemicals that help protect the cells against oxidative damage. These chemicals are called—can you guess?—*anti*oxidants.

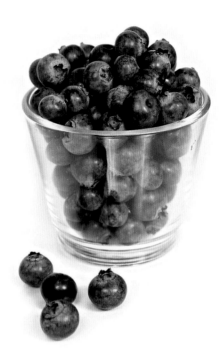

An antioxidant works by exactly the mechanism you might imagine from its name—by fighting oxidation. It donates one of its own electrons to the rogue molecule, essentially rendering it impotent and unable to do any damage. You've probably used the power of antioxidants yourself without realizing it.

Your body has some powerful antioxidants of its own. At the top of the list is one called *coenzyme Q10*, which is found in every cell (and discussed in greater length in chapter 7, on the heart). Another is called *superoxide dismutase* (SOD), an enzyme that repairs cells and reduces damage done by one of the most common (and damaging) oxygen free radicals in the body—*superoxide*. Rounding out this native superstar trio is *glutathione*, arguably the most important antioxidant in the body.

When cholesterol just sits there minding its own business, it is perfectly harmless.

Only when it gets attacked by oxygen free radicals does it become a problem.

But there's one big problem. Our homegrown supply of antioxidants can't keep up with the workload. Our internal antioxidants become less effective as we age, especially when we live in an environment that assaults us with free radicals on a daily basis.

But fortunately, there's help out there.

ANTIOXIDANTS IN FOOD AND PILLS

If you've read my book, *The 150 Healthiest Foods on Earth*, you probably know that one of the biggest benefits of many of the foods I consider to be among the healthiest in the world is that they are absolutely loaded with antioxidants and natural anti-inflammatories. Plants have their own built-in protection against the oxidative damage of the sun, and these built-in protectors function as cell protectors in our bodies. The very pigments that make blueberries blue and raspberries red protect those berries from oxidative damage, and they do the same for you once inside your body. This is probably one of the many reasons for the greater health and longevity of people who regularly consume tons of fruits and vegetables.

ANTI-AGING ACTION PLAN:

Eat Antioxidant and Anti-Inflammatory—Rich Foods

→ Berries (wild blueberries, raspberries, blackberries, strawberries, cranberries, etc.): Consume daily. A serving is ½–1 cup.

→ Apples: True to the old saying, one a day.

→ Prunes: Three times a week or as part of your morning meal.

→ Green leafy vegetables: As often as possible.

→ Brassica vegetables (broccoli, Brussels sprouts, cabbage): As often as possible.

→ Beans (red beans, kidney beans, pinto beans): Three times a week.

→ Wild salmon (especially sockeye): At least twice a week.

→ Tea (all kinds): Daily.

→ Pomegranate juice: Drink 4–8 ounces daily.

→ Spices (ginger, turmeric, cinnamon, cloves, oregano): Use as often as possible.

→ Herbs: Use as often as possible.

→ Cocoa (or dark chocolate with 60–80 percent cocoa content): Weekly.

Avoid These Foods

→ Sugar and high-sugar foods

→ Trans-fatty acids (trans fats)

WHICH FOODS CONTAIN ANTIOXIDANTS

CLASS/COMPONENTS	REPRESENTATIVE SOURCES	POTENTIAL ANTI-AGING BENEFIT
Carotenoids		
Beta-carotene	Carrots, red pepper, sweet potato, kale, spinach	Neutralizes aging free radicals
Lutein, zeaxanthin	Kale, spinach, turnip greens, collard greens	Helps protect aging eyes and may help vision
Lycopene	Tomatoes, guava, watermelon	Helps protect against prostate cancer
Flavonoids		
Anthocyanidins	Berries, dark grapes, cherries	Boosts antioxidant defenses and may help protect aging brain
Flavonols: catechins, epicatechins, procyanidins	Tea, chocolate, cocoa, apples, grapes	Helps protect aging heart
Flavanones	Citrus fruits	Neutralizes aging-related free radicals
Flavonols	Onions, apples, tea, broccoli	Neutralizes aging-related free radicals
Proanthocyanidins	Cranberries, peanuts, wine, grapes, strawberries, apples, cocoa	Helps protect urinary tract and heart from damage
Isothiocyanates		
Sulforaphane	Broccoli, broccoli sprouts, cabbage, kale, cauliflower	Enhances detoxification of toxins, boosts antioxidant defenses
Phenols		
Caffeic acid, ferulic acid	Apples, pears, citrus fruits, coffee (caffeic acid)	Powerful antioxidants; caffeic acid is a carcinogenic (cancer) inhibitor
Sulfides/Thiols		
Diallyl sulfide, allyl methyl trisulfide	Garlic, leeks, scallions, onions	Enhances detoxification of toxins, supports heart and immune function in aging body
Dithiolthiones	Cruciferous vegetables: broccoli, cabbage, collards, bok choy	Supports immune system

Adapted from the International Food Information Council Foundation: Media Guide on Food Safety and Nutrition: 2004–2006.

The most famous of the powerhouse antioxidants are vitamin C and vitamin E, but that's only the beginning of the list. Vitamin A is an antioxidant. Minerals like zinc and selenium are powerful antioxidants, as are dozens, perhaps hundreds, of plant compounds known as *phytochemicals*. Quercetin, for example, a member of the flavonoid family, is found in apples and onions and has tremendous antioxidant activity. So does curcumin, a phytochemical found in turmeric, the spice that makes Indian food yellow. Spices in general are a tremendous source of antioxidants, as we'll see later. And nutrients rarely found in any appreciable amount in food, such as alpha-lipoic acid, are also tremendous weapons in the battle against oxidative damage.

Sometimes a nutrient's "good deeds" depends on being in an environment provided by the rest of the components in the food, and without these, the isolated nutrient doesn't "perform" as well. (An example: The vision-enhancing carotenoids *lutein* and *zeaxanthin* are only absorbed properly when they're consumed with some fat.)

Because of this synergistic effect, it's much more useful to look at the food itself and see how it performs, with all its components, in fighting free radicals. One of the strongest arguments for eating whole foods is that they contain an array of healthy nutrients found in combination with other nutrients, some of which may not even have been discovered yet. Nature has a knack for combining things in a unique way, and those combinations can't always be duplicated with pills. Which does not mean you shouldn't take supplements. It just means you should eat whole nutritious foods as often as possible. (We'll get into supplements in much greater depth later.)

As far as food selection goes, you'll pretty much cover all the antioxidant bases by simply following one of the smartest overall pieces of nutritional advice for anti-aging

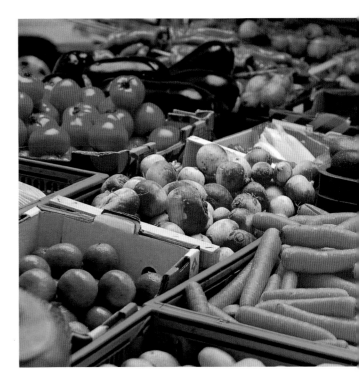

I ever heard, all the more elegant because of its utter simplicity: *Shop so your grocery basket looks colorful.* In fact, if your pile on the checkout counter at the market looks like one of those gorgeous postcards of a European outdoor farmers' market, you're in good shape. You will automatically be eating a ton of high-antioxidant, high anti-inflammatory foods that will help protect you from a virtual encyclopedia of syndromes and diseases associated with aging.

Eat Wild Salmon to Fight Oxidative Damage

Wild Alaskan salmon is the perfect anti-aging food. It's loaded with anti-inflammatory omega-3 properties, and it also contains a powerful and little-known antioxidant called *astaxanthin*, which is what gives salmon its natural red color. (Farmed salmon get their color from artificial coloring and chemicals.)

Wild Alaskan salmon from pristine sources is remarkably free of mercury as well as PCBs, a particularly nasty chemical that has been found in high amounts in farmed salmon. Farmed salmon eat a diet of grains, which makes their fat content much higher in inflammatory omega-6s —not so for the wild kind. Plus, wild Alaskan salmon is free of the antibiotics that are routinely fed to salmon raised in crowded pens on a salmon farm.

Like many health professionals, including Andrew Weil, M.D., Nicholas Perricone, M.D., Joseph Mercola, D.O., and Christiane Northrup, M.D., I recommend the absolute best source in the world for salmon and fish: Vital Choice. I have a link to this terrific company, located in Alaska, on my website, www.jonnybowden.com, and the company even has a *Dr. Jonny Starter Pack*, consisting of my personal favorites. Once you've tasted real pristine Alaskan salmon, you'll never settle for the average kind again.

Check out the recipe at right for salmon from my book *The Healthiest Meals on Earth*, cowritten by my friend Jeanette Bessinger.

Recent research from the Agricultural Research Service investigated the effects of antioxidants on after-meal "oxidative stress." In it, volunteers first drank a shake containing carbohydrates, protein, and fat, but no antioxidants. Sure enough, they produced blood samples with a reduced ability to counter noxious free radicals.

Not good.

"We're learning that antioxidants should be consumed with every meal," says Ronald Prior, a chemist who was the lead researcher on the study. "And if you routinely skip antioxidants in your diet, over time, the excess number of free radicals being produced may begin damaging cellular components, ultimately leading to atherosclerosis, cancer, and other diseases." In other words, all the diseases of aging.

But here's where it gets interesting. The researchers also found something that absolutely qualifies as usable information that you can apply right now in your fight against aging and disease: Consuming *grapes* with that same test meal *prevented* the decline in antioxidant capacity.

Of course, it's not just grapes, though they're high in antioxidants and were used in this research. It can be any antioxidant-rich food or foods—vegetables and fruits being the most obvious. In other research, Prior found that grapes, kiwi, and wild blueberries were high performers when it came to raising blood levels of important antioxidants. Adding high-antioxidant foods, whether a portion of grapes or a couple of servings of vegetables, seems to act as a kind of damage control button even when you eat a bad meal. When you eat those foods as part of a *good* meal, it's even better.

Bottom line: If you can pluck it or gather it—if it's a food you could eat straight from the ground or right off a tree or a bush—it's probably good for you. These are the foods that make up a large part of the diet of virtually every one of the longest-lived and healthiest populations on the planet. I call them the Jonny Bowden Four Food Groups: Foods you could hunt, fish, gather, or pluck.

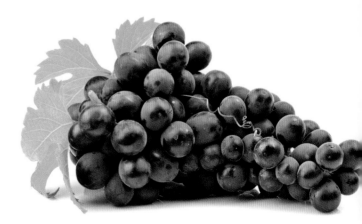

Broiled Salmon with Tamari-Orange Marinade

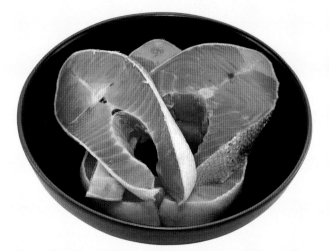

Prep Time: 10 minutes, then marinate for 4 to 6 hours
Cook Time: 10 to 15 minutes

Ingredients

⅓ cup (80 ml) high-quality dry white wine,
such as Chardonnay, or medium sweet wine,
such as Riesling

2 tablespoons (30 ml) low-sodium tamari

⅓ cup (80 ml) orange juice (fresh squeezed is best;
about 1 large juice orange)

3 tablespoons (24 g) peeled and finely grated ginger

¼ cup (25 g) finely chopped scallions

1 teaspoon raw honey

1½ pounds (680 g) wild Alaskan salmon fillet, cut into 4 equal portions,
or four 6-ounce (170-g) salmon steaks

½ teaspoon extra-virgin olive oil

Rinse the salmon gently in water and pat to dry.

In a small bowl, combine the wine, tamari, orange juice, ginger, scallions, and honey and whisk to combine well.

Place the salmon in a shallow glass baking pan, skin-side down if a fillet, and pour the marinade evenly on top.

Cover the baking pan with plastic wrap and refrigerate for 4 to 6 hours or overnight, tipping the dish occasionally to recoat the salmon.

Remove the baking pan from the refrigerator and let it stand at room temperature for 30 minutes. Preheat the broiler.

Lift the salmon out of the baking pan and remove any ginger or scallions to prevent burning. Rub the oil on the skin/bottom side of the salmon and place it on the broiling pan, oiled-side down.

Broil the salmon under high heat for 10 to 15 minutes until the salmon flakes easily with a fork and the flesh inside is firm and light pink. The top should lightly brown and caramelize. (If the salmon browns within the first 5 minutes, move the broiling pan down 1 rack in your oven.)

Yield: 4 servings

From *The Healthiest Meals on Earth* by Jonny Bowden and Jeannette Bessinger (Fair Winds Press, 2008)

OH, MY AGING SKIN

Much of what we consider "aging" skin is really the accumulation of oxidative (free radical) damage.

"The unstable free radical molecules vibrate in the skin, literally poking holes in the collagen fibers of the dermis," explains Michael N. Chang, Ph.D., the former deputy director of medical chemistry at Merck. Collagen is the main protein in connective tissue, and over the years, under continuous assault from free radicals, it basically becomes weaker and weaker, eventually causing the skin to wrinkle. (I discuss the use of collagen supplements on page 208.)

"Every day each skin cell can be exposed to more than 73,000 damaging assaults," says Chang. And it doesn't help that the skin is an external organ. As the first line of defense against any environmental elements, it's often the first and most visually obvious place that we age. In fact, you can think of the skin, especially the face, as a marker for the kind of damage that free radicals are doing inside the body. (Not always a pretty picture, is it?)

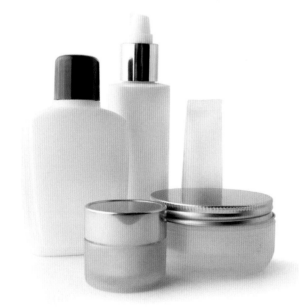

I can tell you about free radical damage on a cellular level from now to doomsday, but because you can't see it, it doesn't seem real. So think of your face as a kind of "visual aid" in this lesson. If you find yourself noticing wrinkles, scars, lines, and the like, consider that the exact same thing is happening inside, where you can't see it. And free radical damage is aging you inside just as sure as it's aging your face—only sometimes with much worse consequences. (A wrinkle on your face may hurt your vanity, but free radical damage to the heart and vascular system will shorten your life.)

It's no coincidence that high-end skin care products are loaded with antioxidants. Antioxidants can easily be absorbed through the skin, which is why the best of these creams can actually help you look better. Antioxidants in the diet and on the skin are a great defense against damage, inside *and* out.

OH, MY AGING EYES

There's not a baby boomer alive who doesn't know this feeling—all of a sudden you can't see items on the menu or read the movie times in the paper or the ingredients on a bottle. Boomers everywhere nod understandingly when a fellow boomer says, "Hold on, I can't see it without my glasses."

Everybody winds up needing reading glasses eventually (at least if he or she wants to read). That's a fact of life that no diet or exercise or lifestyle program can change. Here's why: As they die, all cells are carried away by the bloodstream (or sloughed off in the skin or cut off in the hair). But in the eyes, these cells have nowhere to go, because the lens is in a capsule. As you live longer, more and more cells get trapped inside there and the capsule gets more crowded and stiff. By the time you're forty or forty-five, you can't "flex" the lens, or focus it enough, for close reading. So, you need glasses.

The condition just described is called *presbyopia*, and truth be told, it's no big deal. That's not the aspect of aging eyes we're concerned with. After all, you just whip out a pair of those cool drugstore glasses that every boomer carries around, and you're good to go. There's a far more serious kind of aging disease that affects the eyes—it's called *macular degeneration*.

Macular degeneration is the leading cause of vision loss and blindness in Americans aged sixty-five and older. It produces a slow, or rarely, sudden, painless loss of vision. Symptoms include seeing shadowy areas in your central vision or experiencing unusual fuzzy or distorted vision. When it comes to "aging eyes," macular degeneration is the real problem, much more serious than a minor problem that can be addressed with some fashionable reading glasses.

In 2001, the National Eye Institute conducted the Age-Related Eye Disease Study (AREDS) involving more than 3,600 people. The researchers found that *supplementation with certain nutrients* reduced the risk of progressing to advanced macular degeneration by 28 percent. What you eat profoundly affects the macula, that small sensitive part of the retina responsible for detailed vision. Many experts feel strongly that diet and supplements can be used to treat or prevent its degeneration.

Want to know what those nutrients are? I'm sure you can guess by now: *antioxidants*.

The specific daily amounts of antioxidants and zinc used by the study researchers were 500 milligrams of vitamin C, 400 IU of vitamin E, 15 milligrams of beta-carotene (often labeled as equivalent to 25,000 IU of vitamin A), 80 milligrams of zinc, and 2 milligrams of copper. Since the time of the study, experts now consider the carotenoids lutein and zeaxanthin to be essential to the protection of the eyes, largely through their ability to fight free radical damage in that area.

Since the ARED study came out, published research has shown that omega-3 fatty acids also help prevent macular degeneration. At the same time, consumption of omega-6 fatty acids, the main form of fat in vegetable oils, was associated with an *increased* risk of developing the condition. The reason for this finding brings us to the second major component of every single disease of aging and the focus of the next chapter: *inflammation*.

CHAPTER 2

Put out the Fire of the Second Horseman of Aging: Inflammation

If you've ever stubbed your toe, banged your head against a beam, or gotten a splinter or an abscess on your skin, you know what inflammation is. The affected area gets red and swollen. Why? Because the body immediately sends blood and fluid into the area. White blood cells—also known as *leukocytes*—mobilize to the injury site, surrounding it like an army blocking off an invading force. Specialized white blood cells called *macrophages* initiate defense mechanisms and literally swallow up and immobilize any invading pathogens.

All these activities, which your body does automatically as part of its immune defenses, are collectively called *inflammation*. Inflammation isn't always a bad thing; we actually need inflammatory chemicals in our body, they're an integral part of the body's inborn healing responses.

My great friend Barry Sears, Ph.D., creator of the world-famous Zone diet and author of *The Anti-Inflammation Zone* writes, "Without inflammation we would be sitting ducks in a very hostile world, with no way to repair the damage constantly being inflicted on us. Our internal inflammatory responses let us attack (the) invaders, surround them, and ultimately kill them before they kill us."

The problem is that our inflammatory army is in overdrive.

A WORLD OUT OF BALANCE

We need inflammation to heal—we want those white blood cells rushing to the site of injury trying to put out the potential fire of a microbe invasion. But we *also* need *anti*-inflammatory compounds to act as correctives when there's *too much* inflammation. We need our body's anti-inflammatory army to be just as strong and active and robust as our inflammatory army. "It's the internal

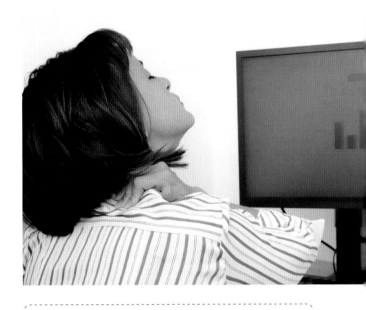

THE SECOND HORSEMAN OF AGING: INFLAMMATION

What it is:

Inflammation is a basic way the body reacts to injury or irritation. Chronic inflammation flies below the radar of your perception and may not cause any pain or symptoms.

Why it's bad for you:

Chronic inflammation is a "silent killer"; it damages the vascular walls and is a factor in every single degenerative disease, including heart disease, Alzheimer's, diabetes, cancer, and obesity.

What you can do about it:

Supplement daily with fish oil, one of the greatest natural anti-inflammatory agents on the planet. Use flax oil in your salad dressing. Eat plenty of vegetables and fruits—all high in natural anti-inflammatories such as quercetin (e.g., apples, onions).

anti-inflammatory response that not only turns off the attack phase of inflammation but also generates the repair processes that lead to cellular rejuvenation," says Sears.

Bottom line: Inflammation and anti-inflammation forces need to be in a constant balance or else we're in trouble.

Now, here's the problem: The inflammatory army doesn't *just* get mobilized whenever there's an obvious injury. It also gets mobilized whenever there's damage to cells—and damaging the cells is exactly what free radicals do!

On the one hand, we have a constant assault from free radicals doing oxidative damage to the cells. On the other, we have the constant response of inflammation to this cellular injury. These processes are going on all the time, slowly wearing down our bodies, contributing to disease, aging, and breakdown.

The problem is that you will certainly notice the pain of inflammation in your knee or hip or joints, but you will probably *not* notice it in your vascular system, where it is doing incalculable damage on a daily basis. Chronic inflammation is a part of diseases as diverse as cancer, Alzheimer's, obesity, congestive heart failure, diabetes, and digestive system diseases. That "silent inflammation" is reducing your odds of long life just as effectively as breathing an invisible, odorless poison gas.

CHRONIC INFLAMMATION: THE SLOW KILLER

Inflammation comes in two flavors—acute and chronic. Many practitioners in the field of anti-aging health believe that most of us are walking around in a state of chronic inflammation. Sears puts it beautifully: "Classic (acute) inflammation hurts," he says. "Silent (chronic) inflammation slowly kills."

According to an excellent article by Kathleen McGowan in *Discover Magazine* ("Can We Cure Aging?"), gerontologists now realize that aging "is actually something our own bodies create, a side effect of the essential inflammatory system that protects us against infectious disease … as we fight off invaders, we inflict massive collateral damage on ourselves, poisoning our own organs and breaking down our own tissues. We are our own worst enemy." Russell Tracy—professor of pathology and biochemistry at the University of Vermont College of Medicine—puts it this way: Inflammation "predicts having heart attacks,

"Classic (acute) inflammation hurts.
Silent (chronic) inflammation slowly kills."

—Barry Sears, Ph.D.

having heart failure, becoming diabetic. It predicts becoming fragile in old age; it predicts cognitive function decline, even, to a certain extent, cancer."

Chronic inflammation is a part of every degenerative disease known to humankind. We're familiar with its role in allergies, acne, and asthma, but what you might *not* be aware of is inflammation's role in obesity, cancer, diabetes, Alzheimer's, and cognitive decline—all the diseases of aging.

Instead of being a transient event, the inflammatory response persists over time, "like an ornery child who can't resist picking at a scab," says science writer Christine Gorman. Eventually, chronic inflammation can and will destroy tissue. And it can absolutely cut off any chances you have for a long, disease-free life.

GET THIS MEDICAL TEST

Here's another place where we've missed the boat in our obsessive focus on cholesterol lowering as a life-extending, disease-preventing strategy. A much publicized 2008 study called the JUPITER study illustrates the point perfectly. It showed that a cholesterol-lowering drug (Crestor) reduced the risk for heart disease by 40 percent. Not terribly interesting, you might think, but consider this: *None of the 17,000 participants in the study had high cholesterol in the first place.*

What they did have were elevated levels of inflammation, as measured by a blood test for an inflammatory compound called *C-reactive protein*. And the cholesterol-lowering drugs, known collectively as *statin drugs*, do lower inflammation. For years, I, and many of my colleagues, have argued that the benefit of statin drugs has little to do with lowering cholesterol. It's *inflammation* that attacks oxidized cholesterol deposits in the arteries, causing the problems that are blamed on cholesterol. Saying statin drugs lower heart disease because they reduce cholesterol is like saying aspirin prevents clotting because it's white.

Any benefit statin drugs may have—and believe me, their benefit is a lot more hotly debated than you might imagine from reading the press releases of the drug companies—comes because they lower inflammation, a far more serious risk for the diseases of aging than cholesterol ever was. I'm not at all sure we need to worry about lowering cholesterol if we want to live longer. I'm *very* sure we need to worry about lowering inflammation.[1]

And drug companies are taking notice. "Virtually our entire research and development effort is focused on inflammation and cancer," said Robert Tepper, M.D., a former clinical professor of medicine at New York University School of Medicine and now president of research and development at Millennium Pharmaceuticals in Cambridge, Massachusetts. "The whole field of inflammation research is about to explode," adds Paul Ridker, M.D., a cardiologist at Brigham and Women's Hospital in Boston.

Inflammatory chemicals come from both internal and external sources. Nearly everything that's an irritant to the system—the air pollution we breathe, the tobacco smoke we inhale directly or indirectly, the some 80,000 chemicals we're exposed to in our environment—has the potential to produce some level of inflammation.

---

1 It's worth pointing out that fully half the people who have heart attacks have normal cholesterol. The drug that lowers the risk of heart attack the most is aspirin, and it doesn't do a thing to cholesterol levels. It does, however, lower inflammation. Something to think about.

For instance, the food we eat can produce an inflammatory reaction. And some foods, such as certain sugars, have the effect of turbocharging our inflammatory production pathways, while some foods have the opposite effect. And here's where the situation gets interesting.

Our bodies make both inflammatory and anti-inflammatory compounds called *eicosanoids* from raw materials that come from the fat in our diet. The *type* of fat you consume affects the eicosanoid production factory. Omega-6 fatty acids, the kind found in vegetable oils such as corn oil, safflower oil, sunflower oil, and the like, are *pro-inflammatory*. Omega-3 fatty acids, the kind found in fish, and fish oil, are the exact opposite. They're the precursors for the *anti-inflammatory* compounds in the body.

Most researchers agree that the ideal relationship of omega-6 (pro-inflammatory fatty acids) to omega-3 (anti-inflammatory fatty acids) fats is about 1:1. And that is exactly the ratio you find in the diet of the hunter-gatherer societies that were so remarkably free of the diseases of aging.[2] This ratio keeps the eicosanoid production factories in harmony, with the body producing a nice balance of pro-inflammatory and anti-inflammatory chemicals.

The importance of this balance to good health and anti-aging can't be overstated. "It is the balance of eicosanoids in your body that is the ultimate key to wellness," Sears says. So when both factories are being adequately fueled—omega-6 fats for the "pro-inflammatory" eicosanoids and omega-3s for the "anti-inflammatory" ones—everything hums along really well.

And the ratio of pro-inflammatory fats to anti-inflammatory fats in the typical Western diet: Fifteen to one.[3]

Think it doesn't matter? Think again. "A high omega-6/omega-3 ratio, as is found in today's Western diet, promotes the pathogenesis of many diseases, including cardiovascular disease, cancer, osteoporosis, and inflammatory and autoimmune diseases," writes Artemis P. Simopoulos, M.D., founder and president of the Center for Genetics, Nutrition, and Health in Washington, DC.

In other words, inflammation is arguably the most significant "engine" driving premature aging.[4] And we're helping it along by overfueling our inflammation factories and undernourishing our anti-inflammatory ones. You couldn't come up with a more perfect prescription for aging badly.

Our food choices make it easier for our tissues to become inflamed, as does lack of exercise and many other aspects of our lifestyle. Our diet is a huge factor in promoting inflammation, as is our method of cooking. But this means there's a lot we *can* do to slow or prevent inflammation, just like there's a lot we can do to slow or prevent oxidative damage.

INFLAMMATION: HOW DO WE MEASURE IT?

One biochemical marker has consistently shown predictive value in determining the risk for heart disease and even death. It's something called *C-reactive protein* (CRP). CRP is a protein that's produced by the liver as part of the

---

2   Yes, you might say, but they died so much younger. True, but they died from exposure, violence, and attacks from wild animals, and all the anthropological evidence suggests that they did not have any early signs of the degenerative diseases that kill most of us in the twenty-first century.

3   That's a conservative estimate that has been demonstrated in research, but many scientists suspect that estimate is low, and it probably is.

4   It's worth mentioning that more than 30 million people worldwide take NSAIDs (non-steroidal anti-inflammatory drugs) on a daily basis. NSAIDs include aspirin and ibuprofen. In the United States, annual sales of NSAIDs and COX-2 inhibitors (another class of anti-inflammatories) exceed $6 billion. And this is just for the inflammation we notice!

immune response to infection or injury. Levels of CRP in the blood increase dramatically, a hundredfold or more, in response to bacterial infections, trauma, and other inflammatory conditions.

The version of this test that's currently used is called the high-sensitivity CRP (hs-CRP) test. That's the test you should demand from your doctor.

You may remember that the people in the JUPITER study I mentioned had high levels of inflammation. How did the researchers know about this inflammation? Simple. They measured the participants' levels of CRP, the most reliable measure of inflammation available. The study participants all had elevated CRP, and their risk for heart disease was lowered *not* because their cholesterol went down (it was normal to begin with) but because their *inflammation* went down. Though experts will continue to debate the true meaning of this study, I'd argue that it's further proof that inflammation is a far greater risk to your health and longevity than cholesterol ever was.

Gerontologists now see aging as a consequence of inflammation "If you talk to many old people, what they are really desperate about is not that fact that they're going

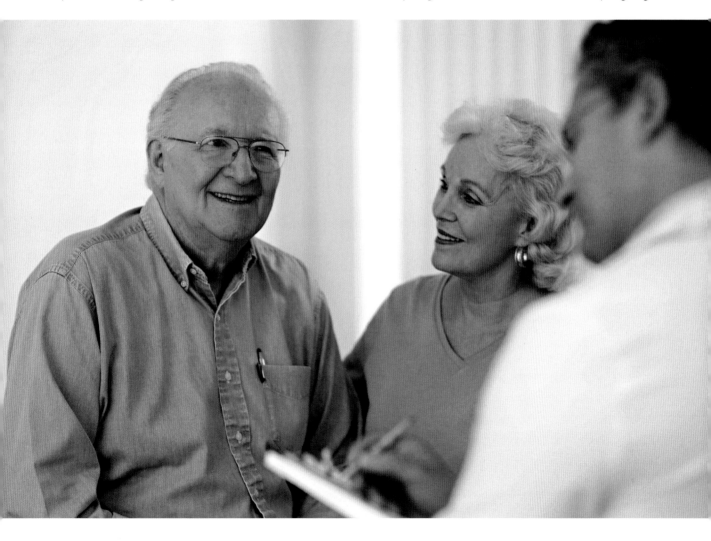

ANTI-AGING ACTION PLAN:

Get an hs-CRP Test to Assess Your Risk of Heart Disease

The liver produces c-reactive protein (CRP) as part of the immune response to infection or injury. It's also produced by muscle cells in the coronary arteries.

Studies show that in the majority of healthy individuals, circulating levels of CRP were found to be below the detection threshold for most standard blood tests, but a new "high-sensitivity" CRP test has fixed the problem. It's the hs-CRP (high-sensitivity CRP) test you should demand from your doctor.

As long ago as the 1990s, Dr. Tracy and his colleagues showed that CRP is an "amazingly accurate predictor of a future heart attack—as good or better than high blood pressure or high cholesterol." And it's not like this test is unknown to mainstream medicine. According to the website of the American Heart Association:

→ A growing number of studies have examined whether hs-CRP (high-sensitivity CRP) can predict recurrent cardiovascular disease, stroke, and death in different settings.

→ High levels of hs-CRP consistently predict recurrent coronary events in patients with unstable angina and acute myocardial infarction (heart attack).

→ Higher hs-CRP levels also are associated with lower survival rates in these patients.

→ Many studies have suggested that after adjusting for other prognostic factors, hs-CRP is useful as a risk predictor.

→ Studies also suggest that higher levels of hs-CRP may increase the risk that an artery will reclose after its been opened by balloon angioplasty.

→ High levels of hs-CRP in the blood also seem to predict prognosis and recurrent events in patients with stroke or peripheral arterial disease.

So, get an hs-CRP test the next time you have blood work done. If your hs-CRP is lower than 1.0mg/L, you have a low risk of developing cardiovascular disease. Lower than 1.0 mg/L is the ideal level.

If your hs-CRP is between 1.0 and 3.0 mg/L, you have an average risk. If your hs-CRP is higher than 3.0 mg/L, you are at high risk for developing heart disease. What can you do? Consult your doctor and start eating an anti-inflammatory diet (see page 51).

to die, but that they are going to be sick, dependent, and have to rely on others," said Luigi Ferrucci, chief of the Longitudinal Study of Aging. Clearly, silent inflammation accelerates the clock.

Inflammation—according to Harvey Jay Cohen, director of the Center for the Study of Aging at Duke University Medical Center—is similar to "little waves lapping on the shore. It's a relatively low level of activity, one that sustained over time wears away at the beach and stimulates other bad events." Inflammatory activity even breaks down skeletal muscle, which leads to the loss of lean muscle mass, one of the hallmarks of an aging body.

In many large-scale prospective studies as well as a number of meta-analyses (studies *of* studies), knowing your hs-CRP significantly improves the predictive value of a blood test when it comes to determining who is at risk for heart disease, the number one life-shortening disease in the United States.

A number of studies have found that the higher your hs-CRP levels, the higher the risk of a heart attack. That's not a good thing for longevity! In fact, according to the American Heart Association, the risk for heart attack in people in the upper third of hs-CRP levels is *twice* that of those whose hs-CRP level is in the lower third. These studies have also shown an association between high hs-CRP and sudden cardiac death as well as the incidence of stroke.

If you want to live long and well, one thing you absolutely have to do is reduce your systemic inflammation. And if you want to see how successful you are at it, get your CRP measured.

WHAT YOU CAN DO ABOUT INFLAMMATION

Fortunately, a great deal of inflammation is under our control. Once again, it all starts with food.

As with antioxidants, the plant kingdom is absolutely loaded with natural anti-inflammatory properties. Some that you should include in your diet are as follows:

- Onions and leeks
- Garlic
- Leafy greens (e.g., spinach, chard, kale)
- Tomatoes
- Bell peppers
- Brassica vegetables (e.g., Brussels sprouts, cabbage, broccoli, cauliflower)
- Beans: all types
- Nuts and seeds
- Spices: ginger, turmeric, cinnamon, cloves
- Herbs: parsley, rosemary, thyme, oregano, mint, tarragon, dill
- Tea: all types

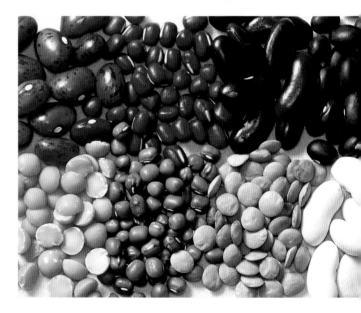

ANTI-AGING ACTION PLAN:

Lower Inflammation with These Supplements

Take These Supplements:

→ Omega-3 fatty acids with DHA and EPA: 2–4 g per day

→ GLA (found in evening primrose oil, borage oil, and black currant oil): 250–500 mg per day

→ MSM (methyl-sulfonyl-methane): 1,000–2,000 mg twice a day

→ Curcumin: This extract from the spice turmeric is one of the most anti-inflammatory substances we know of. Take as directed: 500–1000 mg a day

→ Quercetin: A powerful anti-inflammatory found in apples and oranges and available as a supplement (1000 mg a day)

- Red wine
- Cocoa/chocolate (minimum sugar, maximum chocolate)
- Flaxseeds and flaxseed oil

Wild salmon is also a great source of the two most important omega-3s found in food, as well the superstar antioxidant *astaxanthin*. Grass-fed beef also has omega-3 fats, as do sardines, mackerel, herring, and tuna.

Put this all together and we start to notice an inescapable conclusion: Many of the foods that are high in anti-inflammatory properties are *also* high in antioxidants, providing a weapon against two of the most significant processes in every disease of aging: oxidation and inflammation. And these foods form the bulk of the diets of the longest-lived people on the planet.

One of the most anti-inflammatory compounds on the planet is the class of fats known as omega-3 fatty acids, which are found in fish and flaxseeds. But remember that it's not just the fish oil you want—it's the stuff that's in it. The two fatty acids of greatest importance for the human body are EPA (*eicosapentanoic acid*) and DHA (*docosahexanoic acid*). So, it's not enough to just "take 1,000 milligrams of fish oil." Look on the label for *how much EPA and DHA the fish oil actually contains* and try to take at least 2 (preferably 3 to 4) grams of total EPA and DHA for the best anti-inflammatory results.

When you take large doses of EPA and DHA, it's a good idea to "balance" them with another fat called gamma-linolenic acid (GLA). Many people take supplements such as evening primrose oil, which is an excellent source of GLA. GLA is actually an omega-6 fat, but it's one of the good ones, and it converts in the body to "good" prostaglandins (anti-inflammatory eicosanoids). I suggest taking about 1 gram of evening primrose oil (with GLA) for every 2 to 4 grams of fish oil.

Another supplement that's recommended is MSM (methyl-sulfonyl-methane). I discussed MSM at length in my book, *The Most Effective Natural Cures on Earth*, because of its fantastic effect on pain and inflammation caused by arthritis. It's equally good as an all-around anti-inflammatory compound. My friend Mark Houston, M.D., M.S., recommends 1,000 to 2,000 milligrams of MSM twice a day as part of a supplemental program to reduce inflammation in the body. Remember, the better you are at reducing inflammation, the better your chances of living longer and living well!

How Can You Reduce Inflammation through Dietary Restriction and Lifestyle Changes

- Stay clear of excess processed vegetable oils like soybean, safflower, corn, and canola.
- Stay clear of trans fats.
- Eat more vegetables.
- Opt for low-glycemic (low-sugar/starch) nutrition.
- Exercise regularly and maintain a healthy weight.
- Take a baby aspirin daily if you're over 45.
- Augment your diet with omega-3, curcumin, garlic, ginger, pomegranate, green tea, and lemons.
- Have your hs-CRP levels tested!

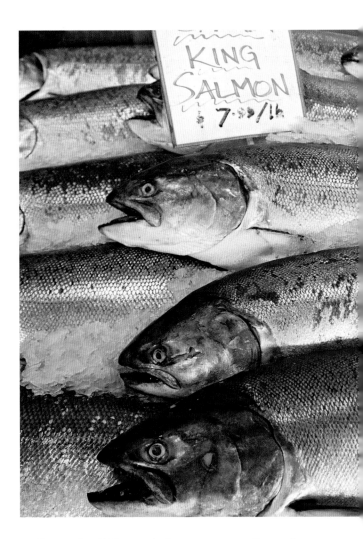

Remember: What we *don't* eat matters, too. Some of the biggest enemies of a long and healthy life are sugar and foods cooked at very high temperatures. And this leads us neatly into a discussion of the third of the "Four Horsemen of Aging," an insidious factor called *glycation*.

CHAPTER 3

Avoid the Damage of the Third Horseman of Aging: Glycation

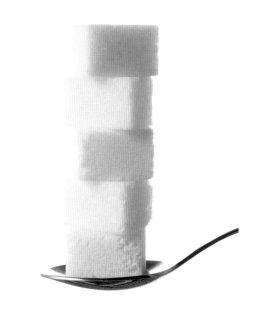

I magine a nice, fluid substance such as almond oil. Imagine the liquid flowing from the amber brown glass container, clear and golden, as you pour it into a cooking pan or drizzle it on a salad or even as you might use it as a wonderful, fragrant massage oil.

Now, imagine what happens if you drop some sticky, pink cotton candy into that lovely, fluid oil.

Not a very appealing picture, is it? But there's no better visual analogy for what happens in your body when proteins—fluid substances just like almond oil—get dirtied up by sugar. The sugar molecules glom onto those formerly glistening, sleek, slippery protein molecules, gumming up the works, jamming up the flow, and generally making a big mess. Aging your body—and all its systems—like nobody's business.

And once the sugar is in the mix, you can't get it back out. The process of sugar "gumming up the works," attaching to formerly sleek proteins and making them sticky, is called *glycation*. It's happening in your body every single day.

Take diabetes, for example, a condition in which the damage from glycation can be seen in clear relief. Type ll diabetes is a disease in which blood sugar typically rises higher than it should, which is why diabetics need to constantly monitor their blood sugar levels. Because diabetics often have uncontrolled blood sugar, they are at greater risk for the aging effects of glycation.

Even in nondiabetics, some of the glucose (sugar) in the bloodstream enters the red blood cells and "hooks up" (glycates) with a protein called *hemoglobin*. Okay, a small amount of "hooking up" can't be helped, and if only a small percentage of hemoglobin is "gummed up," it's no big deal. And remember, once a hemoglobin molecule gets "stuck"

THE THIRD HORSEMAN OF AGING: GLYCATION

What it is:

Glycation is what happens when sugar molecules glom onto protein (or fat) molecules.

Why it's bad for you:

These sticky proteins gum up the works and eventually create AGEs (advanced glycation end products), which are implicated in many of the diseases of aging, including diabetes, cardiovascular disease, Alzheimer's, and cancer.

What you can do about it:

Take carnosine, which is one of the most effective weapons against glycation. It's also a powerful antioxidant.

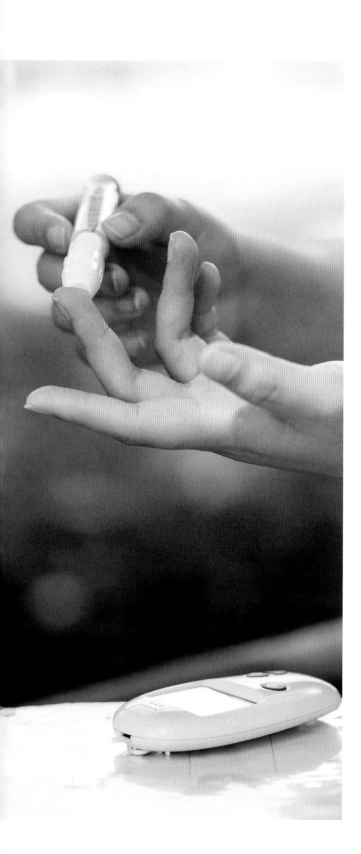

by sugar, it stays stuck! For the life of that red blood cell, about 120 days, that hemoglobin remains "glycated."

In diabetics, there's much more wreckage: more sugar, more glycation. Those sticky proteins can't flow freely through the smaller capillaries and create the problems in circulation that often lead, for diabetics, to blindness, foot amputations, and kidney problems. In large measure, the problems of diabetics can be seen as the problems of *glycation on steroids*—and can serve as a lesson for what we need to do to reduce the less dramatic (but still severely aging) effects of this Third Horseman of Aging.

You can measure that amount of glycated hemoglobin in a blood test called hemoglobin A1c, which is a much more accurate measure than a blood sugar level test is. See, when you prick your finger and measure your blood sugar, you're just getting a *snapshot* of where your blood sugar is at the exact moment you pricked your finger. Blood sugar could be high on Tuesday morning, but totally normal by Wednesday afternoon.

Because hemoglobin sticks around for the life of the red blood cell, any A1c test is going to tell you how much damage sugar has done *over time*—how much damaged hemoglobin is still hanging around. It's like surveying the wreckage after the floodwaters have receded.

Diabetics have high A1c levels (higher than 6 percent)—in fact, an unexpectedly high measurement on an A1c test is often the first way someone finds out he or she has diabetes in the first place. Because of the fact that once sugar has "linked up" with a hemoglobin molecule it stays bonded, the A1c test is a far more accurate measure of what the long-term aging (glycation) effects of high blood sugar are.

HOW A KIDNEY SPECIALIST BECAME A LOW-CARB GURU

One of the leading gurus of both low-carb diets and intermittent fasting is Dr. Jason Fung, a practicing nephrologist (kidney specialist). So how did a kidney specialist become an expert on low-carb diets?

The overwhelming majority of Fung's patients were diabetics, but Fung was unhappy with the state of care in diabetes. He saw little point in continuing to medicate his patients, often with drugs like insulin that had the potential to make things worse by causing even more weight gain. So, he started looking into what makes people diabetic in the first place.

Not surprisingly, he found that high-carbohydrate diets were part of the problem because they were stimuilating large amounts of insulin and leading ultimately to insulin resistance (see page 113 for a fuller explanation). High-carb diets were also providing a ton of sugar, which in turn created even more glycated proteins and AGEs.

Fung became an advocate of very low-carb diets because they limited sugar intake and helped control insulin. He became an advocate of intermittent fasting because it was another way to limit the amount of time the body spent in a high-insulin state. (Remember, insulin is also known as the "fat-storing" hormone.)

In many ways, Fung is a great example of what functional medicine is all about. He didn't just treat the symptoms of diabetes—such as high A1c (glycated hemoglobin)—he looked for why those symptoms happened in the first place and then addressed those "whys" in his treatment plans.

If you're not diabetic, you might be saying, "What does this have to do with me?" And the answer is, *a lot*. Diabetics are hardly the only ones at risk for the aging effects of glycation. Even in nondiabetics, about 5 percent of hemoglobin is glycated. And glycation, with its damaging consequences on all systems in the body, has myriad effects on aging and comes from far-ranging sources in the diet and environment, many of which you can actually *do* something about.

TURN DOWN THE HEAT

One of the ways you can lower the amount of glycated proteins in your body is to be careful about the way you cook food.

Cooking foods at really high temperatures, like those needed for frying, results in what has been called a "browning" effect, which is simply another term for glycation. When you eat that stuff, delicious as it may taste, you're basically eating glycated proteins. Foods cooked at high temperatures are virtual glycation factories, and you are ingesting nasty compounds called AGEs, which are basically the *end result* of glycation. The aptly named acronym AGE stands for *advanced glycation end products*. Your body will make these AGEs, or you can eat them ready-made right out of your frying pan. Let's review how it works:

1. The proteins in your body (or your frying pan) get gummed up by cross-linking with sugars, forming glycated proteins, or glycotoxins.

2. These damaged proteins lose their elasticity and become difficult for the body to break down—they literally become old and inflexible.

3. Damaged glycated proteins then hook up with *other* damaged glycated proteins.

4. When these damaged glycated proteins link together, they form insoluble masses, which in turn generate more free radicals!

And these rather disgusting insoluble masses of linked, damaged proteins—these free radical–generating factories—are what we call AGEs.

AGEs accumulate everywhere—in the skin, the brain, the nervous system, the vital organs, the vascular system—and they do exactly what their name implies. They age you. AGEs play a big role in diabetes, and whether you're diabetic or not, high levels of sugar intake (or foods that convert quickly into sugar, such as most breads and commercial cereals) make it all the more likely that *some* of that excess sugar will wind up binding with proteins and causing glycation, contributing to a whole cascade of aging effects.

ANTI–AGING ACTION PLAN:

Slow Down the Aging Process by Slowing Down Your Cooking

Cooking foods at high temperatures results in what's called a browning effect, another term for glycation, the Third Horseman of Aging.

Here are some good ways to avoid it:
→ Use slow-cooking cookware (such as Crock-Pots).
→ Cook foods in general at lower temperatures, such as simmering at low heat.
→ Don't blacken and don't grill over a high flame.
→ Avoid caramelization.

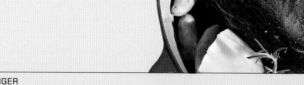

ANTI–AGING ACTION PLAN:

Take Carnosine to Prevent Glycation

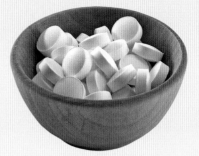

Add 1,000 mg of carnosine to your daily anti-aging regime. Carnosine helps prevent glycation, the Third Horseman of Aging, from happening in the first place. It's also a powerful antioxidant. However, our natural stores of carnosine aren't sufficient, so we need supplementation.

The fact that you can ingest fully formed AGEs by eating foods that have been cooked at high temperatures is no longer in doubt. A recent study published in the *Proceedings of the National Academy of Sciences* strongly suggests that eating foods cooked at high temperatures will increase the rate at which we age, largely due to the fact that such foods cause both chronic inflammation and the formation of AGEs.

Glycated proteins generate the very agents of oxidative damage—free radicals—which in turn create *more* damaged proteins, which then hook up with one another and become AGEs, producing more free radicals, and continuing this awful cycle of destruction and aging. Glycation and oxidation reinforce themselves in the nastiest of vicious circles.

We've now looked at three of the four agents of destruction when it comes to aging. Now, we're going to turn to the fourth horseman of aging, one that, at first glance, appears to be in a different category. But we'll soon see that although this fourth horseman may have more mental, spiritual, and psychological components than the other three, it is no less destructive and damaging to the body on a physical level than the others are.

And what is this mysterious fourth horseman of aging? Read on.

CHAPTER 4

Calm the Silent Killing of the Fourth Horseman of Aging: Stress

I t's popular to complain, "Oh, I'm so stressed out." Indeed, stress has become a buzzword to signal the standard reaction to anything mildly annoying in your life. But stress is a lot more than a mild annoyance. It's a true life shortener.

If longevity is something you want, you need to have a plan of action when it comes to dealing with stress.

There is a common myth that "stress is all in your mind." Fact is, the complicated stress response does *begin* in the brain, often out of conscious awareness, but it doesn't stay there. The stress response is a complicated, multidimensional set of biochemical and hormonal responses and signals that affect virtually the entire body. You can measure blood (and saliva) levels of specific stress hormones—it's not "all in your head!"

The stress response plays an important role in our survival. These built-in mechanisms respond to threats and were designed to save our life in an emergency. The problem isn't with the mechanisms themselves, but the fact that we are no longer following the manual that says "use as directed."

Let me explain.

OUR CAVEMAN HERITAGE

Assume for a moment that you are a calm, happy caveman, resting peacefully on the African Serengeti. All of a sudden, an enraged wildebeest comes charging at you. What do you do?

Well, obviously, you run like hell. Or, you pick up a stick or the nearest object you can use as a weapon and prepare to do battle for your life. But even before your conscious brain registers this, a tiny section deep in the brain called the *amygdala* registers danger even before you're

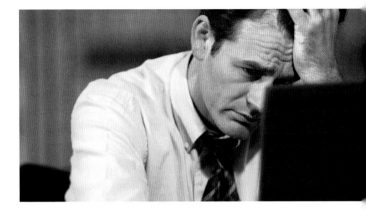

THE FOURTH HORSEMAN OF AGING: STRESS

What it is:
Stress is any physical, mental, or emotional factor that causes mental tension or bodily harm.

Why it's bad for you:
Stress produces hormonal reactions in the body that can shrink parts of the brain, damage your vascular system, and increase blood sugar levels, heart rate, and blood pressure. Stress can exacerbate less deadly but nonetheless important conditions such as skin problems, asthma, and allergies, and it makes recovery from illness much more difficult.

What you can do about it:
Meditation, deep breathing, and/or relaxing are the best antidotes to stress. A full night of restful, recuperative sleep helps correct some of the imbalances created by stress. Remove the conditions that create stress—toxic relationships, for example—or at least balance them with rewarding interpersonal connections, volunteering, time with friends, and gentle exercise such as yoga or qi gong.

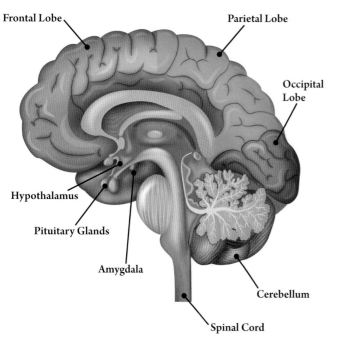

Frontal Lobe

Parietal Lobe

Occipital Lobe

Hypothalamus

Pituitary Glands

Amygdala

Cerebellum

Spinal Cord

consciously aware of it and sends an instant message to the *hypothalamus*. The hypothalamus shoots a hormonal signal to the pituitary gland, which in turn sends a hormonal signal of its own to the intended target of all this rapid-fire communication: a pair of walnut-shaped glands perched atop the kidneys called the *adrenals*.

The adrenals send out powerful hormones, cortisol and adrenaline, which accomplish a number of things. They get your heart racing. They shut off other metabolic operations that might interfere with the energy needed to fight

or run (for example, digestion). In some cases of extreme fear, your body will evacuate your bowels and bladder, because your primitive brain knows you don't need any extra weight while you're trying to scale a tree. Cortisol and adrenaline are known as the *fight or flight* hormones, precisely because that is what they prepare your body to do. If they weren't onboard, you'd continue to lounge lazily on your way to becoming a tasty dinner for the wildebeest.

The stress hormones are like a first gear for the body, turbocharging the engine to prepare for an emergency. But nature meant for the stress response to be used in emergencies. Nature did *not* mean for that pedal to be pressed to the metal all day long.

And here's why: A quick burst of cortisol (and adrenaline) will get your heart racing (so you can run quicker), increase your lung and heart function (same reason), dilate your pupils (so you can see where you're going and what you're running from!), and raise your blood sugar (you'll need it for energy!), all the while turning down the metabolic "volume" on bodily systems that are temporarily superfluous, such as the reproductive and immune systems. But in the long term, cortisol is a big problem.

Although cortisol is always described as a stress hormone, it's actually more of an antidote, or *antistress*, hormone (which is why your doctor will give you a shot of cortisone, a cortisol mimic, when you have a lot of

Stress is a lot more than a mild annoyance. It's a true life shortener.

inflammation). After adrenaline has moved out of the way, cortisol hangs around, trying to put out some of the fires and quench some of the damage that happens as a result of all the hormonal and metabolic changes your body goes through in a state of emergency.

Make no mistake—you need cortisol for survival—it's one of your most important hormones. Problem is, the effects are okay for the short term, but long term, they're an aging nightmare. And when you're in a continual state of stress, cortisol is *always* elevated—not a good thing from a longevity point of view.

For example, high levels of cortisol shrink an important portion of the brain called the hippocampus, which is essential to memory and thinking (we'll discuss the role of stress on the brain in more detail in chapter 8).

In addition, high levels of cortisol also increase insulin resistance, metabolic syndrome, and heart disease, all well-known longevity robbers. Stress hormones lower immunity. And cortisol breaks down muscle and causes your body to gain weight, and not just *any* old weight gain, but weight gain around the middle. Abdominal weight (the well-known "apple shape") is the most metabolically active and dangerous fat on your body, greatly increasing the risk of a whole host of life shorteners, such as heart disease. That's quite a bit of collateral damage if you're trying to live longer and healthier. The bottom line: Continuous, relentless stress shortens your life.

If you've read my book, *The Most Effective Natural Cures on Earth*, you know that for virtually every disease and condition I discussed, stress was a factor. Although stress may not directly *cause* diseases, it *contributes* to many of them and makes almost all of them worse. Simple examples include acne asthma, herpes outbreaks, and allergies—all can be brought on by stress. And even more insidiously,

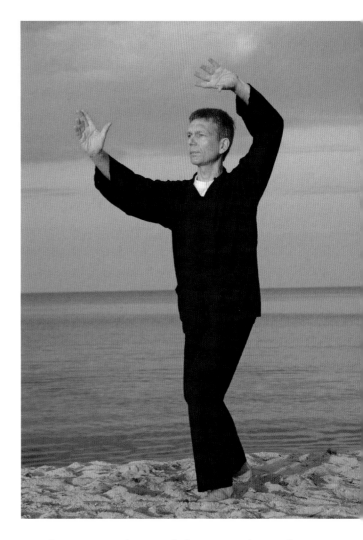

stress hormones produce metabolic activities that are *direct* contributors to hypertension, high blood pressure, and heart disease.

It's important that you understand how essential it is to have a system in place for dealing with, moderating, or eliminating stress. Community, family, contribution, and group membership have a demonstrated relationship to living longer and living well. It's a good bet that these activities exert their anti-aging magic largely because they are ways of balancing and managing the aging effects of stress hormones.

Practice Deep Breathing to Reduce Stress

Take ten minutes out of each day for a deep breathing exercise. Here's how:

1. Sit quietly in a comfortable position.

2. Close your eyes.

3. Slowly and gradually relax all your muscles one by one, beginning at the feet and moving up to the face.

4. Breathe deeply in through your nose and out through your mouth, concentrating only on your breath.

5. As you breathe out, silently say a calming word to yourself. It can be as simple as "joy," "peace," "calm," or even "one."

6. Continue for at least ten minutes.

THE TWO NERVOUS SYSTEMS

Every medical student has heard the joke that the sympathetic nervous system is responsible for the four Fs of behavior—flight, fight, fright, and sex. The *parasympathetic* system is responsible for everything else. It's hard to imagine a single aging process that doesn't *over-engage* the sympathetic nervous system and *under-engage* the parasympathetic one.

Stress turns on the sympathetic nervous system. Big time. Those stress hormones you release when you're in overdrive are *signals* to the body. They mean, quite simply, *something is wrong*. And nothing ages you like "sympathetic overdrive."

WHAT TYPE ARE YOU?

There have been more than a few systems of thought based on identifying people as being *sympathetic dominant* or *parasympathetic dominant*. That sweet, slightly heavy, grandmotherly woman who moves slowly and always has a kind word and a cookie for the neighbor? Parasympathetic dominant. A business tycoon always flying around, screaming into the phone, running late for meetings, and barking orders to subordinates while wolfing down a few Big Macs at his desk? Sympathetic dominant, baby. What else?

Who do you think is going to live longer?

We may not be able to do much about it if we are kind of "hardwired" to be sympathetic dominant. But we can certainly learn to modify the behaviors that send our sympathetic nervous system into overdrive.

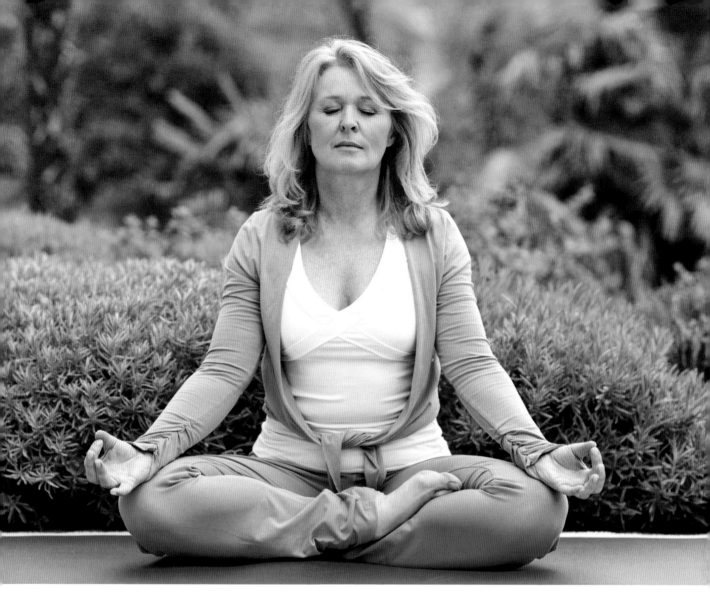

This is where meditation, deep breathing, and calming exercises such as yoga and qi gong come in and why they are such profound anti-aging strategies. They calm down the systems that send out the very messages that cause breakdown in your body and age you from the inside out. It's this engagement of the parasympathetic nervous system and its calming effect on the body (and mind) that helps counter the aging effects of stress. These messages temper the frantic shouting of the sympathetic nervous system and help you live longer and better.

Listen to them. And when they're not talking loudly enough on their own, help them out with activities that turn up their volume—meditating, breathing, relaxing, unwinding, and de-stressing.

That balancing act could not only extend your life—it could also save it.

CHAPTER 5

How Much Influence Do Genes Have on the Four Horsemen of Aging?

Truth be told, genes are misunderstood. Many people think genes are inflexible blueprints for what's going to happen to you, regardless of what you do. There's almost nothing that could be further from the truth. The vast majority of our 30,000-plus genes are dependent upon some *interaction* with the environment (which includes our diet) to *express* themselves.

So, rather than being fixed entities with only one outcome possible, genes are what is called *plastic*—able to be turned on *or* turned off. They work in conjunction with other genes, literally talking to one another. Their ultimate expression depends on complex interactions, both among themselves and, more important for our purposes, with the outside world. Genes respond to dozens, perhaps hundreds, of outside cues that switch them on or off, and many of those cues are firmly within our control.

Consider the genetic marker, 9p21, which I happen to have in a version that makes it much more likely that I will get lung cancer if I smoke cigarettes. But guess what—the influence of that genetic marker on my life is exactly zero if I never pick up a cigarette.

Some genes are turned on or turned off by nutrients. The emerging field of *nutrigenomics* is an exciting area of research that investigates just what effects nutrients and overall dietary practices, such as the number of calories we eat, have on turning on the genes we want to express (such as those for longevity) and turning off the ones we don't (such as those that predispose us to disease). Many of the nutrients we'll discuss throughout this book may exert their anti-aging effects precisely in this way.

Now, don't misunderstand me. Genes undoubtedly play a role in longevity. In a study of fifty-two Italian centenarians, scientists found one particular gene variation to be much more prevalent in people who lived past one

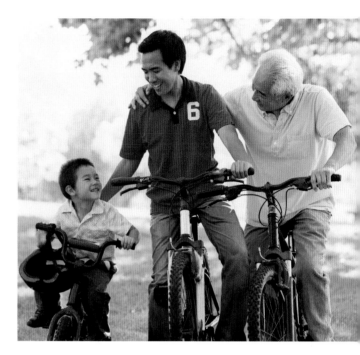

hundred than in people who did not. Possessing this gene increases the chances of living beyond one hundred by 400 percent, according to the researchers. But the interesting thing about it is that you can get this gene either by inheriting it *or* by "creating" it as a mutation that arises during the course of your life. "This introduces the intriguing idea that there may be specific things you can do to *induce* this beneficial mutation, increasing your own chances of living past 100," report scientist Ray Kurzweil and anti-aging pioneer Terry Grossman, M.D., in their terrific book *Fantastic Journey: The Science Behind Radical Life Extension*.

In other words, genes are not destiny.

THE GUN AND THE TRIGGER

In nutrition, we have a saying: Genetics load the gun, but environment pulls the trigger. Except in very few cases (such as the genes for Huntington's cholera or cystic fibrosis), what we *do* probably makes way more difference than

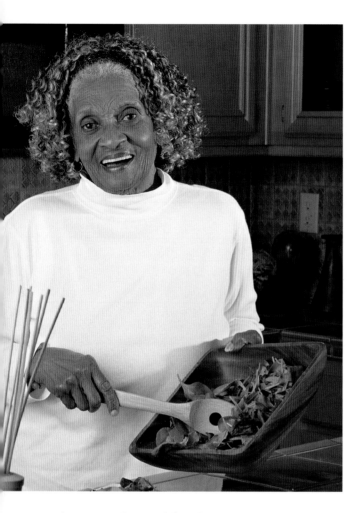

Aging at Harvard Medical School, Sinclair has investigated a set of genes called the *sirtuin* genes, which are considered to be major influencers of how long we live. "The sirtuin genes are the holy grail of medicine and nutrition," says my good friend Mark Houston, M.D. "When you modulate (influence) these genes, they turn on or turn off different metabolic pathways that are designed to promote longevity and health."

One of these genes, called the SIRT1 gene, appears to have an important, if still not fully understood, role in regulating how long we live. When you increase the activity of the SIRT1 gene in animals, it eliminates, or postpones drastically, the diseases of old age and essentially slows down the aging process itself. Leonard Guarente, Ph.D., a biology professor at the Massachusetts Institute of Technology and the discoverer of the sirtuin genes, believes that SIRT1 is activated by caloric restriction (see sidebar at right). Eating about one-third less food than "normal"[2] may "turn on" these longevity genes, in some way that is not yet fully understood.

Sinclair and his team discovered another way these genes can be turned on. A substance found in red wine—as well as the skin of dark grapes and, to some extent, peanuts—seems to have the same effect as calorie restriction in terms of turning the SIRT genes on. The substance is called *resveratrol*—we'll talk more about it in the supplements section (see page 238).

what we were born with.[1] And in any case, we can't control what we were born with, but we *certainly* can control what we do with it.

One of the people in the forefront of the emerging research on what exactly we can do to *turn* on our longevity genes is David Sinclair, Ph.D.

In the world of anti-aging research, Sinclair is a rock star. A professor of pathology and codirector of the Paul F. Glenn Laboratories for the Biological Mechanisms of

---

1   This is why no scientist worth his or her salt talks anymore about the false dichotomy of nature versus nurture. Instead, the discussion is typically framed nature via nurture. It's an interactive model, not an either-or one.

2   "Normal" means the appropriate number of calories for your height, weight, and activity level. If you're currently chowing down seven super-sized meals a day, you'll certainly improve your health by reducing your calories by one-third, but it's better still if you reduce them starting from a reasonable baseline! In fact, if you're eating an appropriate number of calories for your height and weight to begin with, you may be able to get anti-aging benefits by cutting calories by only 25 percent. For example, a man eating 2,500 calories a day would lower that to 1,900 and a woman eating 1,800 would lower it to about 1,350.

EAT LESS, LIVE LONGER

It's a pretty good bet that a diet high in antioxidants, anti-inflammatory properties, and omega-3 fats will stack the odds in your favor when it comes to longevity. But what about the *amount* of food you eat? Could that make a difference?

In 1982, some inventive research scientists decided to investigate the effect of a calorie-restricted diet on longevity and disease. They divided a few hundred male rats into two groups; one group was allowed to eat all the rat chow they desired, and the other group was allowed to eat about two-thirds of what they would have normally consumed when left to their own devices. The results set the stage for some of the most interesting anti-aging research of the past decade.

Here's what happened to the rats: The ones who received the normal diet lived their normal maximum life span of about 1,000 days. And they usually died from cancer, kidney disease, or the deterioration of their hearts. Pretty typical story for a rat, nothing out of the ordinary. But for

the rats fed the limited calorie diet it was a whole different story. These rats lived for about 1,500 days on average—a whopping 50 percent increase in life span. Even better, they avoided much of what we would consider the accompaniments of aging—feebleness, low energy (sluggish behavior), and a grizzled appearance. For example, their coats, which normally would turn gray after the age of two, stayed shiny and white for three and a half years or even longer! And they performed better, running mazes more successfully than their "normal eating" lab mates. Their immune systems were stronger, their rates of diabetes and cancer were far lower, and they had fewer cataracts. When they did finally die, most of them just expired.

They were living examples of what I referred to earlier as a "rectangularized functionality curve." Said Edward Masoro, Ph.D., a physiologist at the University of Texas Health Science Center in San Antonio: "When we look inside them, they're completely clean."

Calorie restriction, at least in rodents, was shown to be a demonstrable anti-aging strategy.

There have now been more than two thousand animal studies confirming these results across species as varied as yeast cells, fruit flies, monkeys, and mice. Scientists have reproduced these dramatic effects hundreds of times under all sorts of laboratory conditions. Because humans live much longer than, say, rats or fruit flies, and because of ethical and practical considerations, there are no long-term definitive studies on calorie restriction and humans. Nevertheless, some people voluntarily practice caloric restriction—they even have their own Caloric Restriction Society (www.calorierestriction.org). And those who do practice calorie restriction are showing the same effects as those seen in the animal studies—less disease, fewer "markers" of aging, and much thinner bodies!

ANTI-AGING ACTION PLAN:

Cut Back on Calories by 33 Percent to Extend Your Life

Eating one-third fewer than your normal number of calories has been shown to extend life and prevent the normal deterioration that comes with aging in every single species studied.

A good place to start is by simply eyeballing the food on your plate, mentally dividing each dish into three equal sections, and then just eating two of them.

In 2003, Sinclair and his research associates published a now-famous paper reporting that plant compounds known as *polyphenols* could activate the human SIRT1 gene as well as extend the life span of yeast. The polyphenol in question is a substance called *resveratrol*, which is found in red wine and the skins of dark grapes (and to a lesser extent, peanuts). Later, Sinclair demonstrated that even if you fed mice a diet known to shorten their life and make them obese, they would still live 15 percent longer when treated with resveratrol. In other studies, he's shown that resveratrol mimics the effect of calorie restriction, effectively slowing down diabetes, cancer, heart disease, and indeed, the very process of aging itself.

Obviously, there are some heavy bets being made on the potential of resveratrol to extend healthy life.

"I think the sirtuin genes and the work that's been done on how to modify [their] expression is one of the major medical breakthroughs of the past several years," said Houston. "For the first time we have the ability to modify the aging process in humans."

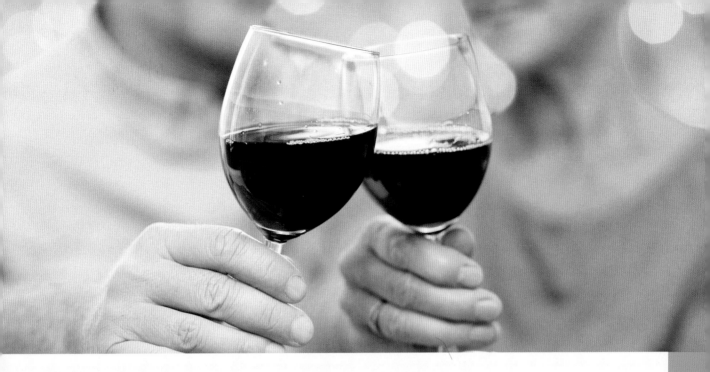

ANTI-AGING ACTION PLAN:

Take 250–500 Milligrams of Trans-Resveratrol Daily to Slow Down the Aging Process

How much resveratrol you need to take to get the anti-aging and life-extension effects shown in the lab is controversial. Certainly, drinking red wine helps, though that may not be appropriate for all people.

"No one knows the correct dose in humans," says Mark Houston, M.D., "but any amount will have health benefits." The smart money is betting that at least 250 milligrams a day should have an effect on aging, though Houston recommends (and takes) more.

One thing is certain: The most effective kind of resveratrol is the trans-resveratrol form. Many of the better products on the market will say "standardized to 20 percent trans-resveratrol." That means a 500 milligram pill delivers 100 milligrams of the potent trans-resveratrol form. You only calculate your dose on the trans-resveratrol component. Life Extension makes a resveratrol supplement that is standardized to 100% trans, meaning if you see 250 mg on the label of one of their resveratrol products, you're getting a full 250 mg of trans. That's very, very rare among supplements, but it's the gold standard, and it's what you should look for.

SECTION II

How to Keep the Key Players in Your Body Fit

·····································

Laguna Woods is a lovely gated community deep in the heart of Orange County, California, located on 2,100 rolling acres of lush greenery just minutes from the Laguna Beach coastline. More than 18,000 people (fifty-five-plus years old) live there, in what the *Orange County Register* has voted the "best retirement community in Orange County."

The average age is seventy-eight.

The residents of Laguna Woods are part of one of the largest ongoing studies on health and mental sharpness in the elderly. Begun in 1981, it's called the *90+ Study*. More than 14,000 men and women age sixty-five or older, including more than one thousand people who have made it to ninety, have had their blood and memory tested, their genetics analyzed, and their activities tracked. Researchers have also performed postmortem analyses on the brains of participants who've died.

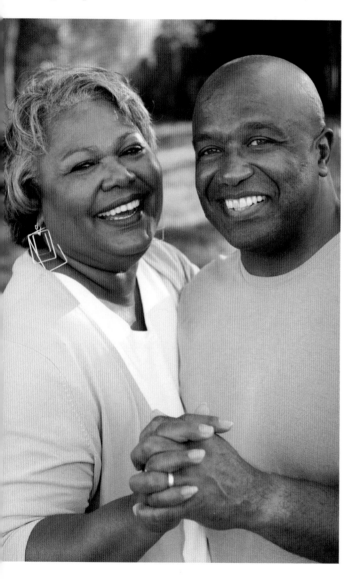

"These are the most successful agers on earth, and they're only just beginning to teach us what's important, in their genes, in their routines, in their lives," Claudia Kawas, M.D., a neurologist at the University of California, Irvine, told *New York Times* columnist Benedict Carey, who wrote a story on the community's fascinating residents.

The 90+ Study is specifically concerned with the aging brain, and researchers are understandably interested in teasing out which factors might be responsible for the fact that, for example, ninety-two-year-old Red Bull–slinging bridge playing Ruth Cummins seems not to have lost a whit of her faculties while many of her contemporaries, at least those who are alive, can't remember their names.

"So far, scientists have found little evidence that diet or exercise affects the risk of dementia in people over 90," writes Carey. "But some researchers argue that mental engagement—doing crossword puzzles, reading books—may delay the arrival of symptoms. And social connections, including interaction with friends, may be very important."

Carey was being cautious. It's now abundantly clear that social connections are *very* important and may even be arguably the most important factor in successful, healthy aging. Many have argued that a strong social fabric may be the single best predictor of longevity and health.

But there's more to successful aging than just preventing dementia.

STRONG IN MIND AND BODY

Although no one would deny for a second that clarity of mind and preservation of memory are high on the desirability checklist for successful aging, life is even better when such an intact and sharp brain is accompanied by a healthy, disease-free body in which the heart beats strongly, the limbs are creak-free, and the owner of said body is able to function autonomously. The owner gets bonus points for possessing the essential qualities of happiness—a connection to others, social integration, a sense of purpose.

In this section, we will look at some of the key areas of the body that can seriously hamper your ability to live well and long should they break down and falter: the heart, brain, immune system, hormonal system, and, taken together, the muscles, joints, and bones.

I've limited this section to the five above-mentioned areas, for several reasons. First, I believe they are the most important, the "heavy hitters" in the game of health. Second, they get the lion's share of attention in the press (you can't throw a rock without seeing an article about heart disease, memory loss, or osteoporosis). Third, they are the areas most people are concerned with when they think about what it takes to live successfully over the long haul.

But let's talk for a moment about the liver, the poor organ that does so much and gets so little attention or respect. The liver is the site of many important metabolic operations. It's where cholesterol is made (and yes, that poor maligned molecule is important for your health). It's where fat is processed (broken down and repackaged into molecules such as *triglycerides*). And—perhaps most important of all—the liver is ground zero for what we call detoxification. The liver breaks down every chemical, pesticide, medication, contaminant, and carcinogen in a two-phase sequence of operations commanded by a critical set of enzymes called the *cytochrome P450 enzymes*.

But here's the thing: Follow all the recommendations in this book and, barring a completely unforeseen event out of your control, the liver (and many of the other areas, including the lungs) will work just fine. Think about it—if your diet is clean and wholesome, you're not taking in a lot of toxins. If you reduce inflammation and oxidation, not to mention stress and glycation, you won't be putting undue stress on your liver. And if you keep your heart, brain, and blood pressure healthy, you'll presumably be taking fewer medications that need neutralizing and elimination. So in many ways, a healthy liver will be a natural and desirable side effect of doing all the things that keep the *other* parts of your system in tip-top shape.

So in this section, we'll talk about how to keep your heart healthy, your brain working, your hormones balanced, your immune system strong, and your muscles, bones, and joints from wearing out prematurely (prematurely being defined by me as "anytime before you die"). Add to this the information in section I on how to reduce the Four Horsemen of Aging—oxidation, inflammation, glycation, and stress—and we've got a working game plan for a long and healthy life!

Let's keep going!

CHAPTER 6

Start with the Eight Pillars of Living Young

You'll notice that the anti-aging tips you find throughout this book fall into some specific categories. I call these "The Eight Pillars of Living Young." They're basically eight areas in which you can exert control over your destiny and ultimately increase the odds of living a long and healthy life with a "rectangularized" functionality curve.

These eight areas are *gut health, food, supplements, detoxification, exercise, sleep, stress reduction, and social relationships*. And because the latest research has shown that virtually every aspect of our health is influenced profoundly by the health of our gut, let's start with that.

1. GUT HEALTH

Who are you, anyway?

Each of us is a collection of ten trillion or so human cells. But along with those ten trillion human cells, our bodies also contain an entire ecosystem of non-human cells living on and inside our bodies. These non-human cells are collectively known as the *microbiome*, and you have between three and ten (!!) times as many of them as you do human cells.

"Which means," says Dr. Rob Knight, "*you* are mostly *not you*." Knight is on the leading edge of research that has the potential to change the way we look at disease, obesity, mood, psychiatric conditions, and overall health. "Intestinal microbes," he writes, "are the gatekeepers of our metabolism."

A consortium of almost eighty universities and scientific organizations are contributing research to the Human Microbiome Project, in an attempt to decode the normal microbial makeup of our bodies. And we are only now beginning to appreciate the profoundly important role those tiny microbes have on just about everything that has to do with our health.

Take weight, for example. Among the hundreds of bacterial species we're all home to, there are two particular species that have a profound effect on what happens to the food we eat. *Firmicutes* are the ultimate in fat-loving microbes. They can convert just about anything you eat into a muffin top. Their kissing cousins, the *bacteroidites*, are the exact opposite. When the bacteroidites get to work on some food you just chowed down on, it's like a school of piranha in a feeding frenzy—they'll incinerate calories almost as fast as you can ingest them.

As you can imagine, if you have more firmicutes than bacteroidites living in your gut, you're going to have a particularly hard time losing weight. Not surprisingly, research shows that obese people have higher levels of firmicutes in their gut than lean people, while lean folks have a predominance of bacteroidites.

Not only that, but higher levels of firmicutes "turn on" the genes that increase the risk for diabetes, obesity, and heart disease. "The relative proportion of these two groups to each other, the Firmicutes-to-Bacteroidetes (or F/B) ratio, is critical for determining health and risk for illness," says integrative neurologist David Perlmutter, M.D.

The notion of the gut being connected to the brain is not new. Dr. Michael Gershon wrote an iconic book about the subject called *The Second Brain* in which he pointed out, for example, that 90 percent of your serotonin—the "feel good" neurotransmitter thought to be increased by antidepressants—actually comes from the gut. Gershon pointed out that even our language reflects the connection—think of expressions like "gut feeling."

One of the maddening things about microbiome research is that the science of *description* has far outpaced the science of *prescription*. We are way better at describing what the microbiome is and what it does than we are at knowing precisely how to keep it healthy.

Everyone now accepts that the microbiome is deeply involved in aspects of human physiology, metabolism, and psychology. We even have some very detailed descriptions of the little buggers. We know, for example, that the microbiota on the skin are very different than, say, the microbiota in the gut. We know that pathogenic microbes can interact with the immune system, causing all kinds of nasty inflammatory cytokines to be fired off like rockets and causing all kinds of collateral damage. And we know that maintaining a healthy microbiome is one of the most important health strategies on the planet, far more important than anyone ever dreamed before a few short years ago.

But just because we're not 100 percent sure of how to create a completely healthy microbiome doesn't mean we're clueless. I interviewed over thirty-five experts on health and metabolism, and here are three actions you could take right now to increase the odds of a healthy gut.

Step One: Eat foods teeming with probiotics.

Probiotics are the class of microbes in our gut that we think of as "good." And knowing what foods contain probiotics is easy—you just have to remember one word: Fermentation.

The very process of fermentation produces probiotics galore, which is one reason that virtually everyone in the integrative health and functional medicine world recommends making fermented foods a regular part of your diet. Examples are yogurt, kefir, the Korean dish *kimchee*, naturally fermented sauerkraut, tempeh, kombucha, and real (fermented) soy sauce. And even if you do take eat these foods on a regular basis (most of us, unfortunately don't), a probiotic supplement makes a lot of sense.

Note: Research from 2018 suggests that the effects of probiotics differ hugely depending on the person, as do the effects of probiotics after a course of antibiotics. Researchers found that there are huge individual differences in what strains of probiotics respond to, suggesting *not* that probiotics aren't important, but that there is still much to learn about individualizing prescriptions and dosages.

Step Two: Go easy on the junk carbs.

Sugar feeds all the bad stuff in your body (from candida to cancer), disrupts your hormonal balance, is inflammatory, and—wait for it—is generally disruptive to the microbiome. Not only that, many of the foods that contain a lot of sugar are wheat-based, which poses a whole different set of problems. High-grain diets are a prescription for gut inflammation, hardly a good strategy for strengthening the integrity of the microbiome.

A diet *high* in fat and *low* in carbs could balance hormones, lower inflammation, and increase the health of the microbiome all at once. Perlmutter, for example, lauded the benefits of a high-fat diet—"Fat is the preferred fuel for human metabolism," he says.

Step Three: Eat foods rich in prebiotics.

Prebiotics are simply food for probiotics. They are usually some sort of fiber, the preferred fuel for gut bacteria (and another reason fiber is so important for your health). The little buggers feast on this fiber and ferment it, turning it into compounds like butryc acid, which nourish the intestinal lining and do other cool things. You want your healthy bacteria well-fed, and prebiotics is the way to do it.

THE REAL DEAL ON FIBER: IT'S MORE IMPORTANT THAN WE THOUGHT

Fiber is essential to the care and feeding of a healthy microbiome. So what is fiber? What does it do? Why do we need it? And why should we care? Let's start with weight loss.

Fiber's not expensive, it's not exotic, and it's certainly not sexy, but when it comes to weight loss, it works like a charm. More than a dozen clinical studies have used dietary fiber supplements for weight loss, most with positive outcomes. When you take the fiber supplement with water before meals, the water-soluble fiber binds to water in the stomach, making you feel full and less likely to overeat. It also suppresses hunger.

Fiber supplements have also been shown to enhance blood sugar control and insulin effects. It has even been shown to reduce the number of calories that the body absorbs—adding up to about 3 to 18 pounds (1.4 to 8.2 kg) a year. And a study in the prestigious *New England Journal of Medicine* found that a diet with 50 grams of fiber benefited type 2 diabetics in a number of ways, including by lowering insulin levels in the blood. For the record, insulin's two common nicknames among health professionals are "the hunger hormone" and "the fat-storing hormone."

Remember, the benefits of fiber aren't limited to weight loss. Fiber is the great modifier of blood sugar, and high blood sugar has been implicated in a baker's dozen of unwanted degenerative disease, including heart disease. Even Alzheimer's is now being called "type 3 diabetes."

Americans currently get a paltry amount of fiber in their diets, estimated at around 10 to 11 grams a day. That's not nearly enough. Current recommendations from major health organizations range from 25 to 38 grams a day (depending on age and sex), but more might be even better.

Here are some great sources of fiber to start including in your diet: any kind of beans (black beans, red beans, kidney beans), chickpeas, lentils, rolled oats, peas, unripe bananas, oatmeal, Brussels sprouts, apples, nuts, blueberries, oranges, avocados (especially Florida avocados). I'm also a fan of adding fiber to shakes and smoothies—try SunFiber, which is tasteless, odorless, mixes well, and is available everywhere.

Unfortunately, nobody eats foods that are naturally high in prebiotics. Or, almost no one. Foods high on the prebiotic list include raw chicory and raw Jerusalem artichoke, not exactly the most popular foods on everyone's menu. One of the best (and most accessible) sources is onion—preferably raw, but cooked works too. Onions aside, it's not all that easy to get a good helping of prebiotics from food, which is why I personally recommend prebiotic supplements. (The one I use is called Oligo30 and is available on Amazon.)

And remember, diet has a powerful shaping effect on the microbiome. And if your microbiome is working against you—say you have an abundance of fat-making bacteria (firmicutes) and a dearth of fat-burning bacteria (bacteroidites)—changing your diet may change the composition of your gut garden and actually be a game changer for your health in general.

Eat as Many Servings of Fruits and Vegetables a Day as You Can—with Emphasis on the Vegetables.

The U.S. Department of Agriculture now recommends between five and nine servings a day, and the Centers for Disease Control and Prevention's slogan regarding fruits and vegetables says it all: "More matters!" Serving sizes are small—about 1 cup—so it's not nearly as hard as you think to get in nine servings. *And potatoes and rice don't count.*

For the health of your microbiome, it's also vitally important that you consume enough fiber every day. I recommend SunFiber powder as a supplement for just that reason. It's odorless, tasteless and mixes with everything, and it's a great way to get an extra 6 grams or so of high-quality soluble fiber in your diet.

2. FOOD: EAT YOUR WAY TO A LONG LIFE

Eat real food.

It sounds so simple yet it's probably the single most powerful health intervention you can do. I've come to believe that the quality of the food you eat trumps the proportion of fat, carbohydrate, and protein. Ask yourself: is this real food? Is this food your great-grandmother would have recognized as food? Is this food that would spoil if you left it outside in the sun? Is this food that you could have theoretically hunted for, fished for, gathered off the ground, or plucked from a tree?

Because really, that matters more than almost anything else.

There are more elements in fruits and vegetables that can extend your life than science has been able to put its collective finger on. Some of their anti-aging value undoubtedly comes from nutrients—antioxidants and anti-inflammatory properties. And some of their anti-aging value is most certainly due to the fiber found in them, which, we now know, is absolutely essential to the health of the microbiome.

People who eat lots of fruits and vegetables tend to have other healthy habits as well, such as eating less of the junk foods that shorten life. Regardless, the effect on aging, disease, and health of a diet high in fruits and vegetables is absolutely incontrovertible and noncontroversial.

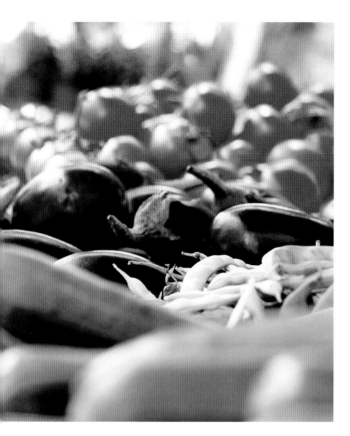

chronic diseases of aging, such as heart disease, cancer, diabetes, and obesity. Ultimately, food is probably the most powerful drug we have in our anti-aging arsenal.

To Juice or Not to Juice: That Is *not* the Question.

The conventional wisdom on juicing is that it's a poor substitute for eating the whole fruit or the whole vegetable. And when you put it in those terms, that's correct. But in my view, that's a short-sighted way to look at it.

First, let's assume you make juice yourself, at home, from fresh fruits and vegetables, eliminating the problem with sugar-laden commercial juices. You're still basically extracting the juice and tossing the fiber—and that *is* a real issue—but it hardly means you shouldn't juice.

In my view, the loss of fiber is a problem but not a deal breaker. If you throw in a mess of vegetables and fruits into a high-quality juicer, you're going to wind up with one of the most nutrient-rich beverages on earth.

Juicing was never meant to be a *substitute* for eating fibrous foods, it's an *addition*. Nothing's stoping you from eating whole fruits and vegetables in addition to your juicing. And the truth is, you can get your fiber in other ways.

There are great fiber supplements on the market to add even more fiber to your diet—my favorite is SunFiber, which is tasteless, odorless, mixes well, and is mainly soluble fiber (the most valuable kind for the microbiome). Fiber supplements like SunFiber can easily be added to smoothies, shakes, or even the freshly made juice I'm talking about.

So overall, I think adding freshly made fruit and vegetable juice is a great idea. It's actually a habit I myself have worked hard to cultivate—I generally make fresh juice at least five times a week.

According to a 2013 report by the Union of Concerned Scientists ("The $11 Trillion Reward"), increasing our consumption of fruits and vegetables could save more than 100,000 lives and $17 billion in health care costs from heart disease each year. According to that same USC report, if Americans ate just one more serving of fruits or vegetables a day, that alone would save more than 30,000 lives and $5 billion in medical costs annually. Low fruit and vegetable intake is estimated to cause about 31 percent of ischemic heart disease and 11 percent of strokes worldwide—amazing numbers!

And if you want to talk anti-aging strategies, a minimum intake of 400 grams of fruits and vegetables a day (not counting potatoes!) would dramatically help prevent

Here's how I make my juice: I basically go to the farmer's market or my local Sprouts, grab everything that looks good, and then experiment. Over the years, I've come up with a few basic templates, but every juice is different and all of them are delicious in their own way. My juice-making lacks consistency but makes up for it in creativity.

Here are two of my favorite go-to recipes—one for a "red" juice and one for a "green" one. Amounts are completely estimated and subject to change with my whims but you'll get the idea.

Jonny's Red Juice Supreme

5–6 apples (My preference is Honeycrisp, but Fuji, Gaia, and Golden Delicious all work well.
Once in a while I'll throw in some Braeburns.)

1 red pepper

1 small to moderate red beet

Carrots (As many as needed to make a total of about a quart [946 ml] of juice—I use the darker, purple carrots when making my "red juice.")

Fresh turmeric (I do this one by eye, so start with a little and work up depending on taste.)

Fresh ginger (Ditto)

½ a lemon, preferably Meyer Lemon (I literally cut the lemon in half and throw the whole half in, skin/rind and all. There's a ton of good stuff in the skin, and you'll never notice it in the mix.)

Jonny's Green Juice Supreme

5–6 apples (See above for suggestions.)

1 green pepper

1 small to moderate golden beet

Carrots (As many as needed to make a total of about a quart [946 ml] of juice—I use white or orange carrots when making my "green juice.")

Fresh turmeric (I do this one by eye, so start with a little and work up depending on taste.)

Fresh ginger (Ditto)

½ a lemon, preferably Meyer Lemon (I literally cut the lemon in half and throw the whole half in, skin/rind and all. There's a ton of good stuff in the skin, and you'll never notice it in the mix.)

Note: Michelle and I like our juices ginger-heavy, but not everyone does. And remember that beets have a strong taste, not to everyone's liking (but to mine!). The point is, if the juice comes out "stronger" than you like, it's an easy fix: just add some water. I've gotten really good at intuitively estimating exactly how much to dilute the juice so that it's perfectly acceptable to the majority of tastes, but you'll figure it out in no time. Just start with a little dilution—no matter how strong the juice came out originally, eventually you can find the perfect dilution for your taste (and the tastes of your family). It's easy. I promise.

3. SUPPLEMENTS: THERAPY IN THE PALM OF YOUR HAND

I like to think of supplements as a technology, a kind of modern-day delivery system for nutrients. The realization that many nutrients in the ideal dosages have an almost pharmaceutical effect has led to wide use of the term *nutraceuticals* for these beneficial compounds. We'll be talking more about supplements later, but for the purposes of this brief intro, I'm going to start with five recommendations. These are the five that almost everyone can benefit from.

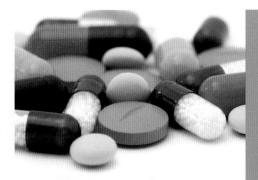

ANTI-AGING ACTION PLAN:

To Reduce Your Risk of Disease, Take More Than an Apple a Day

Take daily:

A Multivitamin

Fish Oil: 2–3 grams of combined EPA and DHA (I recommend Barlean's High EPA-DHA or Barlean's Seriously Delicious Omegas.)

Magnesium: 400–800 mg daily

Vitamin D3: 2000–5000 daily or as recommended by your health practitioner (Any reliable manufacturer will do as long as they use vitamin D3.)

Probiotics: Most important is to get a brand that features these five strains:

→ *Lactobaccilus plantarum*

→ *Lactobaccilus acidophilus*

→ *Lactobaccilus brevis*

→ *Bifidobacterium lactis*

→ *Bifidobacterium longum*

About that multi . . .

The research on multivitamins is mixed. Some studies show long-term benefits. Some don't. Yet, there's enough positive research to convince me they're a good idea. Researchers have found that a multivitamin helped reduce the risk of micronutrient deficiencies and also helped to improve cognitive functioning, including in those ages 75 and older. Studies have also shown that people who regularly take multivitamins have a reduced risk of cardiovascular and cerebral stroke. A 2016 study followed healthy men for 20 years and found that those who used multivitamins over that period of time actually had a statistically lower risk of major cardiovascular events.

Consistent use of multivitamins with minerals may help boost the immune systems of elderly people and play a key role in protecting eye and brain function and maintaining bone mass.

ANTI-AGING ACTION PLAN:

Do the SNACC Detox Program and Take a Break from the Chemicals That Age Us

Here's how to do the SNACC (sugar, nicotine, alcohol, caffeine, and chemicals) detoxification program developed by Elson Haas, M.D.

One week before beginning, eliminate the following in your diet:

→ Sugar

→ Nicotine

→ Alcohol

→ Caffeine

One or two days before starting, eliminate the following:

→ Red meat

→ Milk products

→ Eggs

→ Wheat and baked goods

You eliminate the meat, eggs, and wheat not because many people have low-grade reactions to them. It's a way of starting with an essentially clean slate.

Then, for a week, simply follow this program:

Upon rising:

→ Drink two glasses of filtered water, one glass with half a lemon squeezed into it.

Breakfast:

→ Eat a fresh apple, pear, banana, grapefruit, or even some grapes. Don't forget to chew well.

Fifteen to 30 minutes later:

→ Eat one bowl of cooked whole grains—try millet, amaranth, quinoa, or brown rice. Oatmeal may be okay, but be careful of cross-contamination if you suspect gluten sensitivity. You can sweeten the grain with a couple of tablespoons (30 ml) of fruit juice and feel free to use some organic butter (or butter blended with olive or flaxseed oil).

Lunch:

→ Eat one to two medium-size bowls of steamed vegetables (save the water). Use a variety, including roots, stems, and greens. For example: potatoes or yams, green beans, broccoli, cauliflower, carrots, beets, cabbage, asparagus, chard or kale, and cabbage. Be creative. And feel free to put butter on it; just make it organic.

Dinner:

→ This is easy. Eat the same thing you did for lunch.

Just in case you feel a little fatigued (there's not a ton of protein in this week-long program), feel free to add 3 to 4 ounces (85 to 115 g) of fish, poultry, or beans to the evening meal, or have it between meals. I recommend wild fish from Vital Choice and free-range poultry only. I'd personally feel fine doubling up on the protein (two portions a day instead of one) if you find you feel generally better eating a bit more of it.

And one more thing:

→ Remember that water you collected from steaming the vegetables? Drink it all day long. You can flavor it with some garlic salt or sea salt.

You can do Haas's SNACC program for a week or so, and then add back some of the foods you've been without. Some nutritionists, including the legendary Oz Garcia, Ph.D., have been doing variations with their clients for decades and often recommend that you do a "clean eating" detox four times a year with the season changes.

Adapted from *The New Detox Diet* by Elson Haas, M.D. and Daniella Chace, M.S., C.N. (Celestial Arts, 2004)

4. DETOXIFICATION: TAKE THIS AGE-OLD TIME-OUT

The ability to give our systems a much-needed rest— a kind of "time-out" from the daily assault on our cells of toxic foods and environmental pathogens—is a deeply valuable asset in our quest for a long and healthy life. Fortunately, we have a number of ways of detoxifying, from "cleansing diets" (which are usually just very sparse, nutrient-dense programs of whole foods) to infrared sauna (see my book, *The 150 Most Effective Ways to Boost Your Energy*).

Some critics claim that commercial "detox" products are nothing more than laxatives (sometimes true), while other critics claim that the body is constantly detoxifying anyway (true) and doesn't need any help (false). And finally, some argue that there's no way to effectively measure the toxins we supposedly eliminate through a detox program, and even if there were, there's no way to prove we've actually eliminated them (partially true, partially not).

It may be difficult to document just what toxins are being excreted when we do a "detox", but that doesn't mean we shouldn't try. Since the original edition of this book, I had an opportunity to interview Dr. Joseph Pizzorno about his book, *The Toxin Solution* (highly recommended). Dr. Pizzorno is often thought of as the father of naturopathic medicine in this country, as he founded the top naturopathic medical school in the country (Bastyr University) and is the co-author of the seminal textbook, *Textbook of Natural Medicine*. Pizzorno presented me with a riddle which will probably explain the importance of toxins more than any other illustration I can think of. Here's the riddle.

For decades and decades, sugar consumption in the United States has been rising. Two hundred years ago,

Eat Crunchy Vegetables to Help Rid Your Body of Toxins

A diet high in cruciferous vegetables (kale, cabbage, broccoli) will help with detoxification. Broccoli contains *sulforaphane*, a powerful antioxidant that helps the liver do its job of ridding the body of age-robbing carcinogens and other toxins. (Sulforaphane is now one of the supplements I recommend regularly, see page 208). Eat cruciferous vegetables as often as possible, daily if you can.

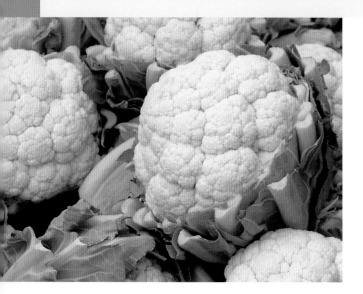

the average person in America, in a typical year, would consume about two pounds (900 g) of the stuff. In 1970, it was up to 123 pounds (56 kg). (Let that sink in for a minute.) And today, we're consuming over 150 pounds (68 kg) of added sugar, per person, per year. So here's the question: Why didn't we have a diabetes epidemic?

I mean, think about it. It's generally accepted that sugar is one of, if not the main, drivers of obesity, metabolic syndrome, and diabetes. But if it was sugar causing diabetes, why didn't the diabetes epidemic begin until 1955?

Dr. Pizzorno explained that it was around 1955 that the number of chemicals in the air, water, and food supply reached a critical mass. Sugar alone didn't "cause" the diabetes epidemic. And toxins alone didn't either. But the combination of the two—well, that's another story. Many of these toxins—found in everyday household products, foods, and the environment—actually poison the insulin receptors, thus contributing to the damage that a high-sugar diet has already done. The combination—from a diabetes point of view—is lethal.

Toxins matter. They interface with your food and your lifestyle to create results that wouldn't necessarily be seen if they weren't in the mix. So take detoxification seriously and think of a detox as nothing more mysterious than a "spring cleaning" for the body.

We can all agree that our bodies, minds, and souls are assaulted with toxins on a daily basis: from the air we breathe, the water we drink, the chemicals in our soil, the medications in our medicine cabinet, the hormones, antibiotics, and steroids in our meat, and the hundreds of other minor exposures we rack up just in the course of daily living. This is not a good situation, and we don't help matters by eating bad food. And finally, I hope we can agree that it might be a good thing to give the body and the mind an occasional rest from the constant onslaught.

Because the liver is the main organ of detoxification for the body, this is a good time to give it a little support. The best supplements for the liver are milk thistle, alpha-lipoic acid, and selenium. I recommend 400 to 900 milligrams of milk thistle, up to 1,200 milligrams of alpha-lipoic acid, and 400 micrograms of selenium as a basic "liver support" formula, with some NAC (N-acetyl-cysteine) and curcumin thrown in for good measure.

5. EXERCISE: AN ACTIVITY FOR THE AGES

All long-lived society on earth are active. Exercise can help you control blood sugar, weight, and blood pressure. It can elevate your "good" cholesterol and reduce your risk of heart disease. It can lower your risk for Alzheimer's disease. A single thirty-minute bout of aerobic exercise can improve mood, measures of positive well-being, and vigor, even in people with major depressive disorder! It can certainly lower stress, and recent research shows that exercise actually helps you grow new brain tissue.

What I want to talk about here is something related to exercise, but quite different: movement. Exercise and movement have much different metabolic consequences.

Let me explain.

Exercise vs. Movement: What's the Difference and Why Does It Matter?

I started my career in health as a trainer at the Equinox Fitness Clubs. No one has a greater respect for the importance of exercise than I do. But most of us have been wrongly led to believe that exercise and movement are the same thing.

In any given day, exercise only accounts for a small part of the number of calories you burn, an even smaller part if you're not exercising a lot. Your resting metabolic rate accounts for about 60 percent of your calorie burn, and most of the rest comes from something called NEAT—non-exercise associated thermogenesis. Here's another word for NEAT: movement.

This is important. Between 15 and 50 percent of your daily calorie burn is associated with ordinary walking around, going to the store, putting away groceries, digesting the food, taking out the garbage, learning to salsa dance, and even washing your hair. Any movement counts. And that extra movement just may have a more profound impact on your metabolism (and your body shape) that exercising intensely.

What's more, if your metabolism isn't primed for it, then intense exercise will be seen by the body as a major stressor and the overall impact on your metabolism will be negative. It's exactly the *opposite* of what we want.

If you are not taking NEAT into account, then you are missing the boat. It's probably the most important contribution to your daily calorie burn, right after RMR (resting metabolic rate, which is the number of calories it would take just to keep you alive in a flotation tank!). This is one of the reasons why policy makers suggest walking 10,000 steps per day. And this time, the "policy makers" got it right.

Modern-day men and women sit for 95 percent or more of their waking day. This has profound implications on health.

SITTING *IS* THE NEW SMOKING

Let's get one thing clear at the outset. There's a difference between too much *sitting* and too *little* exercise. Even if you go to the gym religiously and work out like a demon, you don't get a free pass from the metabolic mischief done by extended periods of sitting.

As great as exercise and activity are, they don't completely wipe away the damage done by spending eight hours a day in a chair.

"Let's say you do 30 minutes of walking five days a week (as recommended by federal health officials) and let's say you sleep for eight hours," exercise physiologist and researcher Stephen Blair, Ph.D., said to NPR in an interview. "Well, that still leaves 15.5 hours a day."

When you sit for extended periods of time, your muscles go silent and the calorie-burning rate drops significantly. Within a single day, your body gets less insulin *sensitive* and more insulin *resistant*—a hallmark of diabetes and pre-diabetes. (One study demonstrated a whopping 40 percent reduction in the ability of insulin to deliver glucose to the cells after only 24 hours of sedentary behavior.) And the enzymes that are responsible for breaking down fat begin to drop.

There are little things you can do that will make a huge difference.

Stand up every so often. Go get a drink of water. Take five-minute breaks and walk around. Try an ergonomic desk chair (or a balance ball) to engage small muscles need to stabilize and balance. If you're on an airplane, walk to the bathroom and back every hour or so.

Anything you can do to break up the long stretches of uninterrupted sitting will make a difference. Remember, we weren't designed for long periods of uninterrupted sitting. It doesn't take a lot of effort to break the pattern. And protecting your body from metabolic damage is well worth the effort.

Why Moving More May Be *More* Important Than Exercise

Recently a rash of research has shown that inactivity may be the biggest risk factor of all for diabetes and heart disease, two of the end-stage consequences of a damaged metabolism.

One recent study published in the May 2013 issue of the journal *Diabetologia* showed that movement was a far better predictor of health than either moderate or even intense physical exercise.

This research, and other studies like it, have led many experts in the health and fitness fields to begin focusing much of their efforts on getting people to *move* more rather than *exercise* more.

But can simply moving more really help with weight loss and be better than exercise?

Yes. If you're wondering how that could possibly be so, consider the fact that numerous studies have shown that intense exercise—while perfectly healthy—can nonetheless cause compensatory reactions that increase hunger and cravings, which work against the very goals you're trying to achieve. And intense exercise causes high levels of cortisol, and this can have a number of damaging effects not typically seen with low-intensity movements like walking.

ANTI-AGING ACTION PLAN:

Reduce Stress with Sleep

Get seven to nine hours of sleep every night. Take the electronics out of the bedroom, remove the lights, and create a dark, warm, and inviting sanctuary where you can actually sleep undisturbed for the full length of time your body needs.

6. SLEEP: LISTEN TO YOUR INTERNAL RHYTHM AND LIVE LONGER

Sleep is a big part of a longevity lifestyle. It's no secret that most of us don't get enough of it. Sleep affects how we work, how we relate to other people, how we make decisions, and how we feel in general. Not getting enough sleep can depress our immune system, raise our stress hormones, and contribute to weight gain.

Prior to electricity, we listened to our biological rhythms, which were in sync with the rhythms of the earth. We slept when it was dark out and awoke when it was light. We spent plenty of time in the sun. We moved around a lot. And when it was dark, we sat around the campfire and went to bed and slept like babies. When the sun rose, we started the day. This, if you will, was the natural order of things. This is the *factory-specified* sleep pattern for healthy humans. It's been wildly disrupted—and we've paid a great price in health and longevity.

Let me explain.

Circadian rhythms are roughly twenty-four-hour cycles in the biological and physiological processes of all living beings. This cycle is incredibly important to human longevity; patterns of brain wave activity, hormone

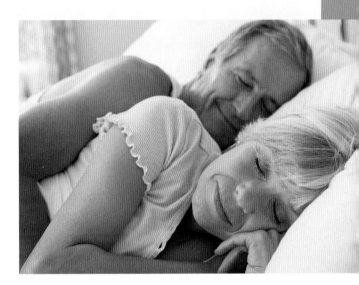

production, and all sorts of other regulatory metabolic functions are connected to this circadian rhythm and intimately connected with the quality and length of our sleep. When our sleep patterns deviate wildly from what we were genetically "programmed" for, countless systems (hormonal, metabolic) inexorably break down and systemic aging accelerates.

Scientists don't fully understand exactly *why* our bodies need sleep, but they know that we do. Sleep generates hormones, such as *human growth hormone*, the ultimate anti-aging hormone (released only in the deep stages of sleep), and *melatonin*, which appears to have anticancer

How can I get more energy?

People are wired and tired, fatigued, running on empty, and dragging through their days. They constantly ask if there's something they can *take*, something they can

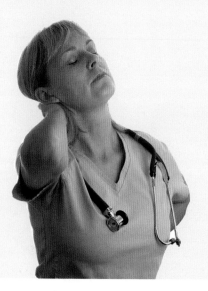

eat, something they can *do* that will give them more of what they are clearly, sadly, lacking: energy.

The *real* reason for the "no energy" epidemic is very simple: it's a lack of sleep.

You need to sleep better and you need to sleep *longer*. So here are three tips for how to do it.

Tip #1: Set the Temperature at 68°F (20°C)...

The body prefers this lower temperature during sleep, and if the room is too hot, you have to "work" to keep the equilibrium and that interferes with good sleep. So keep the room comfortably cool—68°F (20°C) is perfect.

Tip #2: No media.

Take a complete media break for half an hour before hitting the sack. No kidding. This means no television, no email, no computer for *one full half hour* before bedtime.

Tip #3: Keep it Dark . . .

Studies show that even the slightest light in the room can measurably interfere with metrics used to measure good, restful sleep. So keep the lights off—*all* of them.

The bottom line: Sleep matters. More than, perhaps, you realize. Start by doing these three simple steps and watch what happens!

properties. Biochemicals get replaced. And let's not forget that lack of sleep is a huge stressor, causing our bodies to secrete *cortisol*, whose aging effects we've already discussed. In short, not getting enough sleeping can shorten our life and diminish its quality in multiple ways.

And, it's not just the *quantity* of sleep that we get that's important; it's also the *quality*.

Sleep is essential to memory, mood, and cognitive performance, all markers for the youngevity lifestyle. All diminish as you get older unless you take good care of your sleep. Inadequate sleep is linked to increased anger, anxiety, and sadness, all diminishers of the quality (and potentially length) of your life. One study at the University of Pennsylvania showed that when subjects were only allowed to sleep 4.5 hours per night, they exhibited significantly more stress, anger, and mental exhaustion.

7. STRESS MANAGEMENT: IT'S NO LONGER A LUXURY

Stress exacerbates virtually every disease of aging and many others as well (herpes, asthma, allergies, and acne being just some of the more "minor" conditions that stress hormones can aggravate). Stress slows down recovery from serious illness. Stress shrinks areas of the brain that are intimately involved with memory and thinking. It increases the risk of heart disease. It decreases the effectiveness of the immune system. It deeply deserves its designation as one of the Four Horsemen of Aging, and many might reasonably argue that it is the most deadly horseman of all.

Managing stress is not a luxury. And chances are that without even thinking about it too much, you could easily name a dozen things that you personally would find relaxing, enjoyable, and soothing. These dozen things would automatically lower your heart rate, blood pressure, and stress hormones naturally.

Take my advice: Do them.

The longest-lived people in the world may not go to day spas or yoga retreats. But they have constructed their lives in such a way that their stress is naturally manageable. To the extent that you do the same—however that "looks" for you—you will be taking a huge step toward increasing the odds that you wind up living longer, better, and healthier.

8. SOCIAL RELATIONSHIPS (EMOTIONAL INTELLIGENCE)

Whenever researchers have investigated long-lived people, they've looked at their diets, their activity levels, their genes, all sorts of things that pertain to the *individual*. But the absolute universal truth about anti-aging is that *there is no anti-aging without a strong social fabric*. Not one single long-lived society anywhere in the world is absent a set of strong social connections, including family, community, place of worship, and all the rest of the structures that go with living together as a cohesive group.

In looking for a category for this kind of anti-aging behavior, I borrowed a term from psychology—it's called *emotional intelligence*.

I'm going to loosely define emotional intelligence as the sum total of everything in our lives that relates to our

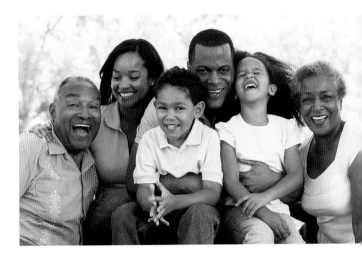

relationships with others, our relationship with ourselves (how we manage our emotions, for example), and our ability to communicate. If we can harness the power of emotions, we can use them to facilitate thinking, problem solving, communication, and connection to other people. All of these have profound implications for anti-aging.

Our thoughts and emotions have powerful effects on our physiology. What we think about can literally affect our blood pressure, our heart rate, and the amount of hormones we release in our bodies, all powerful modulators of aging. Our emotional intelligence is intimately connected to our ability to manage stress. And a big part of our emotional intelligence—its manifestation, if you will—is how we relate to and interact with others.

In fact, if there is one category of behavior that is most associated in the research with anti-aging, it's our relationship with others: being connected to other people, being part of a community, and learning to know and accept yourself. That's emotional intelligence, and it's the most powerful anti-aging tool of all.

Now let's get started!

CHAPTER 7

Keep Your Heart in Shape

At present, heart disease is shortening the lives of millions of people and diminishing the quality of life for millions more. It's currently the leading cause of death in the world, accounting for 12.2 percent of all deaths worldwide, and an even higher percentage, 16.3 percent, in high-income countries. In the United States alone, more than 652,000 people died from heart disease in the last year for which figures are available, more than four times the number of people who died from diabetes and Alzheimer's disease combined and more than five times the number of people who died from accidents.

For many people, the first and only symptom of heart disease will be death. And it's not just men who are dying. Although most women are much more frightened of breast cancer than of heart disease, the sad truth is that heart disease is far more likely to kill them. One out of every two women's deaths in the United States is because of cardiovascular disease.

Heart disease is scary. And at the risk of stating the obvious, if you want to live long and live well, it's best to avoid it.

And a great deal of the risk for shortening your life from heart disease is actually under your control. Few diseases are as preventable, or at least modifiable, by lifestyle choices as heart disease is. Although there are certainly factors that you *can't* control, such as genes, they pale in comparison to the ones that you *can* control.

In fact, a massive amount of data suggests that five simple behaviors can reduce the risk for heart disease: a healthy diet and body weight, moderate physical exercise, no smoking, and limited alcohol consumption.

"We're not asking people to run marathons," said Walter Willett, M.D., chairman of the nutrition department at Harvard School of Public Health and a coauthor of

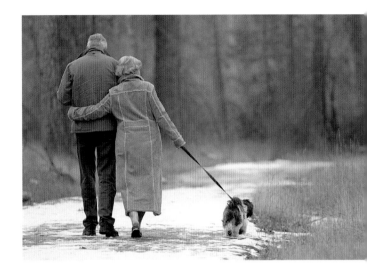

the Nurses Health Study ll. "Everyone could achieve these goals."

A PRIMER ON THE TICKER

Cardiovascular disease includes any arterial disease that affects the blood supply to the heart or the brain (or to the peripheral regions of the body). When the arteries supplying blood to the heart are affected, it's called *coronary heart disease*; when the blood supply to the brain is affected, it's called *cerebrovascular disease* (and the result is usually a stroke).

Although there are two structures in the cardiovascular system that transport blood—the veins and the arteries—they are significantly different from one another. The vein is basically a tube through which blood flows. The arteries, on the other hand, are throbbing, pulsating, living structures that contract, dilate, and have their own version of a muscular system. Although arteries and veins have a similar construction, it's invariably the arteries that are damaged or blocked in heart disease.

The health of your arteries is of prime importance, especially as you get older.

ANATOMY OF THE HEART

The Heart: A View from the Outside

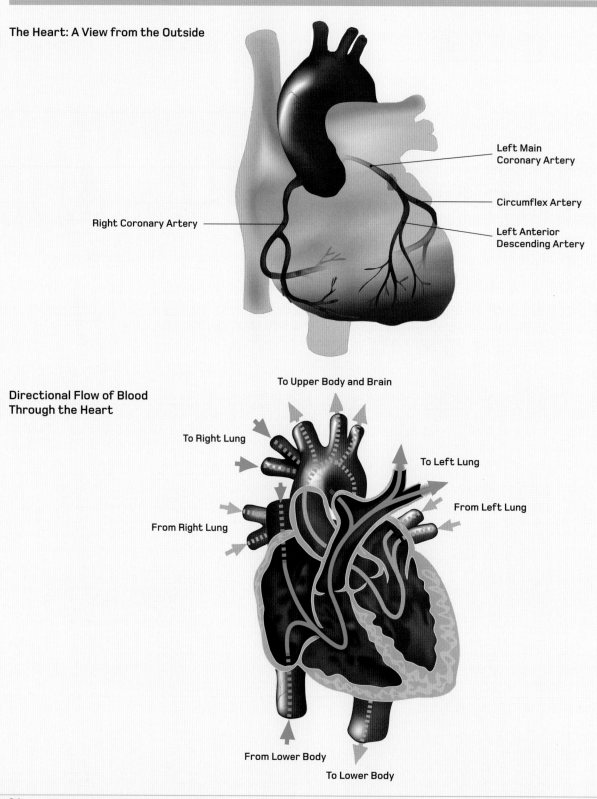

Right Coronary Artery

Left Main
Coronary Artery

Circumflex Artery

Left Anterior
Descending Artery

**Directional Flow of Blood
Through the Heart**

To Upper Body and Brain

To Right Lung

To Left Lung

From Left Lung

From Right Lung

From Lower Body

To Lower Body

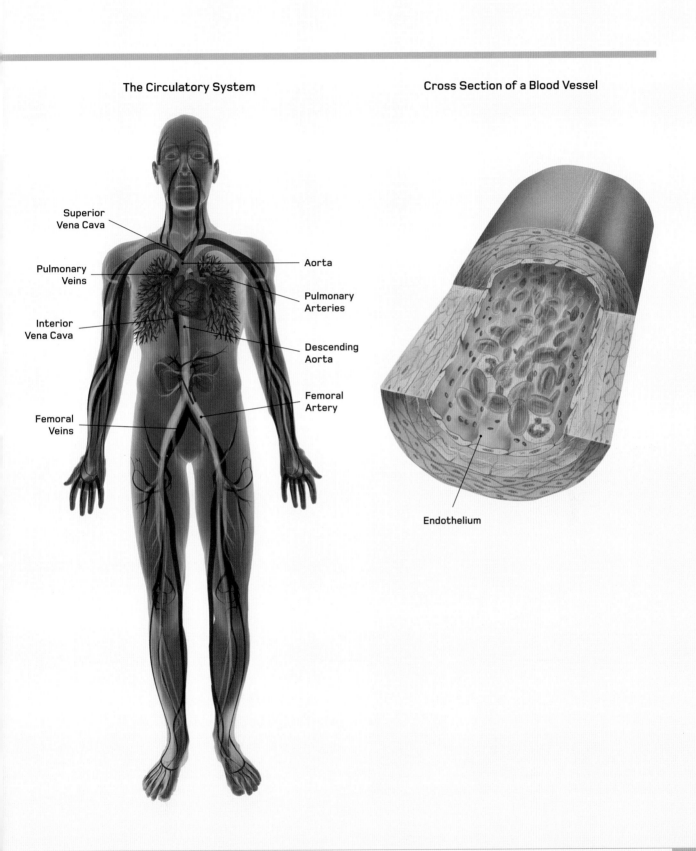

The Circulatory System

Superior
Vena Cava

Pulmonary
Veins

Interior
Vena Cava

Femoral
Veins

Aorta

Pulmonary
Arteries

Descending
Aorta

Femoral
Artery

Cross Section of a Blood Vessel

Endothelium

ANOTHER CORONARY DISEASE MARKER

This is a really good time to introduce a new term: *endothelial dysfunction*.

This is a condition that underlies virtually every circulatory problem and certainly every problem that relates to the aging heart. You've got heart disease? You've got endothelial dysfunction. Not *some* of the time, but *all* the time. In fact, you've got endothelial dysfunction well *in advance* of the hard-core symptoms and traditional signs of heart disease, and if you can do something about it early, you may never progress to heart disease at all.

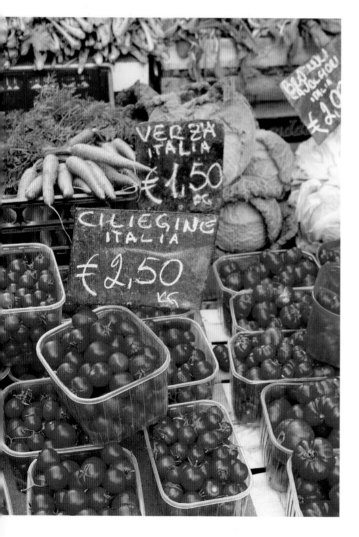

The endothelium is a thin layer of cells that lines the interior surface of blood vessels (such as the arteries and veins). It is like an interface between the blood circulating in the inner tube of the vessel and the walls of the vessel itself. Endothelial cells line the entire circulatory system. But they're anything but passive—they don't just lie there like a rug. Far from it. They secrete substances, including the all-important *nitric oxide*, which helps the arteries dilate. They protect the smooth muscles of the artery from toxic substances in the blood, acting as a kind of protective barrier. They secrete chemicals that protect the artery after an injury, chemicals that send messages to both white blood cells and smooth muscle cells to mobilize quickly and get over to the injury site.

When the endothelium is not functioning well, all hell breaks loose. Absolutely every patient with atherosclerosis (i.e., hardening of the arteries) has endothelial dysfunction. Atherosclerosis begins with inflammation. Endothelial cells respond to that inflammation by activating immune cells. These processes eventually damage the arterial wall and lead to plaque.

With aging, the endothelium starts to be leaky, like an old roof, offering less protection than before. It starts to be less vigilant about letting toxins through. These toxins enter the smooth muscle cells, which then gather at the site of an injury, causing the artery to lose more flexibility. White blood cells start to congregate, and they release pro-inflammatory substances and damaging free radicals (another horseman of aging), which in turn attack the poor aging endothelium even more. The toxins soon penetrate the arterial wall, substances such as cholesterol and triglycerides accumulate and become oxidized by free radicals, and the cycle of damage and aging continues.

When the walls of the arteries that supply blood to the heart thicken, it's the beginning of trouble. That thickening is caused by small lesions in the wall, injuries (minor and not so minor) that get patched over with material that forms into plaque. The plaque itself can restrict blood to the heart muscle, much like a boulder in the middle of the highway can restrict traffic. Worse, if the cap covering the plaque ruptures, the blood may clot and completely obstruct the flow. The result is what doctors call a *myocardial infarction* and what the rest of us know as a heart attack.

The term *atherosclerosis* actually comes from the Greek word *athere*, meaning "porridge," and refers to the soft core of the plaque, which has an oatmeal-like consistency. *Sclerosis* means "hardening." Although there is indeed cholesterol in the plaque, that's hardly the only component, and researchers are beginning to discover that the cholesterol particles have to be oxidized (i.e., damaged by free radicals) before they become a problem.

Oxidated, or damaged, LDL ("bad") cholesterol is taken up by little PacMan-type structures called *macrophages*, which then become known as *foam cells*. Accumulation of these foam cells in the arterial wall leads to the first sign of atherosclerosis, or at least the first sign that's visible, a yellowish spot in the wall that merges into streaks (known as *fatty streaks*). As atherosclerosis progresses, the streaks become larger and more complex, eventually turning into lesions, and finally evolving into fibrous plaque.

Now, you have a real problem. The plaque itself can narrow the arteries, but that's only half of it. If a fibrous plaque becomes unstable, if it breaks or tears, blood clots called *thrombi* can form, further increasing the likelihood of a blockage that can result in a heart attack.

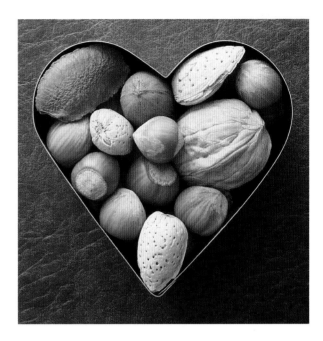

The interesting part of all this is that researchers now understand that atherosclerosis may actually be part of the body's attempt to mount a healing response to injury, an attempt that is initiated by the endothelium. And that injury may come in the form of *inflammation*. This is part of the reason that inflammation has gotten so much attention in recent years; it's clearly a big part of the problem in heart disease. Inflammation may well turn out to be much more important in determining your risk for heart disease than cholesterol.[1] At the very least, it's a factor you need to pay attention to.

The good news is that you can do something about it and probably extend your life in the process. Because endothelial dysfunction *always* involves a measure of inflammation and oxidation, a diet that fights these helps to protect the heart and fight aging.

---

1 I'm being oh-so-politically correct here. The truth is, inflammation is much more important than cholesterol in determining your risk for heart disease, and the sooner conventional medicine accepts that, the better for all of us.

IT'S WHAT YOU EAT

Just as I was writing this chapter, the results of a new study from Greece appeared on my desktop. The study, published in the journal *Risk Analysis*, concluded that knowing what a person eats significantly improves the ability to predict his or her risk for heart disease. In the past, doctors mainly used traditional measures of risk (such as cholesterol), which don't necessarily do a great job of predicting outcomes.[2]

THE FIVE PRINCIPLES OF A HEART-HEALTHY DIET

So what exactly is a heart-healthy diet?

Let's cut to the chase.

1. Increase your consumption of omega-3 fats from fish and fish oil supplements and even plant sources (such as flaxseed).

2. Substitute nonhydrogenated, unsaturated fats for saturated and trans fats. And consume more omega-3 than omega-6 (omega-6 are mostly found in the so-called "vegetable" oils—soybean, safflower, corn, sunflower, peanut, and so on).

3. Eat a diet that is high in vegetables, nuts, fruits, and whole grains and low in sugar and refined grain products.

4. Avoid processed foods.

5. Choose foods, food combinations, and food preparation methods that are low on the glycemic index.

---

2   Full disclosure: Political correctness once again. Cholesterol levels are a lousy predictor for heart disease. Fully half the people who have heart attacks have perfectly normal cholesterol, and half the people with elevated cholesterol do not. Using cholesterol levels to predict heart disease will give you slightly better results than using tea leaves to predict the weather.

One thing to understand is that there is no single magic food that makes a diet heart healthy. It's the combination of low sugar, high antioxidants, high anti-inflammatories, high-quality protein, and omega-3 fats, and the absence of trans fats, that does the trick. And the exact details matter less than the way the parts fit together. That said, there are some superstars among the heart-healthy foods, and you should consider including them on a regular basis if you want to protect your heart and live long and strong.

GO WILD FOR SALMON

The ultimate brain food is also the ultimate heart food—salmon. But not the farm-raised kind, the wild kind.

Farmed salmon has more fat than wild salmon, but a much smaller percentage of that fat is from heart-healthy omega-3s and a much larger percentage is from pro-inflammatory omega-6s. And for variety, herring, mackerel, sardines, and, to a lesser extent, tuna, are rich in the same omega-3s found in salmon! *Note:* Check out the link to VitalChoice on my website—it's where I get all my salmon (and other fish!).

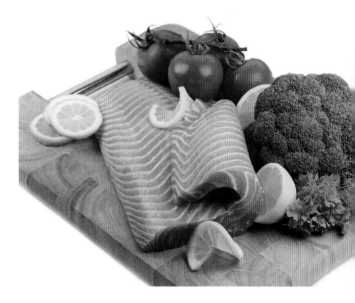

Eat More Beans to Protect Your Heart

Try to include at least four servings of heart-healthy legumes (beans and peas) every week in your diet. Legumes help fight heart disease, contain a lot of fiber, don't raise blood sugar, and are a source of vitamin B. Plus, they're an inexpensive and versatile staple.

Eat them in the morning as many cultures do, sprinkle some on your salad for a protein boost, or create a main-meal soup out of them, such as minestrone.

PROTECT YOUR HEART WITH BROCCOLI

Many studies have demonstrated that a diet rich in vegetables, especially the brassica group, is linked to a significantly decreased risk of stroke and heart attack. In my book *The 150 Healthiest Foods on Earth*, I wrote about a powerful plant compound in broccoli called sulfuraphane, which is known to activate detoxifying enzymes in the liver that may help the body get rid of cancer-causing chemicals.

Eat broccoli as often as possible to keep your heart young. Include broccoli in as many meals as possible—an omelet for breakfast, a salad for lunch, and a side dish for dinner are just a few ideas. The anti-aging benefits are enormous.

BLUEBERRIES: GO WILD, PART II

Eat more berries to protect your memory!

In animal studies, blueberry extracts make old mice behave like young ones.

Research at the University of Maine, Orono, concluded that a diet containing wild blueberries may reduce the risk from cardiovascular disease. Animal research suggests that blueberries have the potential to decrease the vulnerability of blood vessels to both oxidative stress and inflammation. Work by researcher Dorothy Klimis-Zacas, Ph.D., demonstrated the positive effect of a wild blueberry–based diet on blood vessel function in animals. And experiments on both animals and humans have shown that blueberries protect memory!

Make Nuts a Regular Part of Your Diet to Lower Your Risk of Heart Disease

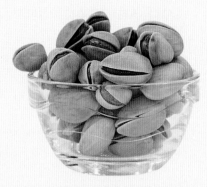

Consume an ounce or two of nuts at least three times a week. The health benefits are numerous: They contain fiber, plant sterols, minerals, and healthy fat, and are a staple in at least one of the longest-lived societies on the planet in Loma Linda, California.

The nuts that contain the highest amount of monounsaturated, or "good," fat are almonds, Brazil nuts, hazelnuts, macadamia nuts, pecans, pistachios, and walnuts. So munch on them as a snack, top salads or soups with them, or mix them with fruit and yogurt.

HEART DISEASE PREVENTION: IT'S NOT ALL ABOUT CHOLESTEROL

You know by now that cholesterol is not the most important thing to worry about when it comes to aging well and avoiding heart disease. Actually, two other risk factors are turning out to be very important. Both are measures of inflammation, and both are things you can do something about immediately. How do you know you have chronic inflammation?

Remember, chronic inflammation doesn't hurt like acute inflammation does. Well, we don't have a *perfect* measure of systemic inflammation, but there are a couple of measures that, as the song says, "will do until the real thing comes along."

Scientists have identified substances in the bloodstream that are excellent markers for systemic inflammation and may turn out to be highly valuable in assessing your risk for heart disease. And though I'd be the last person to say that by bringing these two measures down you're guaranteed to live to one hundred, I'd be foolish not to recommend that you get them down as low as possible. If you have high levels of either of these two compounds, well, as my grandmother used to say, "That can't be good."

You might be interested to know that in addition to heart disease and stroke, excess homocysteine has also been correlated with Alzheimer's disease, osteoporosis, depression, and cognitive impairment.

Most anti-aging doctors that I respect like to see homocysteine levels no higher than 10, and the Life Extension Foundation recommends 7 to 8 as an optimal range.

Drink 6 Ounces (175 ml) of Pomegranate Juice Daily to Help Your Heart— and Your Love Life!

Antioxidant-rich pomegranate juice has been shown to help with erectile dysfunction and may help slow aging and protect against heart disease and cancer. At least five studies have demonstrated a beneficial effect of pomegranate juice on cardiovascular health, including a study that showed a 30 percent reduction in arterial plaque.

Just watch out for added sugars and for the infamous "juice drinks" that can contain as little as 10 percent actual juice!

ASK YOUR DOCTOR TO MEASURE THIS INFLAMMATION MARKER

C-reactive protein (CRP) is a component of the immune system and a substance produced in the liver in response to inflammation. It should be part of every major blood workup.

The high-sensitivity CRP test (hs-CRP) is capable of picking up levels of CRP in the blood at the very earliest stages of vascular disease, and you have a much better shot at treating inflammation early before it ages your body beyond repair. Research has found that high-sensitivity cardiac CRP is able to predict the risk of myocardial infarction (heart attack), stroke, peripheral arterial disease, and even sudden cardiac death among healthy individuals with no history of cardiovascular disease! It can even predict recurrent events and death in patients with coronary syndromes.

And consider this: Increased C-reactive protein is also linked with a greater risk for developing type II diabetes, age-related macular degeneration, and even the loss of cognitive ability in seemingly healthy people. It's also strongly related to major depression in men.

The simple message: Get your levels tested. And if they're high, get them down.

Note: Because there are no drugs that specifically lower CRP levels, the best protection we have right now is to eat an anti-inflammatory diet. The foods recommended in this chapter are a great beginning. Fish oil (and even the omega-3s from plant foods such as flaxseed) may help keep CRP levels in check.

Take These Three B Vitamins to Lower Your Risk of Heart Disease

The toxic compound homocysteine is a risk factor in heart disease and stroke. Get tested for homocysteine levels in your blood and take these vitamins daily to lower your levels if they're too high:

→ Folic Acid: 800 mcg

→ B12: 1,000 mcg (At least—it's best absorbed orally under the tongue or taken by injection.)

→ B6: 100 mg

If your homocysteine levels remain elevated, your doctor may suggest higher doses and may also add the supplement TMG (trimethylglycine), which usually does the trick.

TAKING THE (BLOOD) PRESSURE OFF

Increase in blood pressure is normal and important for survival. Whether you're running from a lion or running a 5K, your blood pressure and heart rate are going to increase, but once things return to normal, they should go back down.

"With hypertension (high blood pressure)," says Houston, "your heart is often or *always* working harder than normal and your arteries are *always* narrow and constricted."

So, why is this not a good thing from the point of view of aging?

When blood comes pounding through the arteries, the one-cell-thick lining (endothelium) gets damaged. "Damage to the endothelium speeds up what's called hardening of the arteries (atherosclerosis), a process that affects all of us as we age," says Houston. "These stiffened, narrowed arteries have a hard time supplying the body with enough oxygen and nutrients, which means the tissues and organs that they serve can be damaged." This is one way that high blood pressure will age you.

High blood pressure damages the heart, the brain, the kidneys, and the eyes. "It causes stroke by weakening and wearing away at the lining of the brain arteries and choking these arteries with plaque," says Houston. "The damaged linings provide a perfect site for plaque deposition and the formation of blood clots."

Here's a chart that shows the relationship between life expectancy and blood pressure for a thirty-five-year-old man.

BLOOD PRESSURE (MM/HG)	LIFE EXPECTANCY
120/80	76
130/90	67½
140/95	62½
150/100	55

THE POTASSIUM CONNECTION

A lot of research suggests that high potassium intake can reduce high blood pressure. Large groups of people with a high intake of potassium have lower blood pressure than large groups of people who don't consume a lot of potassium. And there's research showing that this is true for individuals as well.

Sodium and potassium operate in a kind of seesaw relationship in the body, performing all sorts of metabolic functions, including the regulation of blood pressure. Although we've heard a ton of warnings about too much sodium in our diet, the truth is a bit more nuanced and has to do with the

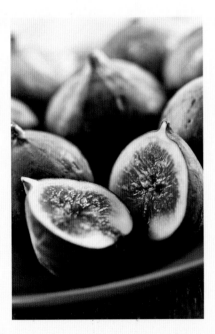

balance between the two. Our Paleolithic ancestors consumed a hearty 5:1 ratio of potassium to sodium in their diet—the average American has that upside down, consuming about a 2:1 ratio of sodium to potassium.

Fruits and vegetables are the best dietary sources of potassium on the planet. Yams, beans, potato skins, Swiss chard, portobello mushrooms, winter squash, and kale are all great sources of potassium, as are apricots, dates, figs, apples, avocados, raisins, prunes, and bananas.

Magnificent Magnesium

In addition to potassium, magnesium may be one of the most helpful nutrients for maintaining healthy blood pressure. One reason: It helps the arteries squeeze and relax as necessary. Plus, it's an essential component of several hundred metabolic processes, including the creation of important hormonelike substances called *eicosanoids* (or *prostaglandins*) that help the arteries dilate (as opposed to constrict). In fact, you can think of magnesium as the "relaxing" mineral; think Epson salts, which are basically high-magnesium baths!

Once again, not surprisingly, magnesium is found everywhere in the plant kingdom. Shiitake mushrooms, navy beans, soybeans,

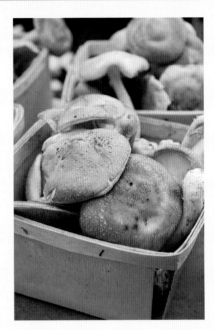

leeks, kale, peppers, spinach, and chard are all great vegetable sources of this wonderful mineral, as are figs, prunes, peaches, apricots, and dates. And nuts and seeds are absolutely loaded with the stuff—pumpkin seeds, flaxseeds, almonds and almond butter, raw cashews, walnuts—if it's a nut or a seed, chances are it's a good source of magnesium.

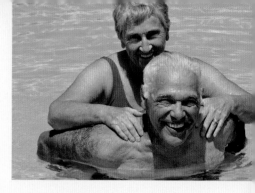

ANTI–AGING ACTION PLAN:

Get Moving to Keep Your Heart Healthy

Exercise doesn't have to be intense to benefit the brain systems that keep the heart healthy (see the section on exercise and movement, page 87). Ping-Pong, tai chi, and ballroom dancing are just a few of the many ways to keep your heart healthy and your body young.

Although you can get cardio benefits from as little as three half-hour sessions a week, the optimal number seems to be the equivalent of thirty to sixty minutes five days a week.

There are risk factors for high blood pressure that you can't change (such as genetics and race), but these are far outweighed by the ones you *can* change. The top of the list is smoking, but right up there with it is poor diet and lack of exercise. Regular exercise lowers blood pressure and the risk of cardiovascular disease. Merely losing weight will bring your blood pressure down.

Exercise will increase blood pressure and heart rate, too, as Houston reminds us, but exercise *also* activates brain areas that allow the brakes to be put on. So when you're exercising, you're actually helping circuits fire in the brain that have the effects of strengthening the "brakes" and protecting your heart from aging. It's not all about the aerobics and the pumping heart; it's also about messages to the brain to keep it flexible and active.

SUPPLEMENT YOUR DIET WITH THESE ITEMS

These are some of the nutritional supplements I think are most important for protecting the heart.

Fish Oil: The omega-3s in fish oil reduce the risk of stroke, lower triglycerides (an independent risk factor for heart disease), reduce blood pressure, and improve blood-clotting mechanisms.

CoQ10: This powerful antioxidant is normally made in the body, but we make less of it as we age. Conezyme Q10 has been used and studied over the years for heart and blood vessel conditions such as heart failure, high blood pressure, and angina. It's one of cardiologist Stephen Sinatra's favorite supplements. People suffering from heart disease often have a deficiency in CoQ10.

L-carnitine: An amino acid–like substance, L-carnitine (also known as carnitine) helps with cellular energy by moving fuel out of the bloodstream and into the energy centers of the cells (the mitochondria). "The more advanced the heart disease, the lower the L-carnitine concentration present and the greater the need for it," says Sinatra. Carnitine comes exclusively from meat (mutton, lamb, and beef).

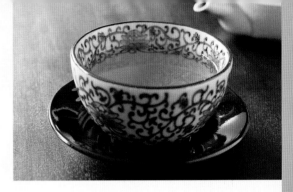

ANTI-AGING ACTION PLAN:

Sip Green Tea to Protect Your Heart

The more green tea people consume, the less likely they are to have coronary artery disease. Japanese researchers found that people who drank five or more cups of tea a day had a significantly lower risk of death compared to the folks who drank only one cup or less a day. The five-cup drinkers had an especially lower risk of dying from cardiovascular disease and stroke.

Five cups a day seems to be the magic number for maximum benefits and heart protection. (Alternatively—or in addition—take an EGCG supplement of 250 milligrams per day.)

Garlic: One of the oldest medicinal foods on the planet, garlic has been the subject of more than 1,200 pharmacological studies. It may influence the genesis and progression of cardiovascular disease through a number of different biological effects, including lowering triglycerides and

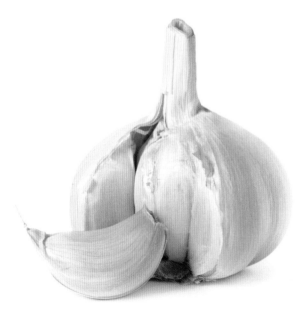

blood pressure. And, because it has other demonstrated medicinal properties, garlic may help knock out pathogens that contribute to inflammation, so it makes sense to make it part of your diet.

Magnesium: When you think magnesium, think "relaxation." Magnesium "relaxes" blood vessel walls, contributing to lower blood pressure. It also helps to lower blood sugar. (Diabetes and heart disease are closely related in terms of risk factors.) Most people in America do not get optimal amounts of magnesium.

CHAPTER 8

How to Keep Your Brain Sharp

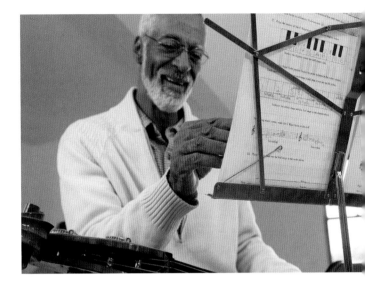

T alking to baby boomers around the country, the single fear I hear repeated most often is not the fear of dying, but the fear of not being able to remember the names of loved ones. Of being infirm and incapacitated and not even knowing what's going on. Of being kept alive, a virtual empty shell of the person you once were.

"Because people tend to forget that their brains are flesh and blood," says Dharma Singh Khalsa, M.D., author of *Brain Longevity*, "they often overlook the physical care and maintenance of their brains." There's an enormous disconnect between the amount of time we spend trying to build and protect our muscles and our skin and even our hearts, all the while virtually ignoring what we can do to protect and nourish our brain.

The brain is responsible for cognitive tasks including attention, thinking, and memory, all of which decline when we age. But hundreds of other unconscious processes, such as the release of hormones, are mediated through signals that originate in the brain, and these processes have profound implications for our health and longevity. The aging brain affects us not only mentally, but also physically. So, anything we can do to keep the brain nourished and fully functioning is going to be a powerful strategy in the anti-aging arsenal.

First, let's get the bad news out of the way: Starting in your early twenties, your brain begins to shrink. It does so at the rate of about 0.2 percent a year, and by your seventh decade or so, it will be about 10 percent smaller than it was in your twenties.

But here's the good news: *It may not matter.*

What *really* matters is the ability of the remaining neurons—and don't worry, there are billions of them— to make connections. In fact, making connections, or reorganizing your brain networks, is the single most important anti-aging strategy for keeping your brain young.

BRAIN BASICS

The average adult has somewhere around 100 billion neurons in his or her brain. (For comparison purposes, you have trillions, that's thousands of billions, of cells in your entire body.) Cells of the nervous system, known as *nerve cells* or *neurons*, are specialists with a particular job description. They have the ability to carry messages to other cells, and the chemical messengers whose job it is to transmit those messages are called *neurotransmitters*.

Neurons share certain characteristics with other cells in the body. They're surrounded by a cell membrane, they have a nucleus (which contains genes), and they have cytoplasm, the jellylike fluid encased inside the membrane where most of the cellular activities occur. Within this cytoplasm are little *organelles*, which are specialized subunits with specific functions. (One of the most important is the mitochondria, little structures that are ground zero for energy production.)

Because the membrane is like the casing for the cell, its health is very important. If the cell membrane is too stiff, nothing, including valuable signaling information, can get

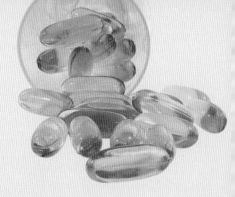

Revitalize Your Brain with Fish Oil

Taking fish oil is good for the cell membranes in the brain. The fatty acids it contains (EPA and DHA) get incorporated into the membranes, making them fluid enough for information to get in and out easily and facilitating cellular communication and, ultimately, a sharp mind! Ideally, take 2–3 grams a day of combined EPA and DHA, the two important omega-3s found in fish oil.

in and out easily, but if it's not stiff enough, the boundaries aren't protected.

THE REAL INFORMATION SUPERHIGHWAY

The ability of your brain cells to form connections with other brain cells is of paramount importance in living long and living well, maybe even more important than the number of brain cells you actually have.

When certain pathways or neurons have deteriorated, making it difficult to "reach" that memory (e.g., remember a name), the adaptable brain can "reroute"—it learns new sequences and develops new networks. That's why the actual physical shrinking, and concomitant loss of neurons, doesn't matter nearly as much as your ability to create these new *networks*, these alternative ways of "reaching" for what you want. "No matter how badly damaged your brain is, it can grow new cells and get more 'thinking power' out of old cells," says Khalsa.

And that's why a mnemonic device, such as remembering that a colleague's name is Peter because his nose looks like a pretzel, is so effective. It's an alternative way to access the memory.

Making new connections is a vital part of anti-aging, both literally (in the brain) and metaphorically (in life), and something that's much more under your control than you might think. When certain pathways or neurons are damaged, the brain simply improvises, using new pathways to accomplish the same activity. It would be as if a tree fell on a hiking trail, cutting off the usual path to the mountaintop. Then, slowly and surely, hikers begin to take an alternate route until a new pathway develops, a trail is laid down, and eventually there's a whole new way to get to the same end point. (Think: a right-handed person learning to write with the left hand.)

The ability to form these new neural networks is one of the most adaptive things our brain can do, and it is one of the keys to protecting the aging brain and keeping it young and active. You can practice network formation. You can strengthen the ability to form new connections, just as you strengthen your biceps by doing dumbbell curls. You can practice network formation and strengthen your brain's ability to do it by living what I call a *life of learning*.

Brain expert Randy Buckner, Ph.D., of Harvard University, suggests that adults take university courses as a strategy to stave off brain aging. And why not? The key is to engage the brain in new activities and new challenging tasks. Personally, I'm addicted to the Teaching Company courses (www.teach12.com). Just for fun, I memorized every U.S. president and can recite them in order, including the years they served. (I'm now a favorite party guest wherever friends play Trivial Pursuit. Want to know how many U.S. presidents were assassinated or died in office? Just ask me!)

It sounds silly, but it isn't. The important thing here is *learning new information.* Think about it: Learning new skills engages the very networks whose health your youngevity depends on. It almost doesn't matter *what* you learn; rather, it matters *that* you learn.

THE LESSON FROM THE CANARY SCAM

Back in the 1930s, one of the most popular pets was the common yellow canary. People loved them because they could sing. But nature wasn't just—it only gave the ability to sing to the male of the species, rendering the females a lot less valuable to the bird-buying population. So what to do about these tone-deaf female canaries? Well, unscrupulous pet store owners improvised. They somehow discovered that injecting the female birds with testosterone, the potent male hormone, temporarily turned the previously undesirable females into a bunch of operatic divas.

Over the past few decades, researchers have investigated this phenomenon more scientifically and discovered that

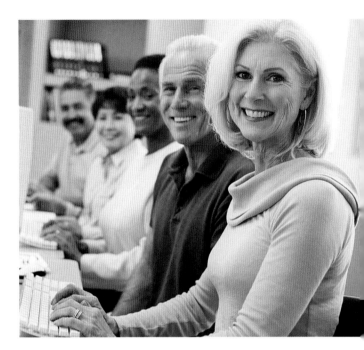

injecting testosterone into female canaries produced an interesting side effect: It caused them to grow new brain cells.

Now, before you throw this into the "so what?" file, consider that the prevailing wisdom at the time was that it was *impossible* to grow new brain cells, that you're born with as many nerve cells (neurons) as you will ever have, and that within the first year of life you start to lose them! The human brain contains about 100 billion nerve cells and a staggering 100 trillion connections, but by late adulthood, those cells are dropping like flies; just in the course of normal use you'll lose about 100,000 brain cells a day (more if you play around with alcohol and drugs). So, the notion that you could actually grow new cells in the *brain* was revolutionary.

"The philosophical implications of this discovery are profound," says Khalsa. "It means that people are not limited to just the brain cells they were born with."

WALK A DAY AND GAIN A SIZE

The work of Arthur Kramer, Ph.D., at the University of Illinois has shown that a simple activity can actually increase the size of the brain. The activity? Walking.

Kramer and his colleagues put a group of sixty volunteers in an MRI machine, which pinpoints changes and abnormalities in body tissues. "These folks were basically couch potatoes," Kramer told me, "healthy but sedentary, and ranging in age from sixty to eighty." Then, the researchers divided them into two groups. One group went into an aerobics program, the other into a "toning and stretching" program.

"We started the aerobics group at fifteen minutes a day at a pretty slow pace," Kramer said, "but after two months they were up to forty-five to sixty minutes, three days a week." And they kept it up for six months. "The other group did some very basic stretching exercises with exercise bands," he said. Good stuff, but not enough to get their heart rates up. Then after six months, the subjects went back into the MRI machine and the experimenters examined their gray and white matter.

The gray matter of the brain is composed of neurons, or *computational units*, while the white matter is the axons, or interconnections, kind of like telephone wires between the neurons. The researchers specifically wanted to see whether any changes in either type of tissue had taken place over the course of the study.

This was a novel approach to looking at the changes in the brain that exercise produces. Although plenty of studies have shown that exercise produces changes in the brain's *functional* abilities (e.g., improved memory, the ability to count backwards, etc.), no one had investigated *structural* changes. Kramer's work was unusual precisely because it focused on the *size* of the brain, not how it functioned. "This was pure anatomy," he told me.

I know you're on the edge of your seat wondering whether the brain actually got bigger, so I won't keep you in suspense: "Both the gray matter *and* the white matter showed increased volume," said Kramer.

In other words, exercise actually *increases* the size of the brain. And, at least when it comes to the brain, size does matter. More good news: It doesn't take much exercise to accomplish this minor miracle. Forty-five to sixty minutes, three times a week, seems to do the trick.

As we'll see countless times in this book, strategies that affect one organ or system in the body often influence others. The body is truly a "global economy" in which benefits spread from system to system without regard for parochial boundaries. In this case, exercise, one of the strongest anti-aging strategies on the planet for the heart (not to mention the bones and the lungs), affects the brain in the same way. "What's good for the heart is good for the brain" has been said by more experts than I can possibly count, largely because it is 100 percent true. Even Kramer's eight-year-old daughter was able to grasp the relationship when she summarized it thusly: "Exercise your heart and get really smart!"

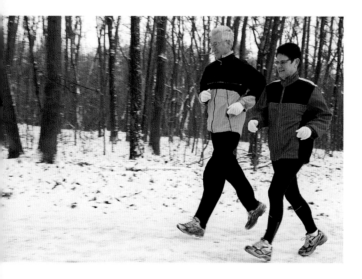

ANTI–AGING ACTION PLAN:

Walk to Build Your Brain Power

Walking is one of the easiest ways to get exercise, so I recommend walking at a moderate pace for thirty minutes every day. All you need is a good pair of shoes. Once you start walking regularly, you can increase the pace and duration of your walks.

Starting in our early twenties, our brains begin to shrink, at a rate of 0.2 percent a year. So by your seventh decade, it will be about 10 percent smaller than it was in your twenties. However, studies show that exercise, such as walking, can actually increase the size of the brain. So get moving!

PROTECT THE BRAIN:
THE CORTISOL CONNECTION

Stress, in the form of the stress hormone cortisol, ages your brain in three primary ways. The first is by decreasing glucose metabolism. When you don't have enough blood sugar, you basically don't have enough fuel to lay down a memory. You may experience putting down the car keys or saying hello to your daughter, but you may not remember doing so. This is probably why short-term memory problems are so common under stress.

The second way cortisol ages your brain is by interfering with neurotransmitter circuits that send information to the brain cells and are necessary for the creation of memories. Under high levels of stress, those memories are, in Khalsa's words, "like downed telephone lines in a storm." They exist, but they can't be accessed.

The third and possibly most insidious way that cortisol ages your brain is by killing brain cells. Cortisol somehow allows too much calcium to get into the brain cells, and the calcium eventually produces free radicals (remember them?), causing oxidative damage and destruction.

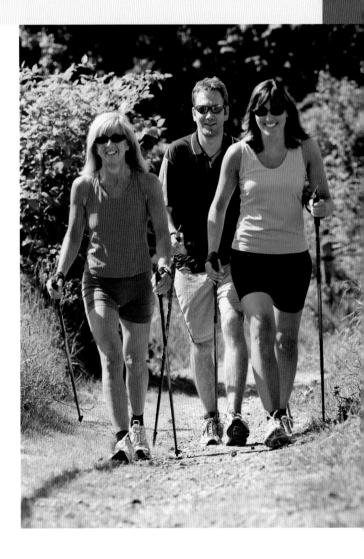

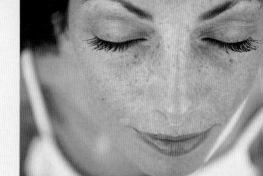

ANTI-AGING ACTION PLAN:

Reduce Stress Every Day by Doing Deep Breathing Exercises in a Quiet Place

Get started in fewer than ten minutes:

1. Lie down in a comfortable position. In yoga, this is called Savasana (corpse pose), which should give you some idea of how relaxed you should be. The pose is used in yoga to practice stilling a hyperactive brain by gaining control over breathing.

2. Your arms should be by your sides, rolled out so your palms are facing up.

3. Your legs should be relaxed. Put support (like a rolled towel) under your knees and allow them to naturally roll outward.

4. Close your eyes.

5. Breathe normally for about a minute. Pay attention to your breath.

6. On each exhalation, imagine that all the points of contact between your body and the floor are softening.

7. After one or two minutes of normal breathing, gradually begin to extend the length of your exhalation. Exhale deeply and slowly.

8. The goal is to inhale fully on a count of four and then exhale fully on a count of eight. In other words, your exhalation should be twice as long as your inhalation.

9. Continue this 1:2 ratio for four to five minutes.

10. Go back to regular breathing for one to two minutes.

Don't get too hung up on the specifics, the counts, or the number of minutes. The idea is to simply breathe in slowly and breathe out even slower and to do it consistently. There are dozens of variations on this theme, including several I've written about in *The 150 Most Effective Ways to Boost Your Energy*. I also wrote about one method called "The Relaxation Response," which I wrote about in *The Most Effective Natural Cures on Earth*. Whatever technique you feel most comfortable with is just fine.

(Thanks to my dear friend, holistic health counselor Jeanette Bessinger of Balance for Life, LLC, for contributing this particular exercise. Visit Jeanette at www.balanceforlifellc.com.)

And just when you thought it couldn't get any worse, consider this: Cortisol literally shrinks the hippocampus, an important brain structure deeply involved in memory and one of the first regions of the brain to suffer damage in Alzheimer's disease. Cortisol does this through what Khalsa calls "the terrible feedback loop," or the destructive cascade. Here's how it works:

There's a ton of research going back to the late 1960s demonstrating the link between high levels of cortisol—one of the most important stress hormones—and the major symptom of brain aging, memory loss. Researcher Sonja Lupien, M.D., found that approximately one-third of fifty-one healthy subjects in a study had sustained high levels of cortisol over a five-year period. This group was consistently terrible at remembering images they had been shown only twenty-four hours earlier. They also took much longer to find their way through a maze that was specially designed to measure spatial memory. Research has shown that even people taking cortisone pills (which turns into cortisol in the body) don't remember word lists as well as people taking placebo (sugar) pills.

Further, in a paper published in 2002, researchers from Beth Israel Medical Center and Harvard Medical School concluded that "stress has a major impact upon neuro-degenerative and mental disorders." They also pointed out that the amount of stress you're under on a daily basis plays a significant role in how susceptible you are to the degenerative diseases associated with brain aging, not to mention the progression of those diseases and their eventual outcome.

And now, it's time for the good news. There is something we can actually *do* to return the cortisol manufacturing plant to its normal hours of operation.

It's called meditation. More effective than any other anti-aging technique for reducing cortisol (and stress) and arresting any further aging of the brain that's caused by stress is simple meditation. And if that's too esoteric for you, deep breathing works just as well.

THE SUGAR–INSULIN CONNECTION

The link between diabetes and Alzheimer's is both well documented and troubling. Several large studies show that people with type II diabetes have double the risk of developing Alzheimer's when compared with nondiabetics of the same sex and age. One study even found that those with borderline diabetes were an incredible 70 percent more likely to develop Alzheimer's than those with normal blood sugar.

Although it's long been suspected that the connection might be due to cardiovascular problems caused by diabetes (resulting in blocked blood flow to the brain and contributing to dementia), other theories are emerging that center around the hormone *insulin*.

Here's how it works: When you eat sugar—or food that converts into sugar easily and quickly (such as white bread and pasta)—your blood sugar rises and your body (specifically your pancreas) responds with a squirt of insulin, a hormone whose many jobs includes escorting that excess blood sugar into the muscle cells, where it can be used for energy. But diabetics usually develop a condition called *insulin resistance* in which this system of regulating blood sugar doesn't work very well. Blood sugar goes up (especially when you eat high-carbohydrate foods), the body tries to protect itself by squirting even higher levels of insulin into the bloodstream, but the cells become resistant to its actions. This requires the pancreas to release even

TRAIN YOUR BRAIN TO REMEMBER!

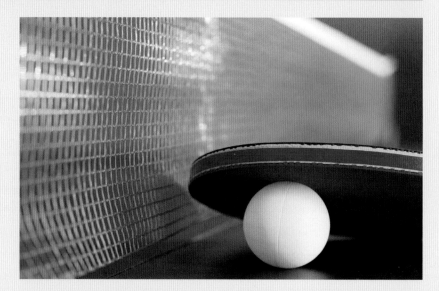

One thing aging can do to brain function is slow down the speed at which you process information. Mayo Clinic researchers investigated whether a computer program might improve the speed and accuracy of brain processing and discovered a fascinating side benefit of the program—it improved memory!

For five days a week for two months, men and women over age sixty-five, all of whom were healthy and none of whom had a diagnosis of cognitive impairment, worked on computer-based activities in their homes. The experimental computer program used six auditory exercises that were specially designed to improve both the speed and the accuracy of processing (such as distinguishing between low- and high-pitched sounds presented at an increasing speed). At the end of the eight weeks, researchers used standardized tools to measure changes in memory (such as the ability to repeat words or numbers after hearing them once).

Those in the experimental group improved twice as much over the course of eight weeks as the group that didn't play with the computer program. What's especially intriguing about this study is that the program really didn't "train" memory. Instead, it trained processing speed, but

it improved memory nonetheless. Best of all, the participants in the experimental group reported that their memory had improved in day-to-day tasks as well.

"The study indicates that choosing a memory-enhancing approach that focuses on improving brain processing speed and accuracy, rather than memory retention, may be helpful," said study author Glenn Smith, Ph.D., of the Mayo Clinic.

And you don't need to wait for technology to come up with the perfect "brain training" program to start doing some work on keeping your mind sharp (not to mention hand-eye coordination). Why not take my friend Dr. Daniel Amen's advice: Pick up a ping-pong racket.

Ping-Pong is an activity tailor made to train your brain's ability to process information quicker. Who knows? That increasingly popular little sport—easily done into your nineties or even beyond—just might be the ticket to keeping your brain young and vibrant for a long time.

more insulin in a futile attempt to get your blood sugar back down where it belongs.

So, now you have high insulin in the bloodstream. Which is not a good thing at all.

What does that have to do with the brain?

Well, a lot actually, and here is where it gets tricky, so pay close attention! Insulin performs a lot of important functions in the brain, most of them *good*. "Insulin in the brain acts on nerve cells to form new connections between brain cells and to resist the dents and dings of aging. It even increases neurogenesis (the formation of new neurons)," explains my friend, renowned brain surgeon Larry McCleary, M.D., author of *The Brain Trust Program*.

But wait, you might think. It sounds like this excess insulin that's carousing around the bloodstream as a result of insulin resistance is actually a *good* thing, right? Insulin resistance means more beneficial insulin for the brain. Every (metabolic) cloud has its silver lining, and all that, right?

Well, it would indeed be a good thing if there were more insulin in the brain. And that is exactly what you would reasonably expect to be the case if there was a lot of insulin hanging around in the bloodstream. What *actually* happens is the exact *opposite*.

With high levels of insulin in the bloodstream, the whole insulin signaling system gets screwed up. The transporters—those little structures responsible for getting insulin from the bloodstream into the brain—start to turn down the volume and become less active, with the result that *less* insulin actually gets into the brain, not more. And this *low* level of insulin in the brain, the direct result of having too *much* in the bloodstream, isn't good for either the brain or memory.

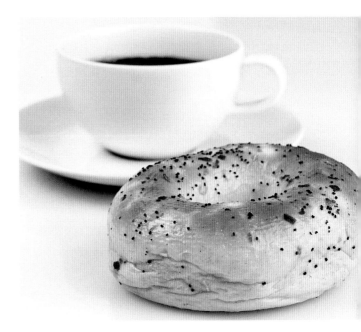

One of the many good things insulin does in the brain is break down a nasty, toxic little protein called amyloid. So one major effect of this whole sugar-insulin "deregulation" (and of the resulting lowered brain insulin) is that less amyloid gets broken down. Amyloid builds up, leading to plaques and causing more inflammation and injury to the brain. It also increases the amyloid plaques that are prominent in the brains of those with Alzheimer's. In the absence of insulin, the amyloid structures bind more readily to nerve cells, which results in—here we go again—*inflammation*! Neurons wind up disconnecting from one another, destroying the very connections that are the basis for all thought. "It's the first step in the degenerative process that eventually results in Alzheimer's disease," says McCleary.

Another feature of Alzheimer's and dementia, indeed of brain aging in general, is the loss of an important neurotransmitter called acetylcholine (more on that later). Acetylcholine deficiency has long been seen as an early abnormality in those who develop Alzheimer's, and it is linked to dementia as well. We need acetylcholine to think and remember. Researcher Suzanne de la Monte, M.D., at Brown University, shows that the enzyme that actually *makes* acetylcholine is regulated by—drum roll, please—*insulin*!

"Insulin is the controlling factor in (many features) of Alzheimer's disease," she says. "If you don't have enough insulin or the ability to respond to insulin is impaired, then neurons will not function well and they will probably die." De la Monte has actually coined the term *type 3 diabetes* to refer to the form of insulin deficiency in the brain that is increasingly linked to brain deterioration (and with the insulin resistance found in type 2 diabetics, made worse by high-sugar diets).

To recap:

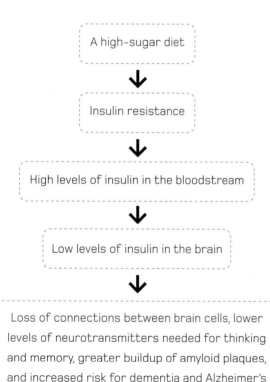

A high-sugar diet

↓

Insulin resistance

↓

High levels of insulin in the bloodstream

↓

Low levels of insulin in the brain

↓

Loss of connections between brain cells, lower levels of neurotransmitters needed for thinking and memory, greater buildup of amyloid plaques, and increased risk for dementia and Alzheimer's

THE HORSEMAN RETURNS

So inflammation has shown its face again, this time as a major player in the aging and deteriorating brain. What about oxidation?

Researchers at Salk Institute and University of California San Diego Department of Pathology wanted to investigate why diabetes seems to predispose people to Alzheimer's disease, so they induced diabetes in mice. The mice suffered damage to the blood vessels, largely due to the overproduction of free radicals. These free radicals caused oxidative damage to the cells that line the brain's blood vessels.

Sugar, long known to be a major culprit in obesity, diabetes, heart disease, and even some cancers, is your worst enemy when it comes to protecting your aging brain.

And you don't have to have diabetes to benefit from getting off sugar (or at least decreasing its presence in your diet substantially). Over the last decade, a substantial amount of research has implicated high blood sugar—and its metabolic consequences—in the development of Alzheimer's. (Alzheimer's is now referred to as type 3 diabetes.) We now know that high blood sugar levels may be to blame for memory lapses, the well-known "senior moment." And research in 2017 showed that people without diabetes can still have high enough blood sugar to have negative health consequences. The lead author of that study, Dr. Erin Walsh, stated that maintaining healthy blood glucose levels can help promote healthy brain aging. "If you don't have diabetes, it's not too early, and if you do have diabetes, it's not too late."

Be a Sugar Detective to Guard Against Premature Aging

Read the label of every food you eat for sugar content. Remember that 4 grams equals 1 teaspoon. A high-sugar diet can prematurely age you, resulting in sending high levels of insulin to the blood stream and low levels to the brain. When it comes to sugar, the less you consume, the better.

My best advice to you regarding sugar is this: Dump it.

Look, I know it's hard. But to the extent that you can do it, eliminating sugar may just be one of the best anti-aging strategies you can use. To the extent that you can eliminate or reduce sugar in your diet, including sugar in the form of high-carb, processed foods—which have the same effects on your brain—you will be doing your brain the greatest possible favor and possibly extending its useful shelf life by many years. What better result could you ask for from an anti-aging strategy?

FEED YOUR BRAIN, EXTEND YOUR LIFE

Let's cut to the chase: Want to start protecting your aging brain big time? Eat fish. At least twice a week, preferably more.

Cold-water fish (such as salmon) contains two critically important fatty acids *docosahexaenoic acid* and *eicosapentanoic acid* (DHA and EPA). People have written entire books extolling the virtues of these omega-3 fats for the heart, brain, and overall human health, but the critical thing to remember for our purposes is that these essential fatty acids are highly concentrated in the brain and are your secret weapon in the fight against aging. (A new baby's brain is about 60 percent fat by weight and most of it is DHA!)

Omega-3s are particularly important for cognitive function (like memory). Research has shown that including omega-3 fatty acids in the diet protects against such brain injuries as stroke caused by plaque buildup and blood clots in the arteries leading to the brain. In fact, eating at least two servings of fish per week can reduce the risk of stroke by as much as 50 percent, according to the University of Maryland Medical Center. The best sources of omega-3s are wild salmon (like the Vital Choice brand linked on my website, www.jonnybowden.com), as well as mackerel, halibut, sardines, tuna, and herring.

Eat One Cup (145 g) of Blueberries Three Times a Week for a Memory Boost

Eat more if you like! Blueberries are the ultimate "memory food." They are loaded with compounds that fight both oxidation and inflammation.

Blueberries can be added to cereal, eaten with yogurt, even sprinkled on green salads. They go great in smoothies. And best of all, you don't need to be limited by their seasonal availability—they're absolutely fabulous frozen. I actually eat them direct from the freezer (mixed with frozen cherries, yogurt or raw milk, and sprinkled with coconut flakes and almonds). Feel free to defrost if you don't like the "faux ice cream" effect!

A DEPRESSED BRAIN IS AN AGING BRAIN

With the relationship between depression and unhealthy aging becoming increasingly clear, consider anything that may help mood and optimism a strong asset in an anti-aging program. Omega-3s fit the bill.

At least one clinical study of patients hospitalized for depression has shown measurably low levels of omega-3 fatty acids (and the ratio of inflammatory omega-6s to anti-inflammatory omega-3s as especially high). Those who incorporated fatty fish two to three times a week into a healthy diet for five years experienced significant reduction in feelings of depression. Omega-3s are clearly mood enhancers, and by reducing depression, they just may extend your life.

One of the best researched foods for protecting the aging brain is blueberries. Blueberries are absolutely loaded with compounds that fight both oxidation and inflammation. They contain plant chemicals called *anthocyanins*, which protect the brain. And special compounds in the blueberries called *polyphenols* actually help neurons (brain cells) talk to each other. Connections can be formed more easily, memories laid down and accessed, and a youthful vitality restored.

LOWER YOUR RISK OF COGNITIVE DECLINE

Can a diet actually protect your brain against one of the most devastating diseases of aging, Alzheimer's? Researchers looked at the eating habits of more than 1,300 people who had no particular cognitive problems as well as almost 500 folks who had what's called *mild cognitive*

ANTI–AGING ACTION PLAN:

Follow the Mediterranean Diet to Slow Cognitive Decline

The Mediterranean diet emphasizes the consumption of vegetables, fruit, legumes, fish, and olive oil. The diet is not low fat, but the amount of junk food and processed carbs is somewhere between very little and zero. There are many terrific books on the Mediterranean diet (although many tend to demonize saturated fat even though current research has debunked the notion that saturated fat causes heart disease).

impairment, a condition that affects about 20 percent of the population over seventy. Mild cognitive impairment is a kind of middle stage between the "normal" cognitive decline of aging and the real serious stuff (e.g., Alzheimer's or dementia). The researchers put each patient into one of three groups, depending on how strictly they followed a Mediterranean-type diet (meaning large amounts of vegetables, fruits, fish, legumes, and olive oil, with relatively small amounts of meat and dairy).

What they found was that the patients who adhered most closely to a Mediterranean-type diet had an almost 30 percent lower risk of developing mild cognitive impairment (compared to those who followed it the least). They also noted that even in those who already had mild cognitive impairment, following a Mediterranean-type diet seemed to slow their decline.

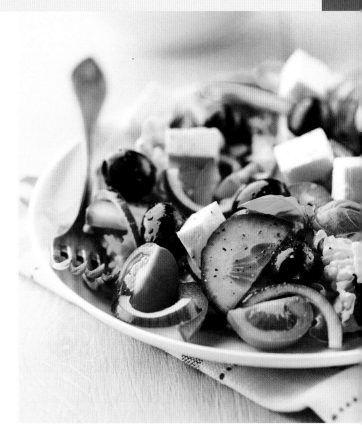

SPICE IT UP AND PROTECT YOUR MEMORY

Want a spice that can protect your brain? Look no further than the stuff that makes curry yellow—turmeric.

I've been a fan of this incredible spice ever since I wrote about it in *The 150 Healthiest Foods on Earth*. Turmeric contains active ingredients called *curcuminoids*, and these have been found to have potent anti-inflammatory and antioxidant properties. They have particular importance to the brain.

The general name for curcuminoids is *curcumin*, and it has been found to prevent the death of neurons (brain cells), reduce oxidative damage, and decrease the formation of inflammatory factors in the brain. And it reduces, or even, amazingly, reverses, the formation of amyloid plaques. Think of curcumin as a kind of natural NSAID (non-steroidal anti-inflammatory drug, such as ibuprofen). In that sense, it works much like omega-3 fatty acids from fish and flaxseed, and that may be part of the reason they are protective against Alzheimer's. Just for the record, the rate of Alzheimer's in the United States is nearly four times that of India, where turmeric is always on the menu.

Research conducted in Singapore took a look at the role of curcumin (turmeric) in the prevention of basic cognitive decline, the kind that supposedly comes "naturally" with aging. The researchers measured decline by looking at scores on a test called the *MMSE* (Mini-Mental

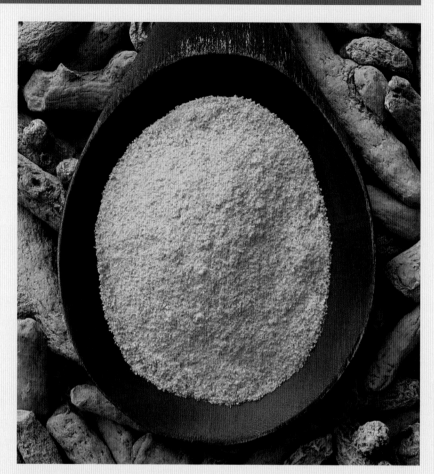

State Exam). The MMSE is a simple, eleven-question test that's pretty standard for measuring cognitive decline. Questions include asking the person to name the date or follow simple instructions such as recalling three objects, counting by sevens, or repeating a simple phrase. The test is quite effective at identifying those with mild cognitive decline. Those who regularly consumed curry scored significantly higher on average compared to those who never, or rarely, did.

Turmeric, the whole spice, contains 2 to 6 percent curcumin. Although curcumin supplements are available, most experts recommend using the whole spice (turmeric) because it may contain a host of related compounds that work synergistically. Turmeric tastes delicious and you really can't overdo it. I sprinkle it on virtually everything, and it's my favorite seasoning for everything from scrambled eggs to soup.

It gets better. The most incredible finding of all was this: Those who followed the Mediterranean diet consistently had a 48 percent lower risk of developing Alzheimer's!

Although there is some variation in the Mediterranean diet depending on which part of the Mediterranean you live near, the foods mentioned in the sidebar on page 119 seem to hold across all regions.

Given that this kind of eating strategy has shown health benefits across a wide range of conditions, and that some of the healthiest and longest-lived people eat a diet not dissimilar from the one just described, it's reasonable to assume that this kind of eating style will protect your brain from aging badly as well as or better than any other dietary strategy on the planet.

PROTECT YOUR BRAIN WITH THESE SUPPLEMENTS

Inside most cells in the body there lives a tiny little structure called a *mitochondrion* (plural: *mitochondria*). The mitochondria are where all the action takes place for energy production in the cell, as well as burning fuel and supplying chemical energy to run the body. Some cells have only one mitochondrion and some have thousands. (Muscle cells, for example, are teeming with the little devils while fat cells—not so much.)

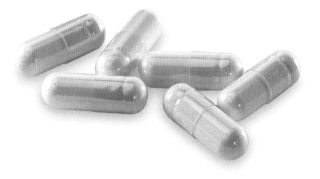

Brain cells have a lot of mitochondria.

The mitochondria play a huge role in aging. When mitochondria are damaged, your energy drops, your heart doesn't function as well, memory declines, muscles start to ache, you don't feel as sharp—the whole nine yards. Result: Your brain gets old, fast.

In a real sense, successful aging is all about avoiding damage to these critical energy-producing structures. Recently, researchers have begun classifying nutrients that have a protective effect on these functions as *mitochondrial nutrients*. Taken alone or, better yet, together, they can significantly reduce the risk of mitochondrial dysfunction, protecting your brain and its various functions well into your ninth decade or beyond.

The major way these mitochondrial nutrients help the brain is by protecting the energy centers of the cell against oxidative damage. One review of recent research, titled, "Can We Prevent Parkinson's and Alzheimer's Disease?" published in the *Journal of Postgraduate Medicine*, concluded that "reducing oxidative stress appears to be a rational choice for the prevention and reduction in the rate of progression of these neurological disorders."

These nutrients act as PacMen toward free radicals and inhibit the damage to brain functioning they can cause. Chief among these mitochondrial nutrients are acetyl-L-carnitine and alpha-lipoic acid, both of which have been shown to protect the brain in significant ways. Other nutrients that work synergistically to keep your brain active and functioning include *phosphatidylserine*, *GPC* (GlyceroPhosCholine), and *ginkgo biloba*.

Let's take a look.

ANTI-AGING ACTION PLAN:

Take Brain-Protecting Nutrients

To Keep Your Brain Firing on All Cylinders, Take These Supplements Daily:

→ Acetyl-L-carnitine: 1,000 mg (500 mg twice daily)

→ Alpha-lipoic acid: 100–300 mg

→ Phosphitadylserine: 150–300 mg

→ GPC (GlyceroPhosCholine): 600 mg

→ Gingko: 120–240 mg

Recommended: Take with 2,000–4,000 mg of omega-3 fatty acids

Note: These dosages are general-purpose recommendations. Individual requirements may vary.

Acetyl-L-Carnitine: Teaching an Old Beagle New Tricks

As noted before in this book, L-carnitine is an amino acid–like compound that is derived from two other amino acids (lysine and methionine). We get it in the diet from red meats such as beef and lamb and we make it ourselves in the liver and kidneys. It's critical for energy production in the cells, including the cells in the brain.

Acetyl-L-carnitine is a form of L-carnitine that is kind of tailor made for the brain. In the acetyl-L-carnitine form, carnitine readily enters the brain, where it may help delay the progression of Alzheimer's, relieve the depression associated with senility and dementia, and improve memory in the elderly. And acetyl-L-carnitine isn't just for those diagnosed with Alzheimer's. It's a powerful brain protector that you can begin taking right now. According to the prestigious (and conservative) *Physicians' Desk Reference for Nutritional Supplements*, preliminary evidence shows that

acetyl-L-carnitine can slow mental decline in the elderly who are not afflicted with Alzheimer's.

Alpha-Lipoic Acid: A Triple Value for Your Supplement Dollar

Alpha-lipoic acid is a remarkable antioxidant—it functions in both water and fat. This "all-access" pass allows it to do its magic act everywhere in the body. Alpha-lipoic acid is also able to revitalize and refurbish two *other* antioxidants: water-soluble vitamin C and fat-soluble vitamin E. When you take alpha-lipoic acid as a supplement, you're really getting triple value for your supplement dollar.

Alpha-lipoic acid as a brain nutrient first gained attention through the work of one of the most respected researchers in nutrition and biochemistry in the country, Bruce Ames, Ph.D. Ames performed a series of experiments in which he gave old rats a combination of acetyl-L-carnitine (see above) and alpha-lipoic acid. The results on aging were remarkable.

"With these two supplements together, these old rats got up and did the Macarena," said Ames. "The brain looks better, they are full of energy—everything we looked at looks more like a young animal." That's not a bad endorsement from a professor of the graduate school division of biochemistry and molecular biology at the University of California!

When researchers analyzed the rats' brain tissue, they found substantially less damage to those little energy furnaces in the cells, the mitochondria. There was also substantially reduced oxidative damage to the hippocampus, the memory center of the brain.

Alpha-lipoic acid's benefit to the brain (and aging) may well come because of its incredible power as an antioxidant. "If your brain is being devoured by free radicals," says David Perlmutter, M.D., author of *The Better Brain Book*, "you will not be able to think clearly, stay focused, or retrieve information when you need it." Perlmutter, a neurologist and nutrition expert, also points out that alpha-lipoic acid is one of the few antioxidants that can significantly boost *glutathione*, arguably the body's most important antioxidant and one that is nearly impossible to get from the diet or supplements because it is poorly absorbed. Alpha-lipoic acid, however, helps you "roll your own."

Phosphatidylserine: Finding Misplaced Keys

When it comes to protecting the brain, membranes matter. Enter phosphatidylserine.

Phosphatidylserine is a member of a class of chemicals called phospholipids, which is a critical component of cell membranes. And it's mostly concentrated in the brain. It's been available as a supplement for several decades and has been shown time and time again to help restore brain function. Phosphatidylserine can improve learning, name recall,

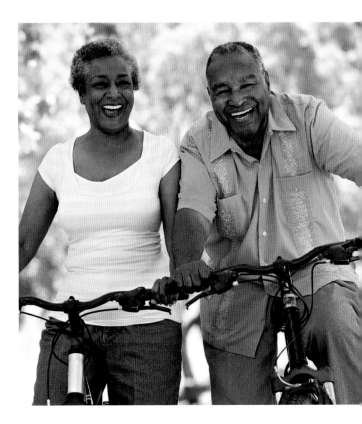

concentration, face recognition, and even the ability to remember telephone numbers and find misplaced objects (like your keys).

One of the main jobs of phosphatidylserine is to help regulate the release of neurotransmitters, those chemical messengers that relay information into and out of the brain cells. Supplementing with phosphatidylserine may have "cognition enhancing activity," meaning it can sharpen your thinking and help slow brain aging, according to the *Physicians' Desk Reference*.

One of the ways it may do this is by acting in the body in a way similar to that of a major Alzheimer's drug called Aricept. See, one of the neurotransmitters most needed for sharp thinking, learning, and memory is called *acetylcholine*. When people have less acetylcholine in their brain, they start to experience the classic signs of the aging

MORE BENEFITS OF RESTRICTING CALORIES: BETTER MEMORY!

Throughout this book, I've alluded to the fact that cutting calories by 25 to 33 percent may be one of the most tested and effective anti-aging strategies of all. In the lab, it's virtually the only thing that's been shown to extend the life of every species tested, from yeast and fruit flies to monkeys.

It may also improve memory.

Researchers in Germany asked one group of elderly volunteers to eat the food they normally ate but to eat about one-third less, primarily by just eating smaller portions. After three months on the diet, they were given a memory test. Compared to two other groups that ate their regular number of calories, the group eating 30 percent fewer calories had significant improvement in memory. "To our knowledge, the current results provide first experimental evidence in humans that caloric restriction improves memory in the elderly," said the researchers.

Why would calorie restriction improve memory? The answer may lay with two of the Four Horsemen of Aging. Scientists aren't sure of the exact mechanism by which calorie restriction helps the brain, but the two most prevalent theories are that calorie restriction reduces inflammation and oxidative damage, both of which are known brain agers.

brain—cognitive impairment and memory loss being among the most common. Acetylcholine is broken down in the brain by an enzyme with a cumbersome name (*acetylcholinesterase*, if you really want to know). If we could somehow slow down the activity of that enzyme, we'd keep more acetylcholine in the brain and our memory and thinking would be sharper. It would be like the Fountain of Youth for the brain.

Aricept works precisely by slowing down the activity of the acetylcholine-destroying enzyme. And so does phosphatidylserine. Several double-blind studies suggest that phosphatidylserine can help maintain a youthful brain in older individuals and may improve memory and learning skill in some. Phosphatidylserine has also shown some ability to slow age-associated memory impairment and general mental deterioration even in non-Alzheimer's dementia.

Biochemist and nutritionist Parris Kidd, Ph.D., states (in his lilting Jamaican accent) that "dietary supplementation with phosphatidylserine can alleviate, ameliorate, and sometimes reverse age-related decline of memory, learning concentration, word skills, and mood."

GPC—Not Your Car's Navigation System

Like its relative, phosphatidylserine, GPC (glycerophos-choline) is a member of the class of biochemicals called *phospholipids*. As a supplement, it has been researched extensively for its effect on mental performance, attention, memory formation, and concentration.

There's a great series of experiments that demonstrate what GPC can do. See, there's a substance called *scopolamine* that causes amnesia. Get yourself some scopolamine and take it by mouth or injection and presto, you've forgotten everything. All information skills, including memory, attention, and learning, just seem to evaporate into the ether. The effect is only temporary, wearing off in a few hours, but for those few hours you pretty much can't remember a thing.

Clever researchers used the scopolamine phenomena to test the hypothesis that GPC might have a protective effect on the brain. For ten days, they gave a bunch of healthy young volunteers a daily dose of either GPC or a placebo (an inert substance). After that, they gave the subjects a nice big dose of scopolamine and sat back to watch the fun begin.

The thing is, the subjects who received the GPC were *significantly protected* from the effects of the drug. Although the drug normally produces amnesia for a full six hours, in the GPC subjects it produced only three hours of forgetfulness and memory impairment. In one test, called the free recall test, the GPC subjects held off the amnesia the entire six hours! And remarkably, even before the administration of the drug, the subjects who took GPC scored higher on a baseline test of word recall. That means the GPC had a positive effect on their brains even before the administration of the drug!

"GPC has a proven track record against age-related decline and other brain damage," says Kidd. "Along with phosphatidylserine, these are the two most clinically proven brain nutrients and both are widely needed, especially since there are no pharmaceuticals available that provide lasting benefit against cognitive decline."

Ginkgo for the Prettiest Brains

I'm a huge fan of my friend Daniel Amen, M.D., who is always pushing the envelope when it comes to brain health (and how to preserve it!). Amen is famous for his SPECT scans, which are pictures of the brain that show where stuff is going on. Amen can read a SPECT scan like a geographer can read a complicated map—he can tell you where the damage is and what impact it's having on functioning.

Amen knows what a healthy brain looks like.

"The prettiest brains I've ever seen are those that are on ginkgo biloba," he told me.

Admittedly, that's not much of a hard science statement, but it contains a lot of truth nonetheless. Ginkgo is a terrific neuroprotector. In Germany, ginkgo biloba extract is registered as an herbal medicine to treat "cerebral

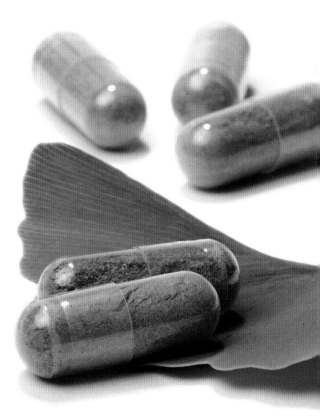

insufficiency," a diagnosis that covers a wide range of conditions. According to the German Commission E monographs—the standard for therapeutic use of herbal medicines—the primary target groups for ginkgo are dementia syndromes. And it's also a powerful antioxidant.

Master herbalist Kerry Bone believes that taking ginkgo on a regular basis might actually help you live longer. When researchers investigated whether ginkgo might help prevent dementia, according to Bone, they found that regular users of the extract had a significantly lower mortality rate from all causes!

Full disclosure: I'm a fan. I take ginkgo on a regular basis, generally about 240 milligrams a day. I like the idea that if Amen ever scanned my brain, he'd class it among the "prettiest" ones he'd ever seen!

VITAMIN B12: THE HOMOCYSTEINE FIGHTER

Okay, my vegan friends are going to hate me, but the truth is you can't get vitamin B12 from plant foods (at least not enough to make any difference at all). And you need vitamin B12 if your brain is going to perform well.

This presents a bit of a conundrum to those of us who wish to live long and keep our faculties. Why? Because to digest and assimilate vitamin B12 you need something in the stomach called *intrinsic factor*. And we make less of it as we get older. (This is why you may have heard of people who take B12 injections; this bypasses the stomach and gets the vitamin directly into the bloodstream.)

Even before B12 gets bound to intrinsic factor, the body has to extract it from food. And we do this with the help of hydrochloric acid, another secretion we make less of as we age. When we have inflammation in the stomach (a condition called *atrophic gastritis*), we produce fewer gastric juices (including hydrochloric acid), and that means less vitamin B12 in the system. Up to 30 percent of adults fifty and older have this condition and may be unable to normally absorb vitamin B12 in food.

Researchers have been interested in the potential connection between vitamin B12 deficiency and dementia for a long time. The connection is long and involved, but B12 deficiency may decrease levels of different substances needed for neurotransmitters—those chemicals that transmit information in the brain—to do their job properly. If your neurotransmitters aren't firing well, it may result in cognitive impairment. Vitamin B12, you may remember, is also one of the three nutrients (folic acid and B6 being the others) that brings down levels of that nasty inflammatory compound called homocysteine (see page 102), the same compound that increases the risk for Alzheimer's, stroke, and heart disease.

Vitamin B12 is so safe and nontoxic that the Institute of Medicine of the National Academies of Science did not establish a recommended upper limit for this vitamin. The Institute of Medicine did, however, recommend that adults over fifty get their B12 from supplements or fortified foods.

Take Vitamin D Supplements Daily to Protect Your Bones and Brain

Vitamin D is a superstar among supplements—and it should be. Research shows that people are becoming more and more deficient in vitamin D, which is needed to protect bones and may help protect the brain and prevent cognitive decline.

However, it's hard to get vitamin D from food, which is why supplementation is important. Take at least 2,000 IUs of vitamin D daily and monitor your levels using the blood test. Many people may benefit from more.

VITAMIN D: THE SUPPLEMENT SUPERSTAR

The U.S. Census Bureau has estimated that nearly 19 million Americans will be age eighty-five by 2050 and that more than half of these will have some form of dementia. Given that elderly populations worldwide are 40 to 100 percent deficient in vitamin D and that the benefits of vitamin D supplements are broad and dramatic, it makes sense for every adult to supplement with this important vitamin. Few foods are natural sources of vitamin D, making supplementation even more crucial as an anti-aging strategy.

VINPOCETINE MAY BE RIGHT FOR YOU

Vinpocetine, an extract of the periwinkle plant, helps improve blood flow to the brain. "In my practice, I have seen vast improvement in patients using the supplement; practically overnight they become more lucid, sharper, and more on the ball," says Perlmutter. But vinpocetine is not

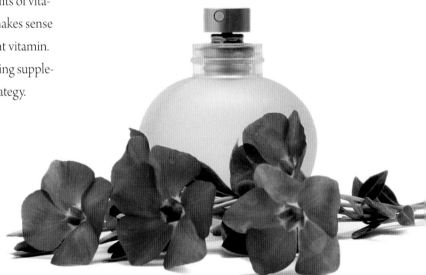

HOW MUCH VITAMIN D IS ENOUGH?

Think you're getting enough vitamin D? Think again.

There is overwhelming evidence that we need far more vitamin D than previously believed. We now know that vitamin D is intimately tied to better physical performance, preservation of muscle strength and physical function, prevention of cancer and heart disease, improved immune function, and happier moods, not to mention being absolutely essential for strong bones.

In the last decade, two major medical organizations—the American Academy of Pediatrics and the Canadian Pediatric Society—have updated their recommendations for vitamin D intake for children. We suspect others will follow suit, and we also suspect that the recommendations will rise over time. Though the increases in recommended daily allowances is a step in the right direction, many feel they don't go far enough.

Michael Holick, M.D., professor of medicine at Boston University School of Medicine and an outstanding crusader for updating vitamin D intake recommendations, has found that 76 percent of the mothers coming into his hospital were severely vitamin D deficient and 81 percent of their infants were as well. Researchers have found that fully one-third of the toddlers in urban Canada have less than the recommended levels of vitamin D, as do 14 percent of toddlers in Boston.

A 2018 study claims that vitamin D does not help bones stay strong and that physicians should reconsider their vitamin D recommendations. This is an important teaching moment.

There will always be studies that say that such-and-such supplement doesn't do what we thought it did, just as there will always be studies proclaiming that the supplement of the moment can cure cancer. Nearly all of these studies are what's called epidemiological or observational studies. (Elsewhere in this book, I explain why epidemiological studies are the redheaded step-sister of real science (see page 17). One point to remember is that these are based on the flimsiest of data and they inevitably produce conflicting results.

The second, most important thing to remember is that one study never decides anything. It almost never "proves" or "disproves"—it suggests and, together with other research, can point in a general direction. The overwhelming preponderance of evidence—in my reading of the research—is positive for vitamin D. And most people don't get enough. That's my story—and I'm sticking to it. Luckily, the facts back me up!

The Dearth of Vitamin D

Why are we so lacking in vitamin D?

One reason might be sun phobia. (Remember, one of the best sources of vitamin D is the sun, which is the fuel that allows our body to manufacture its own vitamin D.) We've been so conditioned to fear the sun that many of us slather on SPF 45 just to go out to the corner grocery store, effectively limiting the major source of "raw material" for vitamin D production.

Meanwhile, studies show that a double digit percentage of Americans have less than optimal levels of vitamin D. And it matters.

Another reason might be the definition of adequate intake. When health professionals believed the main purpose for vitamin D was preventing rickets, they set the bar for adequate intake pretty darn low. So although we might get enough vitamin D by the "old" standards of adequate intake—meaning rickets prevention—we're not getting nearly enough to achieve the many documented health benefits that researchers are now discovering vitamin D has to offer.

And with the highly unpopular cod liver oil being the top source of vitamin D in the diet (followed by nine kinds of fish, none of which has the amount of vitamin D many health experts recommend for optimal intake), it's easy to see why we're so deficient.

Older adults should pay special attention. Research from Wake Forest University School of Medicine in North Carolina shows that older adults who don't get enough vitamin D are at higher risk for disability.

Dosage Dilemma

How much is enough? When the original edition of this book first came out, the Institute of Medicine had just set the "safe upper limit" for vitamin D at 2,000 IUs per day, but as of 2018, it was up to 4,000 IUs. I personally take 5,000 IUs a day, and I live in Southern California and play tennis every day.

Before determining an appropriate dosage, get tested for vitamin D levels. The test one you want is called the 25(OH)D, also known as the 25-hydroxyvitamin D test.

Levels of vitamin D (25-hydroxyvitamin D) below 30 ng/mL are considered deficient. Optimal levels are now considered between 30 and 65 ng/mL, with some arguing for an even higher upper limit of optimal. The Vitamin D Council states that the minimal acceptable level is 50 for children and adults all year-round. (Levels over 100 indicate possible excess.) Integrative and functional medicine docs like to see 50 and above.

If you don't want to wait to have your doctor test your levels, there is now a simple and accurate test for vitamin D recommended by the Vitamin D Council that you can do at home. It's called the Vitamin D Blood Spot Testing Kit and is available through ZRT Labs (www.zrtlab.com) or through a link on the Vitamin D Council's website (www.vitamindcouncil.org).

for everyone; it's primarily useful if you have high levels of homocysteine and/or a history of heart disease or vascular dementia (senility caused by impaired blood flow within the brain).

Vinpocetine has been used in Europe and Japan for more than two decades to treat stroke victims and people suffering from dementia. A 1987 study in the *Journal of the American Geriatric Society* reported that 56 percent of patients treated with vinpocetine made "good to excellent improvement" and scored "consistently better on all evaluations of effectiveness of treatment."

"More than fifty clinical studies have documented that vinpocetine can improve blood flow to the brain, promote better oxygen utilization, increase energy production in the brain, and help prevent blood clots," says Perlmutter. "It is also a potent antioxidant."

Note: Don't use vinpocetine with a blood thinner such as Coumadin.

CHAPTER 9

How to Protect and Maintain Strong Bones, Muscles, and Joints

ere's a riddle for you: What medical condition that almost no one has heard of yet will affect nearly every older person in the world?

The answer: sarcopenia.

Sarcopenia, from the Greek meaning "poverty of flesh," is just a fancy word for muscle loss. It's the gradual loss of strength and muscle tissue that every person experiences to some degree or another as he or she ages. And don't fool yourself—because it's not some minor problem that has no effect on the quality of life, nor is it without significant social and economic costs. In 2000, the estimated health care costs directly attributable to sarcopenia in the United States alone were $18.5 billion. (Just for comparison: U.S. Major League Baseball took in about one-third of that amount, $5.2 billion, in 2006.)

One thing to know about sarcopenia is that it starts imperceptibly, when you're young, around the age of thirty, and progresses throughout your life. (It's no accident that the vast majority of athletic record holders are thirty or younger, a fact that I'm painfully aware of every time I hit the tennis courts.) A second thing to know about sarcopenia is that it can be pretty debilitating. It's not easy to live a robust, active life if you can't open a jar or lift the groceries out of the trunk of the car.

And a third thing to know about sarcopenia is that you can easily prevent it. Okay, maybe that's an exaggeration. Even trained athletes experience some muscle and strength loss, no matter how hard they work out. But you can slow it down so much that the amount of loss won't significantly impair your life or well-being. And—spoiler alert—the solution is simple: exercise.

When it comes to the skeletal system, muscle loss isn't the only thing we need to worry about—there's also bone loss and joint problems. Let's take those one by one.

OSTEOPOROSIS: ONE MAN'S CRUSADE

As far as I'm concerned, there's no one on the planet who can teach us more about aging bones than R. Keith McCormick, D.C., a certified chiropractic sports physician, a former varsity cross-country runner at Stanford University, the winner of the 1975 North American Pentathlon Championship, and a former member of the U.S. Olympic team (XXI Olympiad in Montreal).

One day, while running a track workout, he became suddenly lame with hip pain. Several MRIs and X-rays later, he was diagnosed with severe osteoporosis.

At the ripe old age of forty-five.

"Wow, you have worse bone density than a hundred-year-old woman," blurted the X-ray technician who evaluated his films.

"My first reaction was embarrassment," McCormick says in his book, *The Whole-Body Approach to Osteoporosis.* "How could I have this? I'd eaten well all my life, or at least I thought I had. I'd always drunk a lot of milk. I'd never smoked, drank alcohol, or used any type of drug or medication. I'd never done anything 'wrong.' I'd always

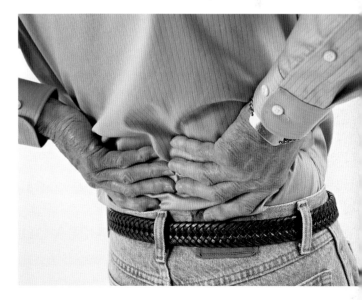

done everything 'right' to be healthy. It just didn't make any sense. Osteoporosis, a disease associated with frailty, was the antithesis of who I thought I was."

Unlucky for McCormick (at least at the time—he continues to compete in triathlons in all distances, including, thank you very much, Ironmans), but very lucky for us.

Why, you ask?

Because McCormick's diagnosis led him to study the disease of osteoporosis with the passion of someone who has a horse in the race—which he does. What he discovered has a great deal to teach us, not only about osteoporosis, but also about aging, longevity, and the interconnectedness of everything in the body. (It's also helped *him* stay in the race.)

"Osteoporosis is not just the weakening of bones," McCormick told me. "It is a weakening of the body's entire physiology. When you have a chronic disease, you have to treat your whole body."

Indeed. And a quick explanation of what goes wrong when bones weaken will illustrate exactly what he means.

The large cast of characters in the drama of bone building makes the New York City phone book look like a grocery list, but these two characters deserve special attention:

The osteoblasts are the cells that form what's called the *bone matrix*, a honeycomb-like structure onto which minerals like calcium are deposited (or absorbed), resulting in nice, hard, mineralized bones. But this is not a one-way street. While minerals continue to be deposited on that honeycomb, other cells called osteoclasts are busy removing minerals in a process called *resorption*. The delicate balance between adding and subtracting, between mineralization (building up) and demineralization (breaking down), between absorption and resorption is called, appropriately enough, *remodeling*.

REENTER THE HORSEMEN

With bones, we again get to see the enormous power of inflammation to wreak havoc in the body. Remember, when you have chronic inflammation your immune system is working overtime. One of the first things the immune system does when it's activated is release T-cells, those sentries of immunity that are summoned whenever the body senses an injury (like inflammation).

"Osteoporosis is not just the weakening of bones. It is a weakening of the body's entire physiology. When you have a chronic disease, you have to treat your whole body."

—Keith McCormick, D.C.

IT'S NOT JUST BONE DENSITY, IT'S BONE QUALITY

Osteoporosis itself doesn't kill people, but fractures can.

Fractures are serious stuff. There are more than 300,000 hip fractures a year in America alone, estimated to go as high as 500,000 by 2040. Someone who sustains a hip fracture is more likely to die than a person of the same age who does not experience this injury. About 20 percent of people who have a hip fracture die within a year of their injury and only about one in four persons have a total recovery from a hip fracture.

At the very least, fractures can significantly reduce quality of life, in some cases forever. "The real concern is breaking bones," writes Gillian Sanson in her excellent book, *The Myth of Osteoporosis*. "The preoccupation with measuring bone mineral density tends to eclipse this obvious and important indicator. You may have low bone density and never fracture; or you may have normal bone density and fracture."

Sanson goes on to point out that the bone mineral density definition of osteoporosis has contributed to the medicalization of aging women. The British Columbia Office of Health Technology Assessment review of the evidence for the effectiveness of bone mineral density testing echoes her concern: "BMD testing is unable to accurately distinguish women at low risk of fracture from those at high risk," the authors write.

Bone mineral density tests may turn out to be very much like cholesterol—an interesting piece of information that has been enormously overrated in terms of its ability to tell us something important about what we really need to know—in this case, our risk of fracture. "Hip fractures that occur between the age of eighty and ninety are invariably linked to factors other than osteoporosis," writes Sanson. "Falling and breaking a hip is most often a marker of generally frail health. A man or woman who remains fit and well is less likely to fracture."

Bone quality—the strength or brittleness of the bone, and its tendency to fracture—is something we should all pay attention to. See page 135 for recommended tests that assess bone quality.

Well, guess what the T-cells do?

They produce a substance in the body that basically instructs bone cells to remove minerals, significantly weakening your bones.

"When we reduce inflammation," says McCormick, "we don't need as much calcium."

Inflammation is intimately connected to the loss of "quality" bone, but it's not the only horseman of aging that plays a role. Remember the stress hormone cortisol? "Cortisol activates receptors on the osteoblasts [bone builders] and shuts them down," McCormick explains.

This leads to an imbalance between mineralization and demineralization; the cells "taking out the trash" are working just fine, but the ones replacing it with new minerals have been put to sleep by stress hormones.

Oxidation, another horseman of aging, plays a part as well. Free radicals, also known as *reactive oxygen species*, stimulate the cells that tear bone down. When there are too many free radicals, the cells that remove the metabolic "trash" from your bones become overstimulated. These now turbocharged cells go into overdrive and you start leaking minerals from your bones. And it all started with

ANTI-AGING ACTION PLAN:

Eat These Foods for Strong Bones

Sardines, broccoli, almonds, prunes, oranges, and onions—these are Keith McCormick's favorite foods for building strong bones. Make them part of your regular diet by eating them every week.

"These are great foods for bone health," says McCormick, D.C. "They provide bioactive compounds that have been shown to increase bone density, and I recommend them to my patients all the time."

oxidative damage from free radicals. This is why antioxidants are a big part of McCormick's recommendation for keeping bones strong (see above sidebar).

McCormick is a particular fan of a powerful antioxidant known as *NAC* (N-Acetyl-Cysteine) because it specifically lowers reactive oxygen species within the osteoclasts themselves. "Every woman should be on 600 to 1,200 milligrams a day of NAC," he told me, "especially after menopause." (Estrogen helps reduce bone resorption; without it, you need even more help keeping the osteoclasts from getting too busy!) McCormick thinks NAC is a good idea for men as well.

And finally, there's our old friend glycation, another of the Four Horsemen of Aging. You may remember our discussion (back in chapter 3) about AGEs (advanced glycation end products), which form as a result of glycation in the body. (Briefly, when excess sugar in the bloodstream gloms on to proteins, the resultant molecules form nasty little compounds appropriately called AGEs that do exactly

what they sound like—they "age" you in the ways discussed earlier.) Those AGEs damage your bones as well.

"The more AGEs, the more brittle bone collagen becomes, because AGEs stick like glue to the collagen fibers," McCormick says. He believes that is why diabetics have a higher fracture rate than nondiabetics, "even though," he adds, "they might have higher bone density."

In his excellent book, *The Whole-Body Approach to Osteoporosis*, McCormick recommends tests for bone health that go well beyond the traditional evaluation of bone density and look at what's going on in the whole body. Although bone density is important, it's far from the whole picture. "It's a natural thing to lose bone, just not too much or too rapidly," he says. "That's why looking at bone density exam results alone isn't good enough. You want to look at bone quality."[1]

---

1 The definition of bone quality is difficult and elusive and beyond the scope of this book, but it involves looking at markers for structural integrity, such as how well put together the collagen fibers are.

Among the various tests McCormick recommends to assess bone quality are the NTX or DPD urine tests,[2] both of which show you how much collagen is being lost in the urine. "That's a reflection of how much resorption is going on," he says. "If it's too much, that's an indication of poor bone quality."

He also looks at blood sugar levels. "The higher your blood sugar is, the more it's likely that you'll make AGEs in your body," he says.

Finally, he recommends a blood test for vitamin D, which makes total sense. Vitamin D is an essential component in bone health and helps ensure that the body absorbs calcium, which, of course, is critical for building strong, healthy bones, according to the *U.S. Surgeon General's Report on Bone Health and Osteoporosis* (2004). Without adequate vitamin D, you can take all the calcium in the world and it won't do you much good. Vitamin D deficiency has often been linked directly to osteoporosis. Research shows that more than 70 percent of women ages fifty-one to seventy and nearly 90 percent of women over seventy are not getting an adequate intake of vitamin D from food and supplements. Low levels of vitamin D are associated with reduced calcium absorption, bone loss, and increased risk of fracture. (For more on vitamin D, see the sidebar on page 128.)

It's interesting that the guru of osteoporosis should reach many of the same conclusions as so many of my respected colleagues who question conventional wisdom when it comes to health ("wisdom" that includes an obsession with cholesterol scores, the demonization of saturated fat, and the advocacy of high-carb diets, to cite just a few examples). His dietary recommendations tellingly contain such bullet points as "go easy on the dairy products," "reduce the grains," "limit refined carbohydrates," and "eat protein" (you can see why I'm such a fan). And, of course, "Eat five to nine servings of fruits and vegetables each day." You can read more about McCormick's recommendations (and the reasons why he makes them) in his book.

ARREST THE ROBBERS

What you eat is critically important for the health of your bones, muscles, and joints, not to mention all the other body systems we've discussed in this book. But when it comes to bone health, it's particularly important to avoid what we call the "bone robbers."

"If you want good bones, you have to limit your alcohol intake, stop smoking, not salt your food excessively, go easy on the sugar, and not consume cola beverages," McCormick says. Sodas in particular are loaded with phosphoric acid, a known robber of calcium. "By eliminating the unhealthy aspects of your lifestyle and diet, you will have better bones."

And what about supplements? Can they help? Absolutely. Here's McCormick's list of the top supplements for bone health:

- Daily multivitamin-mineral
- Calcium: 1,000 to 1,200 mg daily
- Magnesium: 500 to 600 mg daily
- Vitamin D3: 1,000 to 2,000 IUs daily
- Vitamin K: 1 milligram or more daily
- Daily antioxidant supplement:
  - → Fish oil: 2 to 3 g
  - → Flaxseed meal (like Barlean's Forti-Flax): 2 to 4 tablespoons (15 to 30 g)
  - → Probiotics: 3 to 20 million viable cells

---

2 These are standard tests available from any doctor.

But note well: "Calcium and vitamin D, although integral to your skeletal health, may do you little good if your body is … in a constant state of destruction," McCormick says. "Eliminating excess oxidative stress, systemic inflammation, and gastrointestinal dysfunction[3] are far more useful for healing purposes than overloading your body with calcium. Your major objective, instead of simply swallowing a few key nutrients, should be to build up your whole body."

Amen to that!

A PRIMER ON ARTHRITIS AND JOINT PAIN

"Oh, my aching back."

Heard that refrain lately? Said it yourself?

If so, you're hardly alone. One-half of all working Americans admit to having back pain symptoms, and back pain is the second most common reason for doctor visits and the first most common reason for missed work. It's estimated that as many as 80 percent of us will experience a back problem at some point in our lives.

And it's not just the back. All our joints are subject to wear and tear as we age. Once again, inflammation rears its ugly head. In fact, the very term arthritis comes from the Greek *athro* (meaning "joint") and *itis*, meaning "inflammation."

There are more than a hundred different types of arthritis and related conditions, but by far the most common type is *osteoarthritis* (OA), a chronic condition characterized by breakdown of cartilage (the part of the joint that acts as a cushion between the ends of the bones). When cartilage is intact, your joints can move easily (which is

good), but when the cartilage breaks down, there's less of a cushion and your bones wind up rubbing against each other (which is not so good). The result is pain, stiffness, and loss of movement in the joint, typical symptoms of OA. It's not fun to live with.

And it's one of the most frequent causes of physical disability among older adults. Loss of joint function is also one of the major causes of reduced quality of life, potentially limiting people who suffer with it from walking a few blocks, climbing a flight of stairs, or engaging in all kinds of physical activities that they might otherwise enjoy, according to the Arthritis Foundation. It's also expensive. Arthritis and related conditions cost the U.S. economy nearly $128 billion each year in medical care and indirect expenses, including lost wages and productivity. The total annual cost per person living with OA is approximately $5,700.

By age sixty-five, more than half the population has X-ray evidence of OA in at least one joint, most frequently in the hips, knees, neck, low back, or fingers. (Interestingly, only about a third of these folks report actual pain or other symptoms.) And even X-rays don't tell the whole picture because you can have pain without X-ray confirmation of damage. "X-rays are limited in their capacity to reveal how much joint damage may have occurred in osteoarthritis," says Ann Knight, D.C. "You may not see osteorthritic damage on X-rays until there's been a significant loss of cartilage."

It's worth pointing out that of the four classes of drugs most commonly used to treat OA conventionally, three of them are all about fighting inflammation! (The fourth class consists of painkillers.)

So once again we have a major degenerative disease of aging in which the most common symptom is chronic inflammation.

---

3 Gastrointestinal dysfunction is a huge source of inflammation in the body; when the gut isn't healthy, all sorts of problems can occur, including the overstimulation of the immune system.

Although the previously-mentioned drugs fight inflammation, they are hardly without side effects. Some 10 to 50 percent of patients can't tolerate NSAID treatment because of side effects, including abdominal pain, diarrhea, bloating, heartburn, and upset stomach, and approximately 15 percent of patients on long-term NSAID treatment develop ulceration of the stomach and duodenum. A type of NSAID known as a COX-2 inhibitor works by inhibiting an enzyme responsible for inflammation, but it, too, is not without problems. One of the most famous of the COX-2 inhibitors, Vioxx, was withdrawn from the market in September 2004 because of an increased risk of myocardial infarction (heart attack) and stroke.

GET RID OF INFLAMMATION— WITHOUT THE SIDE EFFECTS

So let's review. Arthritis is a condition in which inflammation is always present, usually with accompanying pain. So whatever else we choose to do about it, reducing inflammation has to be the first order of business. We've talked about the most anti-inflammatory substance on the planet—fish oil—more times than I can count, but it's worth pointing out that it's one anti-inflammatory you can take with no danger of side effects.

Another nutritional strategy is to use turmeric—the spice that makes Indian food yellow—as often as possible. Turmeric has myriad health benefits, one of which is that it is highly anti-inflammatory, largely due to the active ingredients in the spice known as curcuminoids. (You can also take that active ingredient in supplement form. It's called curcumin and it's widely available.)

Two other supplements are also useful for arthritis, and both of them are also without side effects.

Glucosamine is a nutritional supplement that can normalize cartilage metabolism, keeping it from breaking down. It's now widely accepted even by the conventional medical establishment as being very helpful for arthritis, particularly arthritis of the knee.

Two studies of the many that have been conducted on glucosamine are worth mentioning in particular. In one of them, 212 patients were put on 1,500 milligrams of glucosamine a day, followed for three years, and compared with a control group given a placebo. The researchers measured changes in the space between the joints and found that those taking glucosamine experienced no loss of joint space (while those on the placebo continued to show progressive cartilage loss). A second study followed 202 patients on the same 1,500 milligrams of glucosamine per day and compared their progress to a matched group of patients who received a placebo. Once again, researchers saw no joint space narrowing in the patients on glucosamine, and once again, those on the placebo continued to see their joints worsen. In addition to these two studies, a

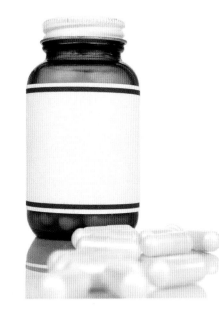

systematic review of published randomized trials whose aim was to determine the effectiveness of glucosamine in OA found that each one of the included studies demonstrated a positive effect.

But preventing cartilage loss wouldn't mean much to the average person if it didn't also decrease pain. "A seemingly overlooked, yet remarkable, finding in both of these trials was the improvement that was seen in joint pain over the years of study follow-up," write University of Utah School of Medicine professors Daniel O. Clegg, M.D., and Christopher Jackson, M.D., in the National Institute of Health's *Encyclopedia of Dietary Supplements*, adding that "sustained lessening in pain of the degree and duration suggested by these trials has never been reported before for any agent in the management of osteoarthritis."

The Natural Standard, an international multidisciplinary collaboration of researchers and clinicians devoted to the rigorous evaluation of research on complementary and alternative therapies, gives glucosamine an "A" rating ("strong scientific evidence") for use in treating knee arthritis and a very respectable "B" rating ("good scientific evidence") for use in treating OA in general.

On a personal note: I have been blessed to be the guardian of many animals over the past fifteen years, who have variously been attended by more than a dozen vets in three cities. I have yet to meet a single vet who does not routinely use glucosamine for animals with arthritic joints. You can't get "placebo effects" (the power of suggestion) with animals. And vets are remarkably free of the political in-fighting that frequently occurs between proponents of natural supplements and the pharmaceutical industry. Vets just use what works.

If you want to use glucosamine for arthritis, and I strongly recommend it, the usual dose is 1,500 milligrams per day,[4] usually in conjunction with chondroitin sulfate (see below). "The safety profile of glucosamine in the published studies ... is uniformly favorable," write Clegg and Jackson.

Chondroitin sulfate is a key component of normal cartilage, but arthritis sufferers have substantially less of it than normal. It draws in precious fluid to the cartilage, protects the cartilage, and stops it from breaking down. Chondroitin sulfate also inhibits certain "cartilage chewing" enzymes, according to chemist and pharmacist Richard Stenlake. A number of studies have reported statistically significant improvement in pain with the use of chondroitin sulfate. Most of these studies have reported important benefits in terms of symptoms (such as pain), function (such as mobility), and reduced medication requirements (such as anti-inflammatories).

"The published medical literature at present suggests that chondroitin sulfate is well tolerated and may be of benefit in alleviating the symptoms of osteoarthritis," write Jackson and Clegg.

The Natural Standard gives chondroitin sulfate an "A" (for "strong scientific evidence") for use in OA. The recommended dose is between 800 and 1,200 milligrams per day, and it's generally used in conjunction with glucosamine (page 137).

Finally, there's one thing you can do that will most assuredly help you reduce the pain of arthritis and will have tremendous collateral benefits as well: Lose weight. For every 1 pound (455 g) of weight lost, there is a 4-pound (1.8 kg) reduction in the load exerted on the knee for each step taken during daily activities. Losing as few as 11 pounds (5 kg) can cut the risk of developing knee arthritis by 50 percent for many people.

---

4 Some research indicates that higher doses, in the range of 2,000 to 2,500 milligrams, may be needed for people who weigh more than 200 pounds (91 kg).

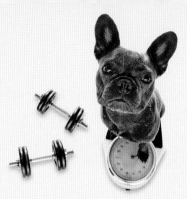

ANTI-AGING ACTION PLAN:

Lose Weight to Take Stress Off Your Joints

When you're carrying extra weight around, you're putting added stress on joints, wearing them down and exacerbating pain. Maintaining a healthy weight nearly always improves the pain of arthritis.

Dozens of research papers have demonstrated that losing even 10 percent of your body weight—a goal considered by most experts to be completely attainable by almost anyone—will significantly benefit your health. It will certainly benefit your joints!

THE SINGLE MOST IMPORTANT ANTI-AGING STRATEGY

So what do all these conditions—sarcopenia, osteoporosis, and arthritis—have in common?

Simple: *They all respond favorably to exercise.* Every single one of them. Exercise is literally the greatest anti-aging strategy in the world—if a drug gave us the reduction in risk that just walking a half hour a day does, that drug would be the best-selling drug of all time!

"Studies have shown that even elderly adults over age eighty who have done active exercise and weight-bearing programs can significantly increase their bone density over a short period of time," says Michael Lam, M.D., M.P.H., a specialist in nutritional and anti-aging medicine. Exercise is the go-to intervention for slowing the negative effects of aging on the entire musculoskeletal system. Exercise builds muscles, countering the effects of sarcopenia, strengthens bones, and is one of the best things you can do for arthritis.

I've mentioned throughout this book that exercise—including just plain walking—is one of five to seven basic

strategies that's been associated with longer and healthier life in just about every study ever done. And, truth be told, if you absolutely hate to exercise, you could start and end with walking and get a lot of benefit from it.

But if you want an even better "insurance policy," add some weight training. I've put together a fairly painless (and effective) manual for how to keep your muscles strong and supple. Performing these seven basic exercises will hit all your major body parts and keep your chest, shoulders, back, arms, legs, and abs perfectly strong and functional for a very long time.

More great news: You only really need to do the series twice a week. That'll keep you mobile, strong, and fit, especially when you couple these exercises with the aerobics I've recommended throughout this book (e.g., walking at least thirty minutes a day) and the stretching exercises I've included afterward (more about those later on).

DR. JONNY'S BASIC PROGRAM FOR MAINTAINING MUSCLE STRENGTH AND BONE MASS

All you need for the exercises below is hand weights (dumbbells), available everywhere. The exact weight will differ from person to person and from exercise to exercise—your legs, for example, are much stronger than your shoulders. Pick a weight with which you can do 8 to 12 repetitions. If you can easily do 12, the weight is too light, and if you can't complete 8, the weight is too heavy. As you get stronger, use heavier weights.

One space- and money-saving trick is to use two water bottles instead of dumbbells. Those plastic gallon-size (3.8 L) bottles you get in the supermarket are perfect because they have handles. Fill the water bottle up just enough to make it difficult, but not impossible, to complete the 8 to 12 reps. You can even use a magic marker to indicate the right fill point for different exercises.

Crunches for the Abdominal Muscles

Lie on the floor with your legs bent, feet flat on the floor, and hands clasped behind your head with your elbows touching the ground. Your head should be in position with the body so that you could hold an apple between your chest and your chin.

Imagine Velcroing your lower back to the floor. You may feel like you're doing a small pelvic thrust slightly forward to accomplish this. Keep your lower back nice and stable in this position.

Curl your upper body forward and up, holding the highest position for a full second before lowering your upper body back down to the ground. Don't pull on your neck when you come up.

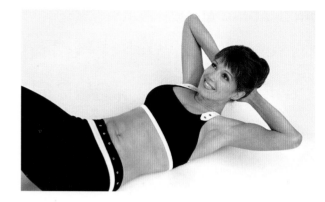

When you lower your upper torso back to the ground, don't return all the way to the "relaxed" position where your weight is supported by the ground, but instead just come down to the point where your upper body is just above the ground and your abs are still contracted. Go back up from this position, so the abs remain tense for the entire time.

Remember to keep your elbows all the way back while doing the movement.

Repeat for as many repetitions as you can manage in good form. The goal is to try for 10 to 20 repetitions.

Note: I constantly used to hear from people who say they're doing "hundreds of crunches" a day. The minute I hear this, I know they're doing them wrong. (I also know there's a good chance they're using momentum rather than strength and are setting themselves up for a lower back injury!) If you do a crunch properly, it's hard! The good news is that when you do them correctly, you don't have to do nearly as many as you think to get good results.

Beginners: Remember that if you can only do one or two, that's fine. You'll work up to more. Don't dwell on what you can't do; concentrate on what you can do.

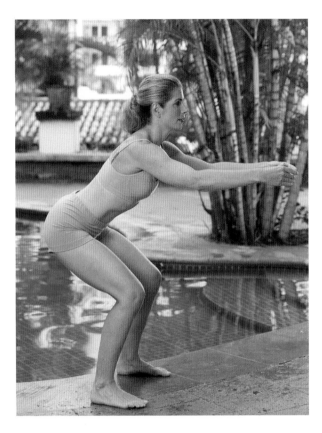

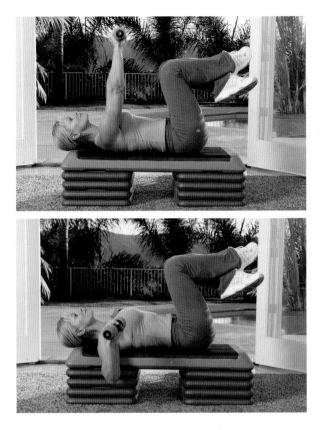

Squats for the Legs and Lower Body

Stand with your arms at your sides. (Do this exercise without weights or hold a dumbbell in each hand.) Keep your feet shoulder-width apart and your head up. There can be a slight arch in your lower back.

Slowly bend your knees while pushing your rear out, until your thighs are about parallel to the ground. Squeeze your thighs and glutes for added contraction. At the same time as you bend, bring your arms up straight in front of you for balance until they're extended straight out at shoulder height, palms facing each other.

Now, come up until you're standing again, dropping your arms back to your sides, and do 10 to 15 repetitions.

Don't lock your knees when returning to the standing position. Adjust your foot stance until it feels comfortable.

Chest Presses

Lie down on a bench, your feet resting comfortably on the floor. (If you don't have a bench, you can use a step or even the floor.) For an added challenge, try raising your feet as in the photos above. Grasp a dumbbell in each hand.

Extend your arms overhead, shoulder-width apart, palms facing out, so that the dumbbells are positioned directly over your shoulders.

Bend your elbows about 90 degrees, gradually lowering the weights until they are above and a little behind your shoulders.

Now, push the dumbbells up with an arcing motion until they're back in the starting position.

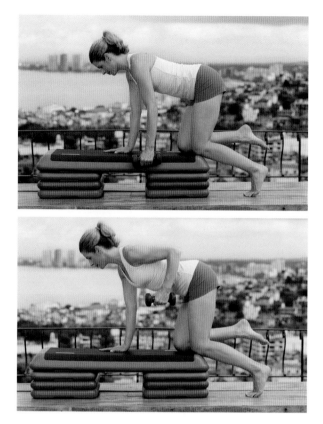

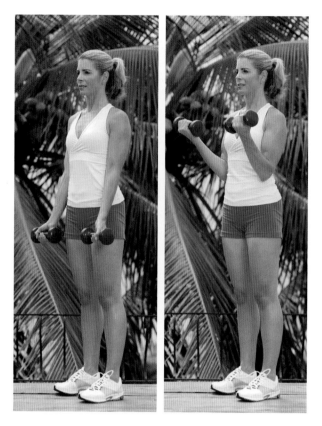

One-Arm Rows for the Back

Bend over and rest your left hand on a bench or stool about 2½ feet (76 cm) high (this doesn't have to be the exact height). Extend your right leg behind you so that you're far enough away from the bench that your back is flat; make sure you don't round your back and instead keep it as flat as possible (you may actually have to arch it a little to keep it in this position). The right arm will be hanging down, straight. Your back should be like a tabletop in this position.

Take a dumbbell in your right hand and bring it straight up toward your hip by bending your elbow and bringing it up behind you toward the ceiling. It should be almost like starting a lawnmower in slow motion. When the weight is about hip level, lower it back down. That's one rep. Do 10 reps and repeat with the left arm.

Biceps Curls for the Arms

Stand with a pair of dumbbells in your hands, palms facing out and shoulder-width apart.

Keeping your elbows stable and next to your sides, raise the dumbbells toward your shoulders and then bring them slowly back down to the original position. Repeat for 8 to 12 repetitions.

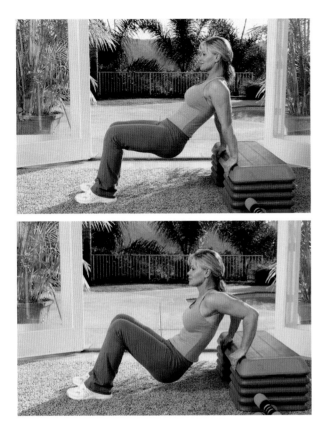

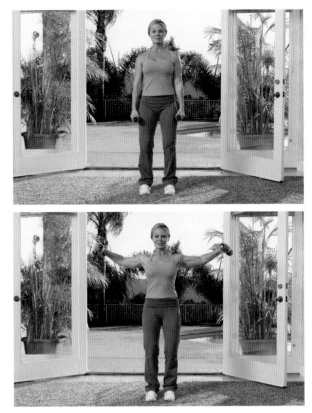

Triceps Dips for the Arms

Sit on the edge of a bench or step, with your hands on the edge of the bench and your fingers facing forward.

Lift your butt off the bench and lower it toward the floor by bending your arms at the elbows. Make sure you stay perpendicular to the ground, back straight. Don't push the hips forward.

Lift yourself back up by straightening your arms, but don't rest your butt back on the bench until you're done. Repeat for 8 to 12 repetitions.

Lateral Raises for the Shoulders

Take a dumbbell in each hand and hold them at the sides of your body, palms facing inward. Stand with your feet shoulder-width apart, knees slightly bent. Don't lean backward.

Raise your arms up and out to the sides until they are parallel to the ground, or "cross" position, and then lower back down. Repeat for 8 to 12 repetitions.

Although this routine won't make you into Mr. or Ms. Olympia, it will do wonders for keeping your muscles from atrophying, and the weight-bearing activity will strengthen your bones and joints. Best of all, a pared-down routine of one set per exercise takes less than half an hour (even with a five-minute warm-up and cool-down added in). And research by noted exercise physiologist and strength researcher Wayne Wescott, Ph.D., shows that merely two weight-training sessions per week is all you need. Just do them on nonconsecutive days so your muscles get a rest in between.

"Research with both older and younger people [produces] an increase in muscular strength of approximately 50 percent after just two months of twice-a-week (weight) training," Wescott writes.

DITCH THE PAIN WITH THESE SUPPLEMENTAL STRETCHING EXERCISES

Although strength-training exercises are great for keeping your muscles and bones young, they won't necessarily get you out of pain. But dozens of other exercises (and stretches) will. The following stretches, courtesy of my good friend Ann Knight, D.C., have specific therapeutic benefits for problem areas of the body. They are designed to strengthen the targeted areas as well as stretch them. Virtually all of them can be done with no equipment and are not very difficult. You can do all of them or just choose the ones that are most appropriate for whatever area of your body feels tight and stiff.

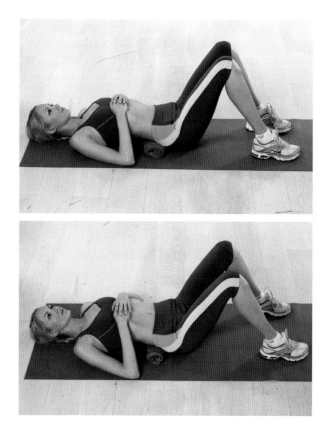

Pelvic Tilt for the Abs and Back

Purpose: To strengthen abdominal and back muscles

1. Begin by lying on your back with you knees bent and feet on the floor.
2. Push the lower part of your back into the floor by tightening your abdominal and buttock muscles. Rotate your pelvis upward without bringing your back off the floor.
3. Hold for 5 seconds and then return to the starting position.
4. Relax for 5 seconds.

Tip: Keep your lower back flat against the floor. You may use a folded towel to support your lower back.

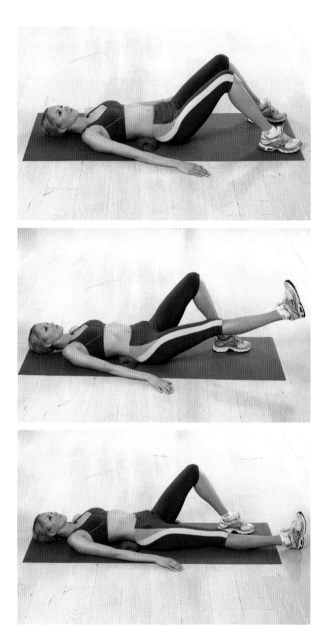

Basic Abdominal Strengthener

Purpose: To strengthen abdominal muscles

1. Lie on your back with your knees bent. Place a towel underneath the small of your back. Keep your lower back pressed against the towel.
2. Tighten your abdominal muscles and hold.
3. In one continuous move, slowly straighten your left leg, pause, and then bring it back to the starting position. Do the same with your right leg. Let your heels slide across the floor.
4. Maintain the tightened abdominals as you alternate legs.

Tip: When you are unable to keep pressure on the towel with your lower back, stop.

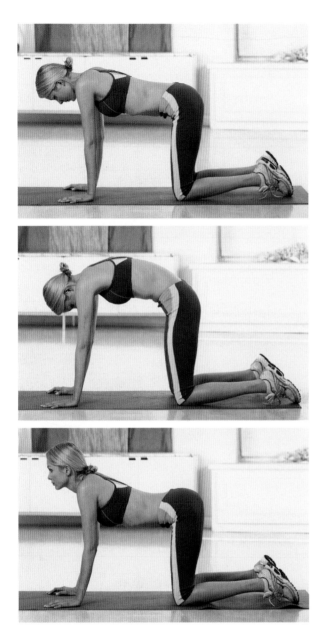

Cat and Camel for the Back

Purpose: To stretch the lower back

1. Start on your hands and knees, with your shoulders vertically above your wrists and your hips above your knees.
2. On an inhalation: Arch your back upward and lower your head. Try to round your spine as much as is comfortably possible. Tuck your pelvis under using your abdominals and buttock muscles.
3. Hold for 5 seconds.
4. On an exhalation: Lift your head upward and push your chest and abdomen toward the floor.
5. Hold for 5 seconds and then repeat, starting with step 2.

Tip: Move slowly, feeling a gentle stretch in your lower back. On an inhalation, avoid compressing your lower back; instead, feel your chest expanding.

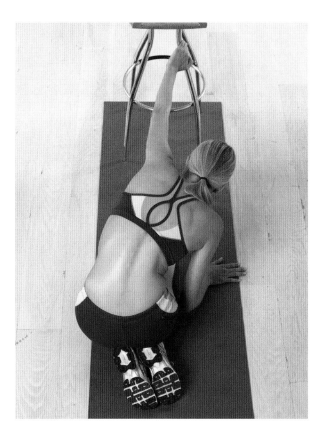 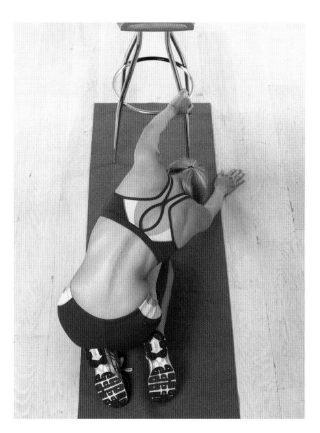

Kneeling Stretch for the Back

Purpose: To stretch the lower back, hips, and sides
(the *quadratus lumborum*)

1. Get down on your hands and knees, reach forward with your left hand, and grasp a secure object.
2. From this position, sit back diagonally toward the left buttock, elongating the left side.
3. The left arm may be internally rotated to increase the stretch.
4. Work on elongation of the left side by dropping the pelvis further diagonally backward and toward the hip.
5. Hold for 5 seconds.
6. Repeat on the opposite side.

Tip: Pull your head slowly.

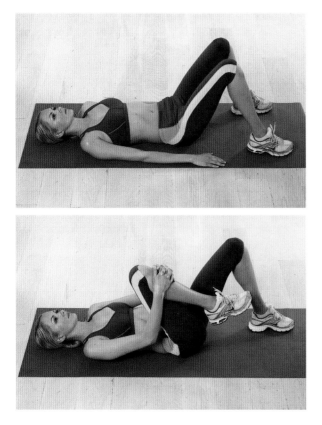

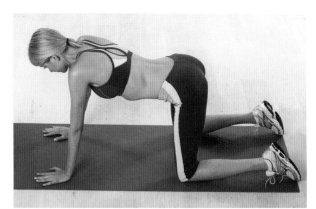

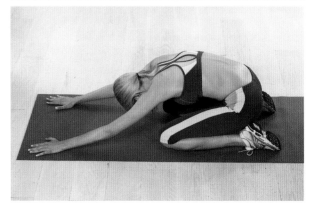

Knee-to-Chest Raise for the Lower Back

Purpose: To loosen and warm up the lower back

1. Begin by lying on your back with your knees bent and your feet on the floor.
2. With both hands, pull (don't lift) your right knee as close to your chest as possible. Keep your left knee bent with your foot flat on the floor. Hold for up to 30 seconds.
3. Repeat using your left knee.

Tip: Don't "lift" your legs with your hands and arms; just pull until you feel a gentle stretch in the lower back. If you have bad knees, put your hands under the knee and pull. To intensify the stretch, straighten the supporting leg.

Prayer Stretch for the Back for the Lower Back

Purpose: To warm up and gently stretch the lower back

1. Start on your hands and knees, with your arms stretched out in front of you.
2. Extend your hips backward and move your face close to the floor. Try to touch your buttocks to your heels.
3. Hold for 10 seconds and then return to the starting position.

Tip: Slide your hands while maintaining your arm position. Keep your back straight.

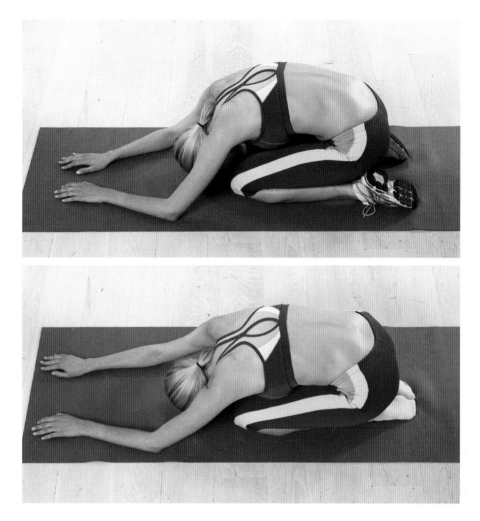

Mid-Back and Shoulder Stretch

Purpose: To strengthen the mid-back and shoulder girdle (the lower trapezius)

1. Begin on your hands and knees, sit back on your heels, and bend forward, resting your forehead on the floor.

2. Pull your shoulder blades down and back. Do not squeeze your shoulder blades together.

3. Hold for 3 to 5 seconds. Repeat 5 times.

Tip: A variation can be performed by lying on your stomach.

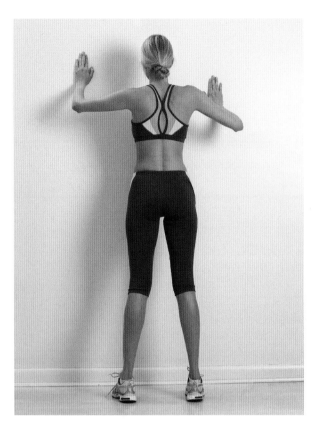
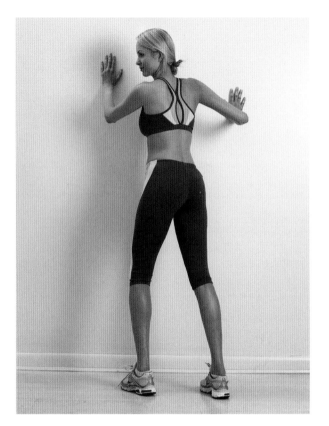

Chest Stretch

Purpose: To stretch the shoulders and chest

1. Start by facing a wall. Reach your right hand straight out to the side, against the wall, just below shoulder height. Place your left hand firmly on the wall at chin height.

2. Bend the left elbow down to bring the right shoulder blade down and back. Maintain this position as the feet turn 90 degrees so they are parallel to the wall.

3. Press your right fingertips against the wall to help turn the chest to the right.

4. Slowly turn your chest further around to the right, opening both sides of the chest and feeling a stretch in the front of the right shoulder and chest.

5. It is important not to allow the right shoulder to elevate during the stretch.

6. Hold for 3 to 5 seconds.

7. Repeat on the left side.

Tip: Do not arch your back during this exercise.

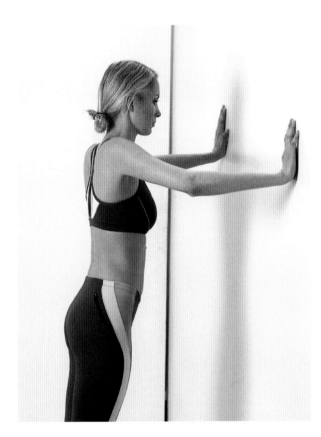 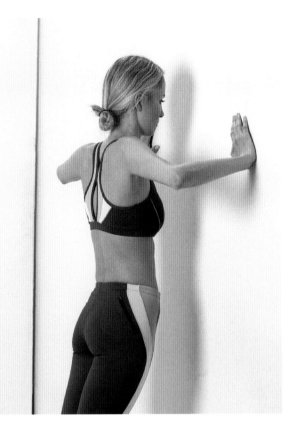

Wall Press for the Back and Chest

Purpose: To stretch the upper back and chest

1. Start by standing at arm's length from the wall. Place both hands on the wall at shoulder height.
2. Squeeze your shoulder blades together and down.
3. Slowly bend your arms and touch your nose to the wall. Keep your spine straight.

4. From this position push your shoulder blades apart, tuck in your chin, and push your mid-back away from the wall.
5. Hold for 5 to 10 seconds and then return to the starting position.

Tip: Keep your spine as straight as possible.

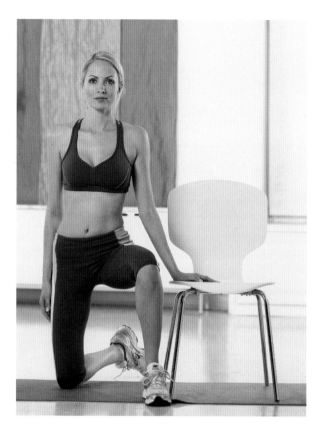 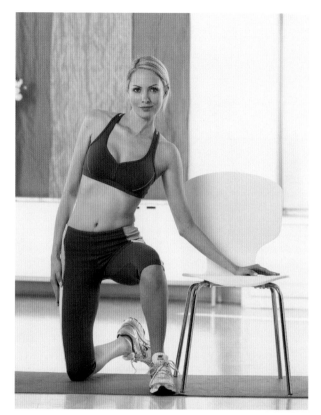

Outer Thigh Stretch

Purpose: To stretch the outer thigh muscle
(*tensor fascia latae*)

1. Start with your right knee on the ground and your left foot on the floor, keeping your knee bent. Rest your left arm on a chair for support. Your right arm should rest at your side.

2. Pull in your stomach and posterior. Tilt the pelvis forward by using the left leg, particularly the hamstrings. Then, shift the hips from left to right, maintaining a strong posterior pelvic tilt, and contract your buttocks. You should feel a stretch on the outside of your right hip.

3. Stretch for a total of 5 to 10 seconds.

4. Switch sides and repeat on the left side.

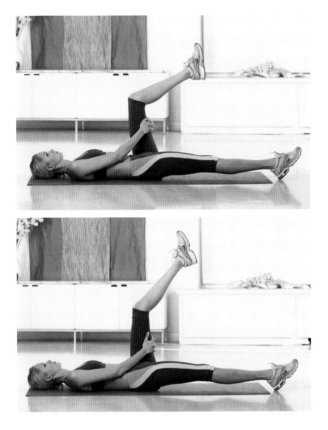

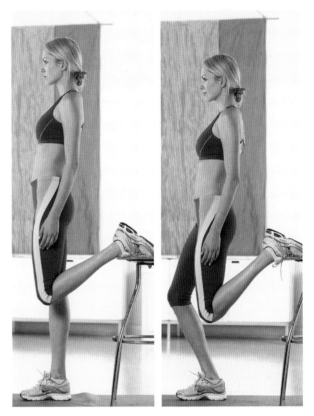

Hamstring Stretch

Purpose: To warm up and stretch the back of the legs
(the hamstring muscles)

1. Begin by lying on your back with your arms at your
   sides. Keep your left leg straight on the floor.
2. Lift your right leg to approximately 90 degrees and
   place both hands behind your right leg.
3. Keep your elbows straight and slowly straighten
   your right knee to feel a stretch behind the right leg.
4. Hold for 1 to 5 seconds.
5. Slowly return your leg to the floor and relax.
6. Repeat with the left leg.

Tip: Use a belt or towel to elevate your leg. You should feel
no pain in your lower back.

Standing Quad Stretch for the Legs

Purpose: To stretch the front of the thigh (the quadriceps)

1. Place your right foot behind you on a bench or
   chair with your knee flexed.
2. Keep your right buttock tight and tucked under
   by tightening your stomach muscles.
3. Bend your left knee and allow your right knee to
   flex or bend further until you feel a stretch in the
   front of the right thigh.

Tip: Do not allow your back to arch!

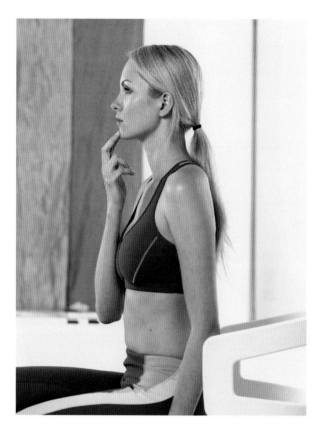 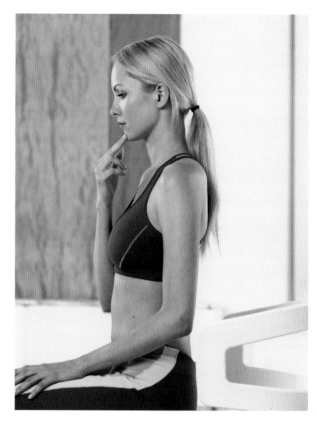

Upper Neck Head Nod for the Neck

Purpose: To stretch the upper neck at the base of the skull

1. Sit upright in a chair and place your fingertips on your chin.
2. Tuck in your chin and draw the back of your head forward and down. You should feel the stretch at the base of your skull.
3. Hold for 3 to 5 seconds.
4. Repeat 5 times.

Tip: Use your fingers to help guide your forward motion.

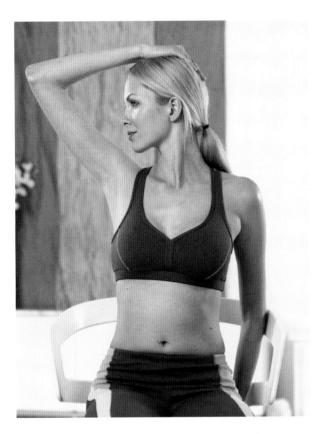
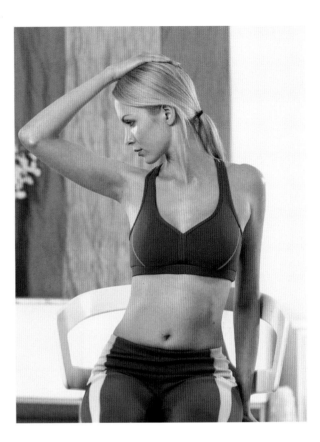

Neck Stretch

Purpose: To stretch the neck muscles (the *levator scapulae*)

1. Sit upright in a chair and turn your head to the right. Place your right hand on top of your head.
2. Slowly bend your neck toward your right shoulder. Do not pull your head; simply allow your hand to support the head and neck in this position.
3. With your left hand, grasp the chair and slowly lean your torso toward the right and slightly forward until you feel a stretch.
4. Hold for 3 to 5 seconds.
5. Repeat on the left side.

Tip: Move your head slowly.

CHAPTER 10

Boost Your Immune System

You've got an amazingly protective mechanism in the body called the immune system. Its job is to fight off, disarm, and defeat the many germs, bugs, parasites, viruses, bacteria, and other problem-causing compounds that you're exposed to on a daily basis. And guess what: The immune system is the perfect place to really get into the nuts and bolts of anti-aging.

Think about it. If your immune system is working great, you're far less likely to succumb to the little things that sideline mere mortals, such as colds, fevers, flu, and the like. You're also less likely to be felled by some of the big-picture degenerative diseases of aging. A healthy, robust immune system won't protect you for eternity, but by keeping it in tip-top shape, you can do an awful lot to "rectangularize the curve," keeping infirmity mercifully brief and limiting it to the very end of a (hopefully long and vigorous) life.

Which is, after all, what we want. And what this book is about.

LOOK TO THE HOST

Remember the last time "something was going around" your office and half the people were out sick? Then you also probably remember that half the people did *not* get sick. And some were probably sidelined for a day or so while others were still dragging around trying to "shake the bug" two weeks later.

In other words, there was a pretty big variance in the reaction, even though the same germs were involved. In fact, it's safe to assume that everyone in the office had probably been exposed. But not everyone reacted the same way. Why?

"Look to the host," said famous chemist and microbiologist Louis Pasteur. The "host" is the *person* who is exposed to the microbe. This is where the action is.

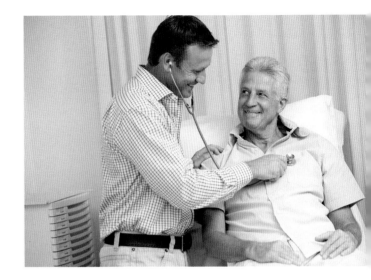

If you want to strengthen the immune system, it helps to understand how it works. Then, as we have with the brain and heart, we can understand where it breaks down and how we might protect it from such breakdown. By doing so, we greatly increase the odds of living longer and in greater health.

Let's get started.

THE HALO EFFECT

As you've probably deduced from reading the above, I'm a big fan of Pasteur's final message to the world. How sick you get depends only *partially* on the germs you're exposed to. In my view, getting sick (and even the process of aging itself) is the product of two variables, the person and the environment. Under the heading of "person" is everything from the food we eat to the lifestyle choices we make, and under "environment" is everything else, from the toxins in the air to the germs we pick up in the office bathroom. These overlapping variables form hundreds of feedback loops, interacting with one another in countless ways, right

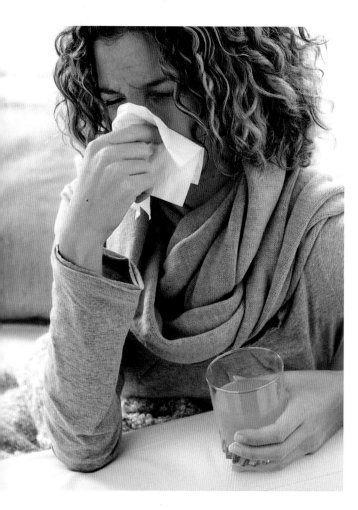

THE IMMUNE SYSTEM: KEEPING OUT THE RIFFRAFF

The number one task of the immune system is to be alert to substances that don't belong—and to dispatch with the riffraff as quickly and efficiently as possible.

All the rest is details.

The best place to start our journey into those details is with a discussion of the lymphatic system. The lymphatic system consists of all kinds of organs, nodes, and ducts that transport a watery fluid called *lymph* throughout the body. Lymph also interacts with the circulatory system (blood) to drain fluid from tissues and cells. (The term *lymph* actually means "clear water"; it's the fluid and protein that's been drained out of the blood.) Lymph also distributes immune cells, delivering the cellular defense army to all the places it needs to be.

The primary lymph organs include bone marrow and the thymus gland, while the secondary lymph organs include the lymph nodes, spleen, tonsils, appendix, and the all-important liver.

In the cellular army of the immune system, the main troops are white blood cells, the technical name for which is *leukocytes*. Their job is to defend against infectious disease and any other foreign invader (or what the body *perceives* as a foreign invader). This last caveat is important, because sometimes the body makes a mistake and thinks something (like pollen or ragweed) is more dangerous than it actually is, mounting a disproportionate attack against a relatively innocuous compound. Sometimes, too, the body gets confused and attacks its own tissues and cells (autoimmune disease). But for the most part, when things are working as they should, the leukocytes identify the bad guys accurately and then dispense with them in a variety of ways. It's in our interest to keep this system healthy and

down to the cellular level. Sickness—and aging—is the *product* of these interactions, not of any one single variable.

In fact, immunity can be *strengthened* by any one of these variables. Although it would be great to have strength and power in all areas of life, from your food to your exercise to your relationships and environment, in truth, excellence and strength in one area can be so powerful that it can often make up for a bit of a deficit in another.

So, we'd all benefit by boosting the quality of all the components that go into strengthening the immune system—our food, supplements, environment, and even spirituality.

vibrant and fully functioning for as long as possible. In fact, a strong, healthy immunity is one of the foundations of healthy aging.

Just to get the cast of characters out of the way, it's helpful to understand that there are many different types of white blood cells (leukocytes). The chart below describes some of the major ones, which, if you've ever looked at your blood test results, will seem vaguely familiar. Now, when you see these names listed you'll know what your doctor is looking at. If, overall, the number of white blood cells is wildly off, it's valuable information about the behavior of your white blood cell army (and hence your immune system in general).

"WE ARE WHAT WE THINK ABOUT"

One of the most exciting new areas of research to emerge in the last few decades is the science of—get ready for a long word now—*psychoneuroimmunology*. Take it apart and it's not so daunting. *Psych* refers to psychology, what you and I might call the mind, with its entire constellation of thoughts and feelings. *Neuro* refers to what happens in the brain when you actually *think* those thoughts and feel those feelings—the release, for example, of neurotransmitters

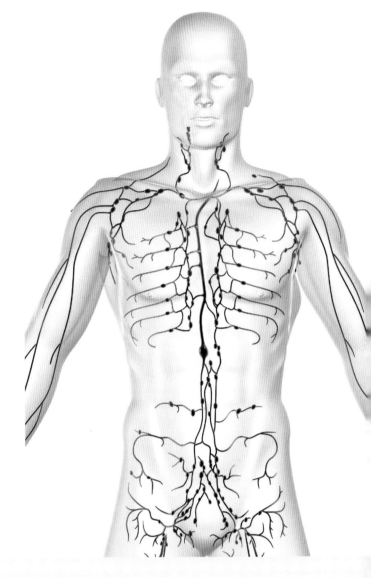

THE LYMPHATIC SYSTEM

Types of Leukocytes (white blood cells)	Approximate Percentage in Adults	Main Target
Neutrophils	54–62 percent	Bacteria and fungi
Eosinophils	1–6 percent	Parasites/also involved in allergic reactions
Basophils	<1 percent	Involved in allergic reactions
Lymphocytes	25–33 percent	Varies according to type

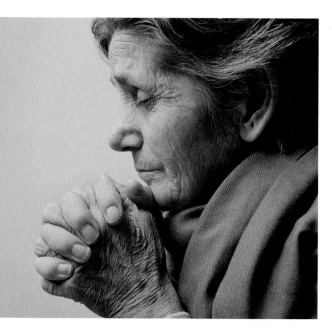

body, it would have shown that specific areas of the brain were lit up and that your body was pumping out increased levels of certain hormones (like cortisol and adrenaline) and certain neurotransmitters (like epinephrine).

The point is that what you *think about* and what you *feel* have far-ranging effects on your body.

As they do on your immune system.

USE LAUGHTER AS MEDICINE

Natural killer cells, or NK cells, are a type of lymphocyte and an important player in mounting an immune system attack on invading microbes. And guess what? Those NK cells actually respond to your mood.

They increase when you're happy!

Yup, strange and counterintuitive as it may seem, when you're feeling good, optimistic, and happy, when you're pursuing your bliss, your NK cells multiply like rabbits. Why? Who knows? But they do. More than a few studies have shown a relationship between, for example, optimism and immune system response—optimists have higher numbers of T-cells and a higher level of NK cell activity.

Now, I'm going to go out on a limb here and assume there are at least a few of you who might think: *"But I'm a confirmed pessimist. So what can I do about my immunity? How much of it is under my control?"*

So glad you asked.

Japanese researchers recently designed an ingenious experiment that should be of interest to you. They made up what they called a "recreational music protocol" and tried it out in a corporate environment. Basically, they taught a group-drumming class. First, the researchers measured NK activity (as well as two important inflammatory markers, *interleukin-1* and *interleukin-10*) in two groups of Japanese

like serotonin and dopamine. And *immunology* is exactly what it sounds like—the study of the immune system.

Put them together and you get the fascinating study of the interaction between the brain and the immune system. And what an interaction it is. As the great biologist and Stanford University researcher Robert Sapolsky, Ph.D., says, "The brain has a vast potential for sticking its nose into the immune system's business."

The real father of psychoneuroimmunology was the Buddha, who basically summed up the whole field of research even before it was invented with these words: "We are what we think about." You probably understand intuitively the connection between thoughts and physiology. Just think back to the last time you watched a horror movie or an exciting thriller. You sat in the theater (or in front of your wide-screen television), probably not moving very much, yet your heart was racing, your blood pressure was elevated, and if some mad scientist had hooked you up to a monitoring device to measure everything going on in your

Boost Your Immune System with these Techniques

Happiness and feeling good actually help multiply your NK cells, important players in mounting an immune system attack on invading microbes. Use these suggestions to help boost your immune system:

- → Be on the lookout for cynical thoughts.
- → Examine situations reasonably, from all angles.
- → Put yourself in other people's shoes.
- → Learn to laugh at yourself.
- → Learn to relax.
- → Practice trust.
- → Learn to listen.
- → Practice forgiveness.

executives. Then, the execs got together and drummed for an hour, while a "control" group of execs spent the same amount of time reading leisurely. Afterward, the researchers measured NK activity again.

The results? The drumming executives demonstrated enhanced mood, reduced levels of the inflammatory markers, and increased NK cell activity. And lest you think that maybe the researchers just happened to accidentally pick happy guys for their drumming group who would have better immunity anyway, they came back six months later and reversed the groups. The previous drummers got to lay back and read for an hour while the previous readers got to drum. Same results—the drummers had improved immunity and lower inflammation.

So you may not be a natural optimist, but there are still plenty of things you can do to boost your immunity (and drumming is just one of them!).

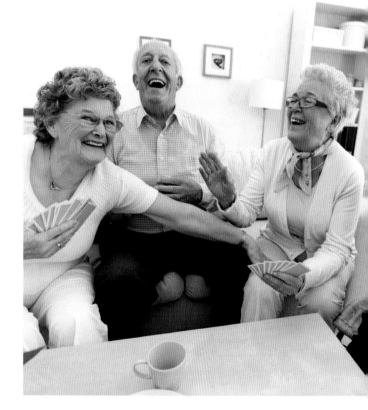

Act as if Life's a Stage and Boost Your Immune Responsiveness

A study done at the University of California, Los Angeles, showed that professional actors spending the day doing a depressing, negative scene had decreased immune responsiveness. However, actors who spent the day on an uplifting, euphoric scene had increased immune responsiveness. How does this apply to you: Fake it till you make it—if you don't feel happy, at least act like you do! Your body will respond accordingly.

Even the mere act of laughing can make a huge difference, something that was first discovered by a writer and editor named Norman Cousins.

If you don't know the story of Norman Cousins you're in for a treat, and I'm delighted to be the one to deliver it. Cousins was the editor of a once-legendary publication called *Saturday Evening Review*. In 1964, doctors discovered that he had ankylosing spondylitis, a condition that's as bad as it sounds—the connective tissue in the spine deteriorates. Doctors gave Cousins a one in five hundred chance of survival.

So here's what he did:

First, he did his own research on all the drugs he was on and found that the drugs were totally depleting his body of vitamin C. Doctors agreed to take him off some of the drugs and inject him with massive doses of vitamin C, especially because Cousins believed this might be his last hope and the doctors didn't have much of anything else to offer.

The second thing he did—pay attention here, folks—was check himself out of the hospital. He reasoned that hospitals were probably the worst place to be for someone who was seriously ill, so he decided to check into a hotel.

The third thing he did was rent a bunch of Marx Brothers movies. (Okay, they didn't have rental back then, but Cousins was pretty famous and was able to get a supply from the distributors.) And then, he literally laughed his you-know-what off.

In a state of euphoria, Cousins basically laughed his way back to health. Within a month he was back to work at the *Saturday Evening Review*, and although he continued to have minor health problems, he lived another twenty years.

Cousins wrote about his experiences in *The Anatomy of an Illness*, considered one of the classic early works in psychoneuroimmunology.

Since then, there's been a ton of research on laughter and the immune system, notably by Lee Berk, Ph.D., and

Stanley Tan, M.D., Ph.D., of the Center for Spiritual Life and Wholeness at Loma Linda University, California. Their studies have shown that laughter reduces blood pressure and stress hormones and increases immune function by raising both T-cell and B-cell numbers. They've also found that laughter triggers the release of endorphins, the body's natural painkillers, as well as the number and activity level of NK cells.

NK cells are also protective against cancer. In one study of seventy-seven women with breast cancer, researchers took a sample of each woman's tumor at the time of diagnosis. They put these samples in test tubes, together with some NK cells taken from each of the women. Some women had NK cells that just kind of lay there and gave up, not doing much of anything. Other women had NK cells that were vital and alive and went on a cleanup mission, indicating a seriously active immune system. Then, the researchers followed up with the women twelve years later. Almost half (47 percent) of the women whose NK cells were fairly inactive had died, but a whopping 95 percent of the women whose NK cells were tigers were still alive.

Other studies have shown that the less active your NK cells are, the more rapid cancer progresses and the more it spreads throughout the body. "Lively immune cells thus seem essential to countering the growth of tumors and the spread of metastases," writes David Servan-Schrieber, M.D., Ph.D. "Everything that strengthens our precious immune cells also impedes the growth of cancers."

The moral of the story is that you may not be able to reprogram yourself to be a complete optimist at heart, but there are definitely things you can do—from making music to watching funny movies, from coloring in books to walking in the woods, from going to a comedy show to taking long, luxurious baths to spending time with friends—that can increase your sense of well-being.

Whatever increases your well-being also increases your immunity. And, incidentally, can extend your life!

THE STRESS CONNECTION

The connection between stress and immunity makes such intuitive sense that you'd think it wouldn't be necessary to demonstrate it scientifically. Nonetheless, a tremendous amount of research has been done and the results are pretty unequivocal.

"A period of stress will disrupt a wide variety of immune functions," says the internationally known biologist and stress physiologist Robert Sapolsky, Ph.D. Among them

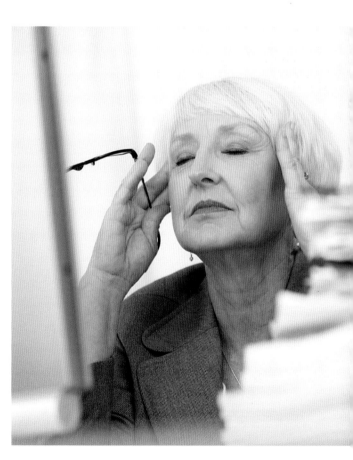

are the formation of new lymphocytes, their release into the circulation, the amount of time preexisting lymphocytes stay in circulation, the manufacture of antibodies in response to an infectious agent, and even the way the lymphocytes communicate "trouble" to one another. These are just a few of the ways stress affects immunity, according to Sapolsky.

Take glucocorticoids. These are hormones produced in the adrenal gland that are chemically classed as steroids. The most important glucocorticoid is cortisol (aka "the stress hormone"), which goes around cleaning up a lot of the mess of inflammation. (This is why your physician may give you a shot of cortisone—the drug version of cortisol—for serious inflammation.) So the glucocorticoids (mainly cortisol) have important, even life-saving, functions in the body. However, they also produce a lot of collateral damage when they're in overdrive, which is what happens when you're in a state of chronic stress. Glucocorticoids can cause shrinking of the thymus gland, an important player in the immune system and the site of T-cell maturation.

"Before it was possible to measure directly the amount of glucocorticoids in the bloodstream, one indirect way of doing so was to see how much the thymus gland in an animal had shrunk," notes Sapolsky. Because the thymus gland is an important part of the immune system, this shrinkage has implications for immunity.

Glucocorticoids also stop the formation of new infection-fighting lymphocytes in the thymus. "They also make circulating lymphocytes less responsive to an infectious alarm," says Sapolsky, and cause lymphocytes to be yanked right out of circulation. "Most impressively, glucocorticoids actually kill lymphocytes," he says.

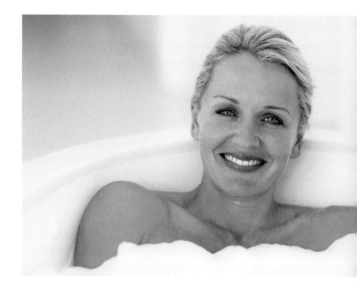

The interesting thing is that a little bit of stress actually gives a temporary boost to the immune system function. All stress isn't bad, and some small doses kind of "prime" the system, making it more rugged and able to take on bigger challenges. The problem arises with long-term, chronic stress. Remember from chapter 2, on inflammation, we talked about how adaptive it is to have a "turbo" pedal like stress hormones that help prepare the body for immediate action: fight or flight? Without the ability to turn those hormones on in response to an immediate stressor, you'd probably die. The problem is when the pedal is to the metal all the time.

Chronic, unrelenting stress ages us, exacerbates all the major diseases, lengthens the time we're sick when we're sick, and ultimately, left unchecked, can kill us altogether. Unfortunately, that's the kind of stress most of us live with, whether it be from traffic, commutes, family issues, job insecurity, unmet deadlines, lack of sleep, poor diet, environmental toxins or, more than likely, a combination of some or all of the above. The point here is simple and clear: Take stress seriously. And build some sort of steam escape valve into your daily life, whether it be in the form of deep breathing exercises, meditation, yoga, qi gong, tai chi, a warm bath, or a walk in the woods.

Those activities may seem like ones you "don't have time for," and if that's the case, let me describe an old *New Yorker* cartoon for you: A profoundly out-of-shape man is in the examination room with his doctor. The doctor gives him some simple advice about exercising a half hour a day. The man snaps that he hasn't got time in his busy schedule for something like that. At which point the doctor wryly replies: "Well then, can you find 24 hours a day in your busy schedule to be dead?"

Enough said. Find ten to thirty minutes a day to do something that lowers your stress and makes you feel good. That's it. Case closed. To quote the famous Nike slogan: "Just do it."

HOW SUPPLEMENTATION CAN HELP YOU

We are about to make a completely unscientific statement that will get us banned from the society of smart academics who only believe double-blind studies.[1] You ready? Here goes: *Many people who take vitamins on a regular basis don't get sick very often.* Whether that's because they're healthier to begin with or because the vitamins in some way support their immune system is an open question, but the fact is that there are probably many people reading this book who are nodding their heads in agreement. Vitamins aren't the only thing that can keep you healthy, but they may help. And I can tell you from personal experience that when I get sick—which is rarely—I have my "go-to" cocktail of

immune-support nutrients that I find shorten the duration and intensity of anything I happen to come down with.

We'll save you a long discussion of the science behind multivitamins, but the Chandra, Bogden, and Foote references on page 251 will satisfy even the most skeptical reader about how a nutritional insurance policy—i.e. a multivitamin—can strengthen the immune system.

For now, we can say a few incontrovertible facts about nutritional deficiencies and the immune system:

1. Nutritional deficiencies make it easier for bacteria or a virus to invade the body.
2. Nutritional deficiencies have an effect on the bacteria or virus once it has established itself.
3. Nutritional deficiencies increase the susceptibility of secondary infection.
4. Nutritional deficiencies make convalescence longer.

According to no less a mainstream organization than the Cleveland Clinic, supplementing your diet with a balanced multivitamin is essential. Read on for a list of the most important nutrients and herbs for immunity, any of which are worth taking on a regular basis.

GIVE YOUR IMMUNE SYSTEM A BOOST WITH ZINC

Zinc is present in every tissue, organ, fluid, and secretion of the body. In fact, it's present in every living cell. It plays a huge role in immunity (not to mention cell division, DNA synthesis, growth and development, and the activity of about a hundred different enzymes). And because the body has no specific storage sites for zinc, you need to consume it on a daily basis.

Many of us don't.

---

1 Don't misunderstand us. We're big fans of double-blind studies, we just know that the absence of proof isn't proof of absence. The NYC fire department has never done a double-blind study to show that water puts out fire, but they're pretty sure it works.

ANTI-AGING ACTION PLAN:

Get Your Immune System In Sync with Zinc

Take a multivitamin with at least 15 milligrams of zinc every day. When you feel an illness coming on, boost your zinc intake to 50 milligrams daily.

Studies show that zinc supplementation helps fight illness. The body can't store zinc, so taking a daily supplement is important.

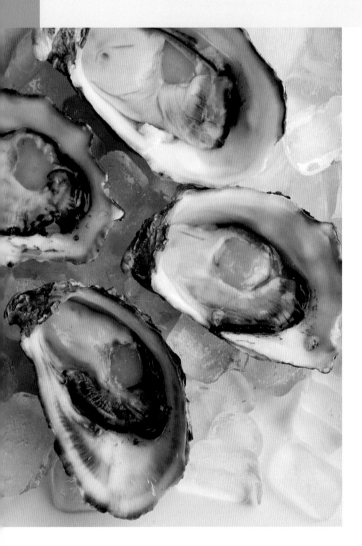

Sure, cereals and grains contain zinc, but that zinc is bound to phytates[2] which makes it unavailable for absorption by the body. Alcohol and other drugs may also reduce zinc absorption (or increase zinc excretion). And we really don't have consistently reliable measures of zinc deficiency, so we have to make guesstimates from our dietary intake. The average zinc intake of Americans from food is a measly 13 milligrams a day for men and 9 milligrams a day for women. Yes, that just about meets the minimum daily requirement set by the Food and Nutrition Board at the Institute of Medicine, but barely. The symptoms of zinc deficiency include hair loss, delayed wound healing, apathy, and low energy.

And it definitely includes depressed immune function.

According to the conservative *Physicians' Desk Reference for Nutritional Supplements*, "zinc deficiency has been shown to impair immunity in many ways." The question then becomes a philosophic one: What exactly

---

2 Phytates are a storage form of potassium found in plants; they bind to minerals and make them unavailable for digestion and assimilation. For this reason, they're sometimes described as "anti-nutrients."

is deficiency? Is it having less than the bare recommended daily allowance that will allow you to escape major disease? Or is it any amount that's less than optimal?

I'm going with the latter.

The body requires zinc to develop and activate T-cells. Low zinc levels are associated with increased susceptibility to pneumonia and other infections in the elderly. And even mild to moderate degrees of zinc deficiency can impair macrophage functions (the PacMen of the immune system), as well as NK cell activity.

The best food source of zinc is oysters. Six medium oysters give you 76.7 milligrams. Beef is another excellent source; 3 ounces (85 g) of cooked beef shanks gives you 8.9 milligrams, a distant second to oysters but still far ahead of everything else. Red meat and poultry provide the majority of zinc in the American diet, and with many people becoming vegetarians, there's reason to be concerned that we're consuming less than the optimal amount of this important immunity nutrient.

GREEN TEA AND GREEN TEA EXTRACT

Much research has pointed to the protective effects of green tea on the human body, including the ability of compounds in green tea (called catechins) to inhibit the growth of tumors. In fact, the evidence that green tea has a protective effect against cancer is so compelling that the chemoprevention branch of the National Cancer Institute has initiated a plan to develop tea compounds as cancer-chemopreventive agents in human trials. It's now fairly well established that green tea may help prevent a number of different cancers in humans, including bladder, colon, esophagus, pancreas, rectum, and stomach cancer. One Chinese study suggested that the mechanism for this anticancer activity included cellular immune function and noted that animals treated with green tea extract had significantly greater NK cell activity.

If "all" it did was help prevent cancer, green tea would be assured a place on the table of every meal designed to promote longevity. But its résumé is hardly limited to fighting cancer (as if that weren't enough!). In a 2004 article titled "Effects of Green Tea Intake on the Development of Coronary Artery Disease," researchers writing in the Japanese medical publication *Circulation Journal* concluded that "the more green tea patients consume, the less likely they are to have coronary artery disease."

Other research has shown that green tea helps fight oxidation and glycation, two of the Four Horsemen of Aging. It appears to help with stress as well. Green tea contains a substance called theanine, which is helpful in improving mood and increasing a sense of relaxation. Green tea also lowers a nasty compound in the blood called *fibrinogen*, which can contribute to clots and strokes. Finally, in several animal studies, green tea has demonstrated the ability to lower blood sugar, and regular consumption of green tea can be a great help in the quest to maintain a healthy weight.

OLIVE LEAF EXTRACT: A BOUNTY OF GOODNESS

Open any basic nutrition textbook and you're sure to find a paean to the healthy Mediterranean diet, which features a generous amount of olive oil. But according to *Nutrition Research Reviews* in 2005, the Mediterranean diet's healthy effects can be attributed not only to the high relationship between unsaturated and saturated fatty acids in olive oil but also to the antioxidant property of abundant plant chemicals in the olive called *phenolic compounds*.

ANTI-AGING ACTION PLAN:

Extend the Olive Branch to Your Immune Cells

Take one to two capfuls of a high-quality olive leaf extract daily. (I personally recommend Barlean's Olive Leaf Complex, which has been around for years and is the industry standard.)

Olive leaf complex can help prevent the spread of viruses and may stimulate immune cells. It also eats up free radicals and fights oxidative damage.

The use of olive leaf for medicinal purposes goes all the way back to the ancient Egyptians. They believed that the olive leaf was a symbol of heavenly power, and they used the extracted oils from the leaf in the mummification rituals of their kings.

Olive leaf extract is a rich source of some of the most important phenolic compounds on earth, such as *oleuropein, hydroxytyrosol, tyrosol, rutin, luteolin, catechin,* and *apigenin,* which are believed to be responsible for most of the leaf's pharmacological effects. Olive leaf extract also contains various trace elements vital to good health, such as selenium, chromium, iron, zinc, vitamin C, beta-carotene, and a wide range of amino acids.

Olive phenolics have a powerful ability to eat up free radicals and are a tremendous weapon in the fight against oxidative damage. They also show a strong synergistic behavior when combined, as occurs naturally in the olive leaf, and concentrated, as in olive leaf extract. The most active flavonoids, rutin, catechin, and luteolin, exert antioxidant effects almost two and a half times greater than those of vitamin C and E and are comparable to those of

lycopene, according to in vitro tests. The powerful antioxidant effect produced by high-quality olive leaf extract may also be due to the synergy of flavonoids, phenols, and a high oleuropein content.

Olive leaf extract can be a powerful weapon in the battle between your immune system and invading microbes. Compounds in the olive leaf have long been used to help fight illnesses brought on by microbes. The first formal mention of olive leaf, an account describing its ability to cure severe cases of fever and malaria, occurred in 1854, when the *Pharmaceutical Journal* carried a report by one Daniel Hanbury, according to James R. Privitera, M.D. The report contained the following simple healing recipe:

"Boil a handful of (olive) leaves in a quart (946 ml) of water down to half its original volume. Then administer the liquid in the amount of a wineglass every three or four hours until the fever is cured."
—*Pharmaceutical Journal,* 1854

This method became popular in England for treating sick Englishmen returning from the tropical colonies, according to Hanbury. He believed that a bitter substance in the leaves was the healing ingredient. That substance in olive leaf extract, since identified as oleuropein, has been found to be particularly helpful in resisting bacterial damage. In fact, early research by the drug company Upjohn found olive leaf extract to be effective in treating infection by a large number of viruses, as well as bacteria and parasitic protozoans.

One of the active ingredients in oleuropein is a substance called *elenolic acid*. Research shows that elenolic acid has an uncanny ability to inhibit the growth of viruses. And one form of elenolic acid, calcium elenolate, fights not only viruses but bacteria and parasitic agents as well, studies show.

PROBIOTICS: GOOD FOR THE GUT

If you've never heard of probiotics or you're not entirely sure what they are, let me introduce you, as they play an important role in immunity. (If you're reading the book sequentially, you've already heard about probiotics in the section on gut health in "the eight pillars of living young" [page 77]. If not, let us introduce them to you now.)

Your gut functions by providing a colony of live bacteria that help you digest and absorb important nutrients while helpinging to alleviate intestinal inflammation.

The gut is like a garden with both weeds and flowers. The *weeds* are the bad bacteria, such as *Candida albicans*, or yeast, which, when they overgrow, can create all kinds of problems in the body. The *flowers* are the good guys—healthy bacteria that protect your gut, help you digest food, and improve immunity. Those "good guy" bacteria we call probiotics.

In addition to helping you digest and assimilate nutrients needed for a long and healthy life, probiotics also make a serious dent in the ability of one of the four horsemen to age your body—inflammation. "A lack of probiotics in the intestinal tract allows bad microbes to grow and release toxins that cause intestinal inflammation," explains Allison Tannis, M.Sc., R.H.N., author of *Probiotic Rescue*. "Probiotics may also help the immune system become strong enough to fight off viral infections."

Note: A recent set of studies published in the journal *Cell* (2018) showed something we've known for a long time: The *effects of different strains of probiotics are different depending on the person.* Some people "recolonize" their gut with probiotics very easily—some do not. (The researchers called them, respectively, "persisters" and "resisters.") One of the two studies also suggested taking probiotics during the same period of time as you take antibiotics—something many of us (including me) have advised people to do for years—may *not* always be the best advice.

This new research does not in any way diminish the importance of probiotics in gut health. It just shows (once again) that we have a lot to learn about personalized medicine—in this case, choosing the right strains of probiotics for the right situations. There's no doubt in my mind that we'll get there in a few years and have a much more precise idea of how to prescribe probiotics with more precision so that they can do the most for each individual patient.

MIXED ANTIOXIDANTS

No matter how well you design your diet, you can still augment it with supplemental antioxidants, according to the Cleveland Clinic website.

Vitamin C, for example, though it may not necessarily prevent colds, definitely shortens their duration. It also increases antibodies, *phagocytosis* (the ability of the PacMen to eat up the bad guys) and *chemotaxis* (the speed with which white blood cells get to the infection or injury site). "The concentration of vitamin C in immune cells is twenty to a hundred times higher than in the rest of the blood," says Robert Rountree, M.D. "People who take vitamin C supplements see a measurable increase in NK activity within twenty-four hours."

Selenium, one of the most important microminerals on the planet, is associated with higher rates of survival in AIDS patients and lower rates of cancer in general.

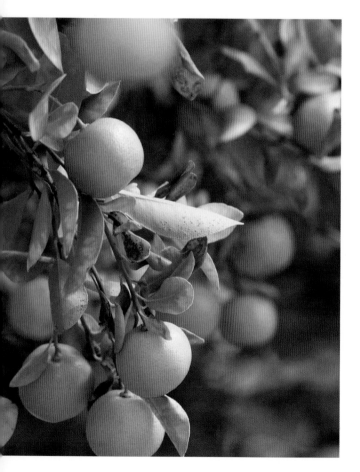

According to Bert Berkson, M.D., Ph.D., selenium acts like "birth control" for the hepatitis C virus. It's important stuff!

On **beta-carotene**, the Cleveland Clinic has this to say: "You should add beta-carotene in a dose of 25,000 international units (IU) twice per day. Beta-carotene is one of the most potent nutrients and can protect the body from oxidative stress. Populations that have diets high in beta-carotene have a lower incidence of certain forms of cancer." (Most experts now recommend "mixed carotenoids" rather than beta-carotene exclusively.)

Vitamin E is one of the most important antioxidants on the planet, and it's especially critical for older people experiencing the typical slowdown in immune function, according to Rountree. In a study at the U.S. Department of Agriculture's Human Nutrition Center at Tufts University, eighty-eight people aged sixty-five and older were given either a placebo or vitamin E supplement daily for four months. At the end of the four-month period, researchers reported an increase in both T-cell and B-cell activity among the vitamin E takers. The people taking vitamin E also had a more vigorous immune system response to tetanus and hepatitis B vaccines, meaning their ability to produce antibodies had improved. "If you supplement the elderly with vitamin E, you can enhance their immune response," said lead researcher Simin Meydani, D.V.M., Ph.D.

The general antioxidant protection formula I like best comes from my good friend Robert Rountree, M.D., whose excellent book, *Immunotics*, provides an in-depth exploration of many of the issues discussed in this chapter. "[Antioxidants are] a building block of a healthy immune system," he writes. "Everyone should take a daily antioxidant supplement, but it is especially important for people over fifty and endurance athletes."

ANTI–AGING ACTION PLAN:

Take an Immunity Cocktail

Sprinkle a spoonful of powdered probiotics on yogurt or fruit and consume every day. The powder has virtually no taste and blends quite well into yogurt dishes. In my house, we put some Greek yogurt (higher in protein but lower in probiotics) on top of fruit (blueberries and cherries are my favorite), sprinkle with powdered probiotics, and then top with some flaked coconut and slivered almonds. Mix it up and enjoy!

Alternately, take probiotic capsules. Look for a formula that contains the following five strains:

→ *Lactobacillus plantarum*

→ *Lactobacillus acidophilus*

→ *Lactobacillus brevis*

→ *Bifidobacterium lactis (or B. animalis)*

→ *Bifidobacterium longum*

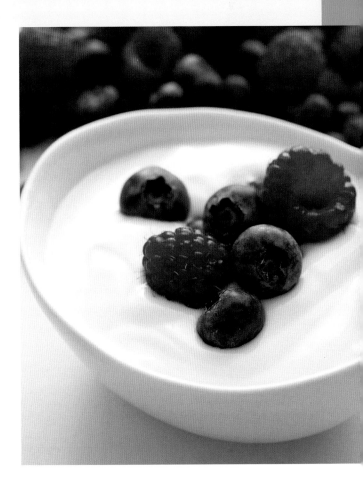

Just as health experts now recommend mixed *carotenoids,* as opposed to just beta-carotene, we now strongly recommend that your vitamin E be from mixed *tocopherols.* Vitamin E actually has eight different components, and most early studies (and many health food stores) only sell vitamin E as "alpha-tocopherol" (one of the eight fractions). Emerging research is clear that *alpha*-tocopherol is not a particularly effective form of vitamin E and pales in comparison to *gamma*-tocopherol, which seems to do all the heavy lifting. Get a high-gamma formula or at least one where the vitamin E comes from "mixed tocopherols." Don't buy vitamin E supplements that are exclusively alpha-tocopherol.

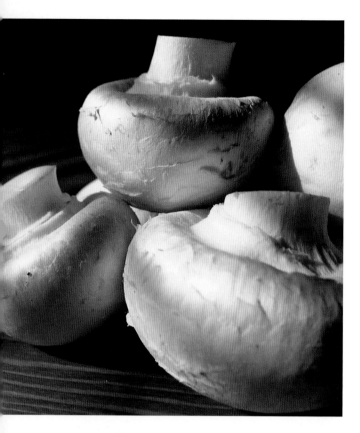

to Rountree, shiitake works for people at high risk for colds and flus, while reishi can help the body cope with physical or emotional stress. Maitake is the most potent, but also the most expensive. "Maitake is my choice for cancer prevention and chronic hepatitis," he says.

Garlic is a wonderful immune system booster. It has antimicrobial properties and is able to kill or stop the growth of various types of bacteria. It also increases NK cell activity and stimulates T-cells. "For more than twenty years, garlic has been a mainstay of my medical practice," says Rountree.

IMMUNITY AND AGING

So here's the bad news: All things being equal, as we age we have a reduced ability to fight off infection and other health challenges.[3]

In elderly people, the body's usual, innate response to infection, such as heating up with a fever, doesn't happen automatically. Twenty percent of adults over the age of sixty-five with serious bacterial infections don't have fevers at all, according to Edith Burns, M.D., associate professor of medicine at the Medical College of Wisconsin. "At this age [the body] probably still has the ability to generate fevers and other immunity weapons, but the central nervous system is simply less sensitive to immune signals and doesn't react as quickly or efficiently to infection," she writes.

Elderly adults are also less capable of producing lymphocytes. And the cells that they do produce are less vigorous and effective. The duration of antibody response is shorter in older adults, and fewer of them are made.

While the recommended nutrients (see page 173) constitute a "greatest hits" of the best supplements for immunity, it's very far from a complete list of immune-supportive compounds. You should also consider the following:

Quercetin is a member of the flavonoid family and found in apples and onions. It's known for it's powerful anti-inflammatory effect and also for its ability to block the action of many known cancer-producing substances. "Quercetin has strong antiviral activity, particularly against herpes, so I recommend it to people with serious viral infections," says Rountree.

Mushrooms have been used medicinally for centuries and are terrific immune boosters. Each of the "big three" has a special purpose, though they may overlap. According

---

3 Of course, the key phrase here is "all things being equal," and the purpose of this book is to make sure all things are not equal; rather, that you've stacked the deck in your favor, increasing the odds that what usually happens in the course of aging will either not happen (loss of memory, for example) or happen significantly less or significantly later (if at all).

Take Antioxidant Supplements Daily for Immune System Support

Your daily supplements should include the following:

→ Vitamin E (from gamma-tocopherol or mixed tocopherols): 400 IU

→ Vitamin C: 1,000–2,000 mg

→ Zinc: 25–50 mg

→ Selenium: 100–200 mcg

→ Mixed carotenoids: 15,000–30,000 mg

In fact, warns Burns, elderly adults, particularly those older than seventy, are more likely to produce autoantibodies, which attack parts of the body itself rather than attacking infections. Autoantibodies are factors in causing rheumatoid arthritis as well as atherosclerosis.

Then there are the psychological components of immunity. "Older adults often experience loss and stress, and suppressed immunity has been associated with bereavement, depression, and poor social support," writes Burns.

Again, there's much you can do to increase the odds that your body will maintain healthy and robust immunity well into your ninth decade and beyond. Stress reduction and an active social life, the focus of the last section in this book, are certainly at the top of the list. Removing toxins, pesticides, and other physical stressors from your diet is another, as is eating a whole foods diet with plenty of protein and omega-3 fats. And exercising on a regular basis is another strong booster of immunity and general health. A recent study looked at all the available evidence on exercise and immunity and concluded that "aerobic exercise is a friend of the immune system," helping to balance diminished adaptive responses and reduce inflammation.

And what does Burns, a mainstream doctor with academic ties who specializes in geriatrics, have to say about vitamins and supplements?

"In both healthy and nutritionally deficient older adults, vitamin and dietary supplements have been found to enhance the response of the immune system."

CHAPTER 11

What You Should Know about Hormones

"**I**t's my hormones!" says the woman suffering from a host of monthly related maladies sometimes known as PMS. "It's his hormones!" says the parent, describing the bafflingly stupid behavior of a teenage boy risking life and limb in the latest version of some extreme sport.

Are they right?

Hormones have been blamed for everything from groping backseat encounters in the teenage years to the purchase of a red Porsche at age fifty-five. But the idea that "it's all about hormones," like many clichés, has some grounding in fact. Hormones are absolutely essential messengers that tell cells, organs, tissues, muscles, and bones what to do. They are drivers of behavior and physiology. Many of them diminish with aging. And it's a reasonable question to ask how hormones change as we age, which ones change, how those changes affect our longevity, and what, if anything, we can or should do about it.

Let's start with one hormone over which we actually have some control. Compared to the sexy stuff (like testosterone and estrogen), it doesn't get a ton of attention from the media, but it's almost impossible to overstate its importance.

I'm talking about insulin.

INSULIN, LONGEVITY, AND HEALTH

In 1992, researchers collected data on people who were both mentally and physically fit and were at least one hundred years old. They looked carefully at the factors these folks had in common to see whether they might turn out to be predictors for a long and healthy life.

They came up with three.

The first was low blood levels of triglycerides, a kind of fat found in the body and blood, high levels of which put

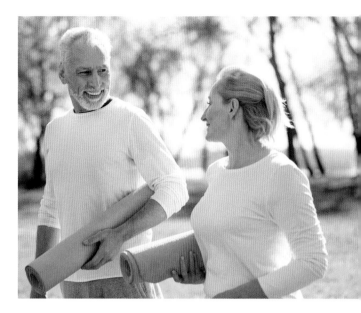

you at risk for heart disease. The second was high blood levels of the so-called "good" cholesterol, HDL, the kind of cholesterol thought to be protective against heart disease. And the third was a low level of fasting insulin.

Let's take a look at this last factor.

Insulin: Sensitivity versus Resistance

Although there's not a whole lot you can do (short of recommended hormone replacement therapy) to change your levels of important hormones like testosterone and estrogen, there's a *tremendous* amount you can do to modify your insulin levels. The cells' sensitivity to insulin—a property called (big surprise) insulin sensitivity—is turning out to be one of the most important predictors of overall health. "If there is a single marker for life span," says Ron Rosedale, M.D., author of *The Rosedale Diet*, "it's insulin sensitivity."

Insulin sensitivity? Aging?

Yup.

To understand this incredibly important phenomena and its effect on metabolism and longevity, let's start by looking at the metabolism of a five-year-old kid. Why? Because, theoretically at least, a five-year-old hasn't screwed up his metabolism yet. After all, if you want to know how something is supposed to work, it's good to look at how it performs before it gets screwed up. Hence, our mythical five-year-old.

So our five-year-old kid comes home from school and he eats an apple. The apple causes his blood sugar to rise just a bit, which is perfectly normal—when you eat food, especially carbohydrate and to a lesser extent protein, your blood sugar goes up. (It actually doesn't rise when you eat fat, but that's another discussion.) That slight rise in blood sugar is a good thing because our mythical five-year-old is now going to go outside and play. He's going to run, jump, slide, bike, and do all the things kids do—or at least what they did before the days when the times became more dangerous and video games replaced sandlot softball and jungle gyms.

Now, when blood sugar goes up, even a little, the pancreas jumps into action and releases a hormone that is the star of our discussion—insulin. Insulin has many jobs in the body, but first among them is to get that excess sugar out of the bloodstream and escort it into the muscle cells, where it can be used for energy. This is an important job, because excess sugar in the bloodstream is damaging to long-term health. And getting that sugar into the muscle cells not only removes it from the bloodstream, preventing damage and aging, but also delivers an important fuel to the muscle cells, which are going to need it if our kid's going to make it through his strenuous afternoon playtime.

So far, so good.

Eventually, insulin peacefully escorts that sugar into the muscles, and the muscles gratefully accept it and burn it, thus fueling our kid's activities. Gradually, his blood sugar returns to normal, even a little below (because he's been so active), which is a good thing because now it's dinnertime.

That's also pretty much the last time you'll see things work that well, at least in modern Western society.

Let's fast-forward thirty to forty years.

You wake up in the morning, probably tired and groggy from not having slept enough. Your stress hormones are immediately elevated as you ponder a ridiculously crowded day in which there's hardly enough time to do half the things you need to get done. You fly out of the house on the way to work, stop briefly at the local coffee emporium to grab a calorie-laden, sugar-loaded caffeinated beverage, perhaps accompanied by one of those 900-calorie healthy-looking "low-fat" muffins that also happen to be loaded with sugar and carbs. Now, your blood sugar is through the roof. The pancreas jumps into action: "Oh my God, this dude just ate the equivalent of five Ding Dongs," it mumbles to itself while it starts pumping out insulin like crazy to deal with the enormous sugar load.

Insulin dutifully begins shoveling that excess sugar into the muscle cells, but this time the muscle cells are having none of it. "We don't *need* all that sugar," they say. "This guy is going to sit around at the computer all day and when he gets home, he's going to veg out on the couch. What do we need all that fuel for? Go take it somewhere else!" In technical terms, the cells become *resistant* to the actions of insulin—insulin resistance, get it?—and they lock their doors and essentially say, "We gave at the office."

What to do, what to do?

Well, insulin's got to take that sugar somewhere, so it starts knocking on the doors of the fat cells. "Hey, let us in! We've got all this sugar for you." And guess what? The fat cells are more than happy to open their doors (at least in the beginning. After a while, even they get resistant, leaving all that sugar to float around the bloodstream, causing all sorts of mischief). Eventually, insulin gets the sugar out of the bloodstream so effectively that your blood sugar plummets and you're starving. Now, it's 11:00 in the morning and you'll kill someone if you don't get a candy bar.

Welcome to blood sugar hell.

Of course, that's just the beginning. Once on this terrible roller coaster you're caught in a cycle of low blood sugar, mood swings, cravings, carb overeating, and the resultant inevitable fat around your middle (or thighs, butt, or hips). I talk about this in detail in my book *Living Low Carb*, but the point here is that this phenomenon is about much more than unwanted weight gain. It's also about aging. And here's why.

Remember glycation? Let me refresh your memory: It's one of the Four Horsemen of Aging, and it happens when excess sugar gloms onto proteins in the blood, eventually causing them to become sticky and gooey and gum up circulation.

Excess sugar. Like the kind that's floating around in your bloodstream, all dressed up with nowhere to go. The kind that hooks a ride onto innocent proteins, like teenagers hopping on the outside of buses looking for a thrill ride.

From the point of view of aging, the results are disastrous.

Proteins that have become "glycated" (sticky with sugar) are too big and gummy to get through small blood vessels and capillaries, including the small vessels in the kidneys, eyes, and feet (which is why so many diabetics

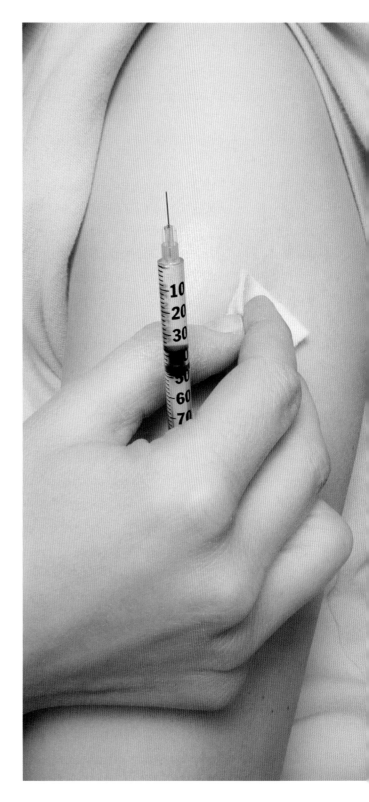

are at risk for kidney disease, vision problems, and amputations of toes and feet). The sugar-coated proteins become toxic, making cell machinery run less efficiently, damaging the body and exhausting the immune system. When cells become insulin resistant, the result is you now have way too much sugar in your bloodstream, which is a disaster just waiting to happen.

All this would be bad enough, but because of your elevated sugar you also have elevated levels of insulin, which is not a good thing from a longevity point of view. Insulin does many things besides acting as a sugar wrangler. For one thing, it sends a message to the kidneys to hold on to sodium, which drives your blood pressure up, increasing your risk for heart disease. For another, insulin turbocharges the activity of a particular enzyme (with the unwieldy name of *HMG-coenzyme A reductase*, or *HMG-CoA reductase*) that runs the cholesterol-making machinery of the body. So high levels of insulin basically signal the liver to ramp up the production lines on cholesterol. Meanwhile, high levels of sugar in the blood increase the production of triglycerides, another serious risk factor for heart disease. And elevated insulin makes losing weight

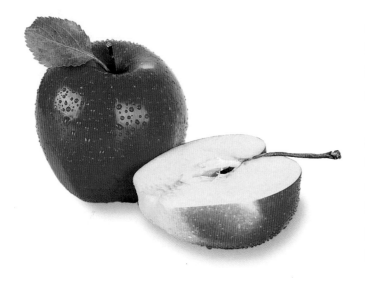

fiendishly difficult—not for nothing is it nicknamed "the fat-storing hormone."

High-sugar diets are also a risk factor for cancer; cancer cells thrive on sugar, consuming far more of it than normal cells. Sugar is pure ecstasy for cancer cells, which chow down on it like hungry rabbits in a lettuce patch. Although the evidence is mixed, emerging research suggests a link between high-sugar diets (technically known as *high-glycemic diets*) and different types of cancer—not exactly a great thing from the point of view of aging well!

Thoroughly depressed? Don't be. This one is easy to fix.

The absolute, number one, easy-as-pie, quick fix for insulin resistance is—wait for it—a low-carb diet. In fact, a low-carb diet (and don't panic, I'll define what I mean by that in a minute) may be a fix for a number of issues that concern those of us who want to live long and well. With its reduced intake of processed carbs and sugar, a low-carb diet will drop your triglycerides like a rock, thereby reducing at least one major risk factor for heart disease. And there's no faster way to bring blood sugar down to normal levels or keep insulin in its "happy" zone, where it can work for you instead of against you.

Now is it starting to make sense why the 1992 researchers found low fasting insulin to be one of the trademark blood measures of healthy centenarians? And why the famous Baltimore Longitudinal Study of Aging found the same thing?

The opposite of the dreaded insulin resistance is *insulin sensitivity*. Insulin sensitivity is *good*. You *want* your cells to be responsive to insulin. In fact, you want them super-responsive, you want them listening like crazy and opening their doors when insulin comes knocking. This keeps glucose (sugar) metabolism working, keeps sugar from getting too high in the bloodstream, keeps the muscle cells fueled, and means that your pancreas doesn't have to work too hard overproducing insulin because a small amount gets the job done quite well. This is a perfect scenario for living longer!

And you can accomplish that with a few lifestyle modifications.

Number one with a bullet: exercise! Here's why.

Every time you move around you create a demand for fuel. Your cells literally open up and say to insulin, "Come on in, the water's fine!" That allows insulin to remove excess sugar from the bloodstream and dump it into the receptive (sensitive) muscle cells, which are eager to have it.

Number two, and probably just as important: adjust your diet.

First, cut out the sugar. The more sugar you eat, the higher your blood sugar goes up, and the more insulin you secrete. For most people, this is a disastrous scenario. (I say "most" to allow for the few, lucky individuals on the planet who can eat all the sugar they want and not have it hurt their health. And in any case, even if such people do exist, I guarantee you're not one of them. Neither am I!)

Second, reduce foods that the body treats as sugar. Unfortunately, it's not just plain ordinary white sugar that plays havoc with your metabolism and contributes to aging. It's anything the body *thinks* is sugar. The body treats most white foods—potatoes, breads, starches, rice, cakes, you name it—as nothing more than sugar, which is pretty much what they turn into once they leave your mouth and enter your stomach. One of the many reasons people who eat fewer carbs have such good results is that they eliminate many of the foods that put you on the hellish blood sugar roller coaster. (A great deal of research has shown that people on low-carb diets not only lose body fat and overall

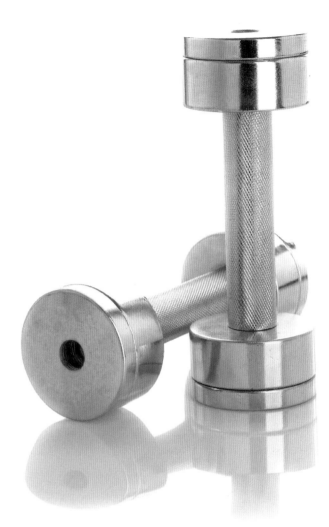

weight, but lower their triglycerides and often improve their cholesterol ratios as well.)

A low-carb diet does not have to mean the stringent first stage of the Atkins Diet (not that there's anything *wrong* with that). Remember, the average American consumes more than 300 grams of carbohydrate a day. You don't need anything like that amount. You can be a pretty active athlete on one-third of that amount, and many people flourish at even lower levels. And forget all the garbage

Balance Your Diet with the Jonny Bowden Four Food Groups

Here are my four food groups: food you can hunt, fish, pluck, or gather. Make that the mainstay of your diet and you'll live a very long time. These foods are part of a low-carb, low-glycemic diet that won't raise your blood sugar and thus keep you off the blood sugar roller coaster.

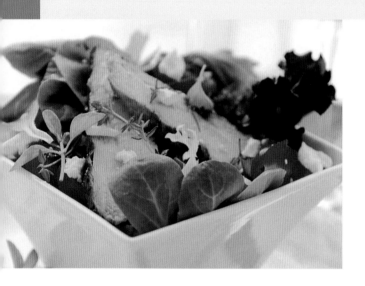

you've heard about "needing carbs for energy." Most carbs that we eat will sap your energy, not add to it. The body's main source of fuel is fat, and we can get by quite nicely with fewer carbs—although how *much* less is an individual question and one best answered by another book (see my book *Living Low Carb*).

When I talk about this stuff in person at workshops, I usually put a PowerPoint slide up that has a person with a megaphone with the following talk balloon coming out of it so it comes across loud and clear: "He's not talking about

fruits and vegetables!" So let me be clear: *I'm not talking about fruits and vegetables (especially vegetables!)*. When I talk about reducing carbs for longevity, I'm talking about *barcode carbs*: processed cereals, pastas, breads, cakes, crackers, all that stuff. Eat all the vegetables you want and add some healthy, low-sugar fruits, such as berries, apples, grapefruit, and the like. Send back the breadbasket at dinner (believe me, you don't need it) and get a second portion of salad or soup. There, wasn't that easy?

Insulin is one incredibly important hormone over which we have a lot of control. But what about the sexy stuff alluded to earlier, those other hormones that get the lion's share of attention in the media?

Let's take a look.

THE KETO DIET

In the years since the original edition of this book was published, the ketogenic diet—also known as the keto diet—was enjoying an unprecedented amount of attention. (As I write this section, I'm sitting in a stateroom on a cruise ship—I'm presenting two talks on the 11th annual

Low Carb and Keto cruise.) And since keto diets are the ultimate tool when it comes to lowering insulin resistance and because they have such wide-ranging health benefits, it's worth spending a few minutes discussing what, exactly, a "keto" diet is.

When the first edition of Dr. Robert C. Atkins's book the *New Diet Revolution* came out in 1972, one of the central features of the diet was nutritional ketosis. Atkins actually called ketosis " … one of life's charmed gifts. It's as delightful as sex and sunshine, and it has fewer drawbacks than either of them." Hyperbole? Maybe a little. Meanwhile, advocating for ketosis got Atkins in a ton of hot water with the medical establishment who believed that ketosis was only something that happens in starvation (untrue). Furthermore, many doctors thought "nutritional ketosis" was the same as a life-threatening condition called diabetic *ketoacidosis* (also untrue). Diabetic ketoacidosis is as different from nutritional ketosis as dolphin (the edible fish) is from Flipper the bottle-nosed dolphin.

But times have changed. Ketogenic diets are an accepted treatment for childhood epilepsy and are used at hospitals (such as Johns Hopkins) around the country. Ketogenic diets are being used successfully for weight loss, notably at the Duke University clinic run by Dr. Eric Westman. And at Tampa University, professor Dominick D'Agostino and his team have been working with the Navy to research the performanc-enhancing effects of ketogenic diets on Navy Seals. Professor Jeff Volek—one of a handful of the most credible and respected scientists doing peer-reviewed research on the keto diet—has worked with ultra-marathoners and tri-atheletes who are on the keto diet and swear it has improved their performance.

So what Exactly is a Ketogenic Diet?

A ketogenic diet is a diet with so little carbohydrate in it that the body is forced to use fat (instead of sugar) as its primary fuel source. Clearly, this has advantages for weight loss, but it apparently has other advantages as well. Since ketogenic diets are by definition high in fat (and moderate in protein), they don't jack blood sugar up, and therefore the demand on the body for insulin is greatly reduced. When insulin is no longer elevated all the time—they way it frequently is on a high-carb diet—the cells begin to regain their sensitivity to insulin and insulin resistance begins to fade. As we've seen, insulin resistance is a factor in a baker's dozen of degenerative diseases, so anything that increases insulin sensitivity (reducing insulin resistance) is a pretty terrific thing for health and longevity.

Ketones—also known as ketone bodies—are produced as a by-product of fat-burning. And they are an absolutely terrific fuel for the heart, the muscles, and the brain. And let's remember that cancer cells thrive on sugar—it's really their only fuel. So when you reduce sugar in the diet (and the bloodstream), you're essentially depriving cancer cells of the fuel they need to survive and spread. Ketogenic diets are now being proposed as an adjunctive cancer therapy. Anecdotally, some well-known people in the health and fitness space—namely superstar trainer Vinnie Tortorich—have credited a ketogenic diet with keeping their cancer in remission. And noted researcher (and TED lecturer) Dr. Terry Wahls has pioneered ketogenic diets for multiple sclerosis and is currently conducting trials of her particular form of the diet—known as the Wahls protocol—for MS patients.

So, the ketogenic diet is essentially a "very low carbohydrate high fat diet", (abbreviated LCHF), one that produces a state known as nutritional ketosis. People who follow keto diets usually monitor their ketone levels with devices that allow them to measure ketones in the blood, the urine, or, more recently, through the breath. In their excellent book *The Art and Science of Low Carb Living*, Professors Jeff Volek and Stephen Phinney—two of the most respected researchers on keto diets—define "light nutritional ketosis" as a ketone level of between .05–1.0 mmol/L and "optimal ketosis" between 1.0-3.0 mmol/L.

My personal opinion is that ketosis is a wonderful nutritional intervention for a variety of conditions, but that one doesn't have to be in nutritional ketosis 24/7 to get the benefits of the diet. You can—as many people do—

go "keto" a few times a year, as a metabolic reset. (My friend, the philosopher, personal trainer and naturopathic physician Dr. Jade Teta, advocates this approach.) It's also possible to "flirt with ketosis", just by eating a low-carb high-fat diet (which is what one of us—Jonny—does, at least most of the time). The diet may not always put you in nutritional ketosis, but it will almost certainly have a positive effect on your blood sugar and insulin.

Note: For those who might want to try a keto diet for a time, a good resource is *Keto Clarity* by Dr. Eric Westman and low-carb/keto blogger and podcaster Jimmy Moore.

THE SEX HORMONES

With sex hormones (like testosterone and estrogen) and aging we're presented with something of a chicken-and-egg conundrum. Changes in hormone levels might well be the result of underlying changes that are associated with unhealthy aging rather than the cause. "Often, it is not possible to establish cause-effect relationships," write Jeffrey Bland, Ph.D., and David Jones, M.D., "but it is clear that changes in (hormones) throughout life are associated with significant changes in physiology and vitality."

The Truth about Testosterone

Ah, testosterone. The much-maligned engine of male behavior, the one blamed for everything from grand theft auto to soccer riots. Never has one hormone gotten such a bad, and undeserved, rap. True, without it, we'd probably be spared the sight of football fans with painted faces waving big spongy fingers in the air, and the entire sport of NASCAR might not exist, but truth be told, testosterone has another, gentler side, and its decline has serious implications for aging well.

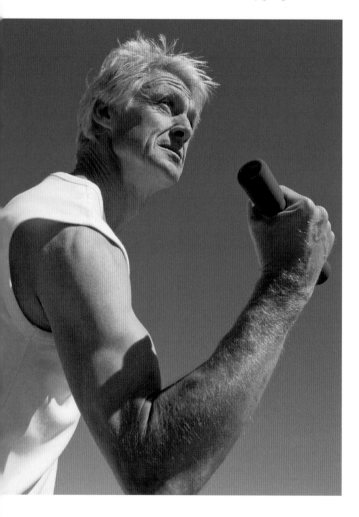

Testosterone, the principle male sex hormone, is what's called a *steroid hormone*. It's primarily secreted in the testes of men and the ovaries of women. It's classed as an *androgen*, which means it controls the development and maintenance of masculine characteristics. It figures prominently in libido, energy, and well-being.

The bad news is it starts to decline around age thirty. So why should you care?

Andropause: a concept whose time has come.

We all recognize that during midlife, females undergo profound changes in their physiology. No one disputes that these changes result in a variety of negative symptoms including (but not limited to) weight gain, loss of energy, memory issues, loss of focus, less clarity of thought, mood changes, and overall decreases in well-being. These "slow down symptoms" are certainly not limited to women, as most middle aged men will tell you. Until recently, we simply didn't address these issues in males. But the good news is that the days of turning a blind eye to the ravages of time may soon be a thing of the past.

Evidence clearly indicates that men with declining testosterone levels are at greater risk for a number of chronic diseases and have an increased risk of death as a result. As recently as 2018, new research found that low amounts of the hormone were associated with chronic disease, even among men forty years of age and younger! And a study funded by the National Institute on Aging and the American Heart Association showed that men older than fifty with low levels of testosterone have a greater risk of dying from all-causes combined than a matched group of their peers with appropriate testosterone levels. And who knows what specific health benefits might have been demonstrated had the researchers looked at men with optimal testosterone levels! It's actually remarkable that men who merely passed the very low bar of having "appropriate for your age" testosterone levels still lived longer than those who were "deficient." We can only imagine how long men with optimized testosterone levels would live.

New research suggests that one in four men in America over the age of thirty has low testosterone, and it's likely that most don't even know it. The worst part is that only 5–10 percent of them are being treated for it! What's more, there's been a generational decline in testosterone levels to the tune of about 1 percent a year. That means that in all likelihood a sample of sixty-five-year-old men reading this book in 2018 would have testosterone levels 15 percent below those of sixty-five-year-old men in 2003.

The condition takes a significant toll on men's lives. Among men polled, 97 percent said low testosterone had a somewhat or very negative impact on the sexual aspect of their lives, and 90 percent said it adversely affected their self-esteem.

Low testosterone is associated with a broad range of physical, psychological, and sexual symptoms, including decreased energy and mood, fatigue, loss of muscle mass, depressed libido, and erectile dysfunction. In addition, low testosterone has been associated with other serious medical conditions, including diabetes, cardiovascular disease, and metabolic syndrome.

It's not an accident that there's a booming business these days in male hormone replacement therapy. Testosterone makes you feel good. It also makes it easier to gain muscle and lose body fat. People on testosterone replacement therapy commonly report feeling more youthful and more energized.

But the story is far more complicated than just a testosterone deficiency. That's because doctors almost never see

WHAT ARE "NORMAL" LEVELS, ANYWAY?

Let's be clear—neither of us puts much stock in what's considered "normal" levels of sex hormones. Normal "for your age" testosterone levels are, in our opinion, wildly different from optimal "for your age" levels.

Most labs compare your measured testosterone level to what's considered the "normal range", but the range that's considered "normal" is astonishingly wide, ranging from 280 ng/dL to 1100 ng/dL. What's more, that range covers all men from twenty-one to sixty-five years of age. Let that sink in for a minute. That would be like saying everyone from age two to eighty-two requires between 20–200 grams of protein a day. It would tell you nothing about the ideal amount to consume at various stages of life.

In the case of testosterone, a twenty-seven year old male and a sixty-four year old male would both be considered to be "normal" if their testosterone levels fell between 280-1100. If the twenty-seven-year-old man happened to have a level of 300, the lab wouldn't even flag it as a problem. And if this has you scratching your head, you're not alone! Us too!

You can see the issue with that reasoning. The long-term health implications for a younger man with low levels of testosterone would certainly not be the same as a sixty-five-year-old man with the same levels.

As a prescribing physician, Dr. Beth Traylor has treated thousands of patients over her many years in practice. During the past fifteen years as a senior physician at Cenegenics Elite Health, she has had the opportunity to see the positive impact of balancing hormonal levels in men of all ages.

On the other end of the prescription pad, Dr. Jonny has been the recipient of such a prescription for almost twenty years and feels strongly that hormone replacement therapy is one of the most significant health promoting interventions he's ever done. For years, his very healthy testosterone levels (between 900–1100) have been far from what's considered "normal for his age."

a single, isolated deficiency. As early as a male's mid-thirties, a number of hormonal values begin to decline, not just "T."

Consider this interesting study published in the *Archives of Internal Medicine*. Researchers tested levels of testosterone as well as two other important hormones (DHEA and IGF-1) on 410 men. The men were then divided into four groups, with the lowest quartile being deficient in all three hormones. A deficiency in any one hormone increased the risk for dying a little, but men with deficiencies in all three hormones had more than double the risk for dying. The moral of the story: hormone deficiencies rarely are single-hormone problems, and multiple deficiencies are way worse.

Cancer and Testosterone

When I (Jonny) tell people about my own hormonal replacement program, I'm often asked if I'm worried about cancer. The answer is no—or at least I don't worry about it any more than I would if I weren't on testosterone. Unfortunately, many traditionally trained physicians have, for decades, scared people into thinking that testosterone therapy increases the risk for prostate cancer. But this does not appear to be true.

A recent analysis of no less than 18 published studies looked at the relationship between male sex hormones and prostate cancer risk. In the study, the *Journal of the National Cancer Institute* looked at studies from 1988 through 2007, which included over 3,800 men. They measured various male hormonal parameters and compared those in the highest hormonal group to those in the lowest hormonal group to see if there was a difference in terms of cancer risk.

There wasn't. The conclusion of the researchers was that blood levels of sex hormones were not associated with any increased risk for prostate cancer.

That said, let's be clear about something. Men on testosterone replacement therapy require careful long-term follow-up and regular monitoring of lab values. This includes monitoring free and total testosterone, DHT (dihydrotestosterone), estradiol (the a metabolic byproduct of testosterone), and PSA levels. Most "Low T" clinics do not—repeat not—closely follow these measurements, which is why we never recommend them even though we do recommend testosterone therapy when appropriate.

But the key to doing T therapy right is to have someone trained in how to properly administer and monitor all the important metrics. Sadly, this is not the case when it comes to Low T clinics. In our experience, it's also rarely the case with general practitioners unless they've received additional training and have expertise in the field of hormone replacement. I have a lot of friends who are top cardiologists, but I don't ask their advice if I have a shoulder injury from tennis. Medicine is highly specialized and testosterone replacement should be done by physicians trained in it, not by physicians who are adding it on to their practice like Botox, because it's a nice additional income stream.

Remember, testosterone is a lot more than just the male "sex hormone," though no one disputes that's a plenty important job. Testosterone actually modulates metabolic function in a number of diverse tissues and organs. It's target organs include the brain, where it affects mood, cognition, and libido; the muscles, where it increases strength and muscle mass; the bones, where it improves bone density; the bone marrow and kidneys—where it induces red blood cell and stem cell production; the liver, where it stimulates the synthesis of important proteins; and of course, the male sex organs which are of course responsible for libido and sexual performance. That's quite a resume.

The good news is that even low dose testosterone replacement therapy is being shown to be beneficial. The largest ever to date prospective study of testosterone replacement therapy in heart failure patients showed that there were significant functional and symptomatic improvements in patients with moderate chronic heart

"Lower levels of testosterone are associated with greater risks for coronary heart disease and diabetes."

— David Leonardi, M.D.

failure. Testosterone, once (wrongly) believed to be detrimental to the heart is now being shown to be protective! Androgens (male sex hormones) actually have anti-inflammatory effects and help to open up (vasodilate) the coronary arteries!

Other more obvious potential benefits for the general population include improvement in libido and erectile function for men, improved mood, decreased depression, increase in muscle strength and size, increase in bone mineral density (and therefore a decreased risk of fracture).

Both of us feel strongly that when testosterone therapy is administered properly to a deficient individual, it is a safe and effective means of improving overall quality of life and sense of well-being.

Can supplements raise testosterone?

No.

Now understand—some supplements may raise total testosterone levels a soupcon, but they do not raise it enough to make any real difference in how you feel.

The fact is you can only raise testosterone reliably and effectively one way—with testosterone replacement therapy.

My personal opinion is that testosterone therapy is an effective anti-aging treatment that can significantly improve well-being, energy, and mood as well as body composition and libido.

And it's not just for men. Let's remember that testosterone doesn't just improve libido for men—it does the same thing for women. That's why physicians trained in age-management medicine routinely include very small, physiologic amounts of testosterone in the hormone-replacement programs of their female clients.

THE ESTROGEN CONTROVERSY

Years ago, I attended a daylong seminar by the famous nutrition educator (and biochemist) Jeffrey Bland, Ph.D., who has taught health practitioners about nutrition for twenty-five years. The title of the event was "Female Endocrinology," and we were there to learn about the subject of women's hormones.

Bland started the day with the following statement: "Well, we're here to talk about female hormones, and we only have eight hours, so it's important that we get started because there's an awful lot to cover." Pause for effect. Then, deadpan, "If we were going to be talking about male hormones, we'd be out of here in forty-five minutes."

Female hormones are, to put it mildly, a complicated subject. But, like all hormones, they play a major part in the aging process and can dramatically affect a number of parameters (from the bones to the heart to the brain).

Take menopause, for example. Menopause is the permanent cessation of the female reproductive cycle. Technically, menopause is the date, fixed retrospectively, from which twelve months have passed when a woman experiences no menstrual periods, but in common usage menopause is used to refer to the whole of the transition period (which can take many years) from regular monthly cycles to the complete cessation of monthly periods. (When I was growing up, it used to be quaintly called "the change of life.")

A full discussion of menopause, with all its psychological, physical, and social ramifications, is several light years beyond the scope of this book, and it has been written about extensively (and sometimes brilliantly) from a number of different points of view. What I want to concentrate on here is the hormonal component and its implications for aging well.

Up until 2002, it was absolutely routine that hormone replacement was *the* answer to menopause. Every woman who became menopausal was put on HRT (*hormone replacement therapy*). Doctors believed it protected bone density, protected the heart, even protected against Alzheimer's.

So what happened in 2002?

Well, to answer that question you have to go back to the fall of 1997, when a landmark study called the Women's Health Initiative began. That study, known as the WHI, looked at more than 16,000 healthy, postmenopausal American women between the ages of fifty and seventy-nine. The purpose of the study was to evaluate the use of HRT by healthy women for the prevention of disease—to study the effect of HRT on all those things doctors believed it was good for, including the bones, heart, and brain. The study was scheduled to be completed eight years later in 2005.

It was stopped in 2002.

Yes, researchers stopped the study because the hormone replacement therapy under investigation appeared to increase a woman's risk of breast cancer as well as heart disease, blood clots, and strokes. (Note the emphasis on the word "appeared.") The media had a feeding frenzy, reduced a complicated issue to a few dramatic (and frightening) sound bites about hormones causing cancer, heart attack, or stroke, and thousands of women immediately ceased their use of hormone replacement therapy.

Okay, now listen up. The truth of what researchers found in that study, and who specifically those results apply to, is far more complicated.

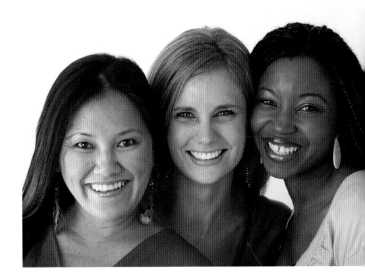

As time went on and the data was picked apart, it became apparent that the effects of these replacement hormones differed greatly depending on whether you were an older woman who was long done with menopause or a younger woman just beginning menopause. To this day, opinion remains divided over how to balance the benefits of a few years of hormone replacement with the possible risks, though it seems to be accepted that the risks vary depending on the age of the woman, her health history, other lifestyle issues, and countless other variables.

If we tried to summarize all the data on hormone replacement, brain health, well-being, depression, heart health, and bone health, we'd be here all day, probably all month. (If you're interested, *The Hormone Decision* by Tara Parker-Pope is a great place to start.)

But we do want to make three important points about female hormones and aging. The first has to do with the issue of "bioidenticals." The second has to do with the method of delivery. The third has to do with the timing.

Let me explain.

Synthetic versus Natural Estrogen

There has been much debate over "natural" or *bioidentical* hormones. The Women's Health Initiative, along with all the other major studies on hormone replacement, used pharmaceutical drugs that many doctors believe act the same as the hormones the body makes. (These drugs were also taken orally, an important point we discuss later on.) The most common of these drugs are Premarin and Provera, both of which are made by Wyeth, which funded the WHI in the first place. (The actual drug used in the WHI was Prempro by Wyeth, a combo drug that consists of both Premarin and Provera in one capsule.)

So, here's the thing. Premarin contains hormones that belong in a horse. There's no other way to say it. Premarin is just not natural in the human body. Proponents of bioidentical hormones argue that it's highly unlikely that they would produce some of the increased risks to women seen with Premarin and Provera (Prempro). Of course, we don't know this for a fact, but it sure does pass the smell test. Virtually every doctor I talked with who deals responsibly with hormone replacement therapy and aging uses only

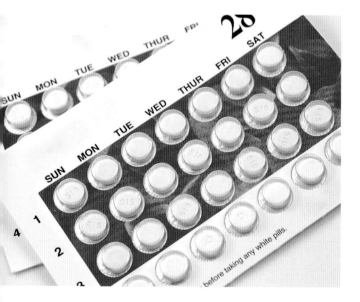

bioidentical hormones and wouldn't be caught dead writing for oral synthetic hormones on their prescription pad.

The debate over whether bioidenticals are safer or different than the pharmaceutical drugs derived from the urine of horses will continue, but it may turn out that those on both sides of the debate are neglecting one important point. In fact, this point is so important that I continue to be amazed that it has not taken center stage in the debate. What is this critical point?

Simple. The method of delivery.

Why the Method of Delivery Matters

When your conventional doctor gives you a prescription for hormone replacement drugs like Prempro, Premarin, or Provera, most likely these drugs come in the form of pills that, of course, you swallow. When your integrative, anti-aging doc gives you a prescription for a bioidentical hormone, it typically comes in the form of a cream or a patch that you put on your skin. This method of delivery (called *transdermal*, meaning "through the skin") may make all the difference in the world. Some hormones are also available as vaginal suppository or ring forms, and technically, those too are in the transdermal form as they are, after all, absorbed through the skin.

When you swallow an estrogen pill, the entire dose hits the liver. "Everything from the intestines goes from the portal vein to the liver before it goes anywhere else," explains Leonardi. "It's been shown that when you flood the liver with estrogen, you increase the production of clotting protein." Indeed, five of the six problems that occurred in the WHI—heart attack, stroke, blood clots in legs, blood clots in lungs, and dementia—are directly or indirectly related to blood clots.

To make matters worse, oral estrogens may interfere with thyroid function by increasing chemicals (thyroid-binding globulin) that make thyroid hormone less available. And oral estrogens are pro-inflammatory.

So even if you were to grant the questionable argument that synthetic hormones are the same as bioidentical ones, you can't disregard the fact that oral hormones have a different effect than transdermal hormones do.

Oral estrogens promote inflammation, making it not so surprising that there were additional heart attacks and strokes in those taking them. Transdermal forms of hormones bypass many of the issues we're worried about with oral hormone replacement.

The "method of delivery" issue hasn't escaped the attention of researchers. In 2007, an important study from France, where transdermal estrogen is far more common than in the United States, compared patients on oral estrogen with patients on transdermal estrogen. The study found that oral estrogen therapy was associated with a fourfold increase in the risk of conditions associated with clotting (including pulmonary embolism) while transdermal estrogen presented no increased risks. The study also found that the type of progesterone used by women taking combination estrogen-progestin hormone therapy made a significant difference as well.

In our view, if you're a candidate for hormone replacement therapy, transdermal hormones are the way to go.

The Timing Question

One of the most important take away points we have subsequently learned from the WHI is that *when* hormone therapy is initiated in the menopausal transition is very important.

Recent analysis of the data suggests that the earlier hormone replacement therapy is started, the safer it is. This just makes sense. The younger you are, the healthier your blood vessels and the lower the risk of cardiovascular disease.

With all that being said, the question remains whether taking hormones at all is necessary for successful, optimal, youthful aging.

On that all-important question, there continues to be passionate debate.

Virtually all of the physicians interviewed on this subject agree that the quality of life in their menopausal patients has been enhanced by hormone replacement therapy.

In the early stages, the relief from the hot flashes and night sweats that can disrupt sleep are dramatic. Later, menopausal women will certainly benefit in terms of relief from vaginal dryness and urinary incontinence and help to strengthen bone in later years.

Yet, some are more cautious. "When you look at centenarians in the so-called 'blue zones' you see that their longevity is all about the food they eat, the nontoxic environment they live in, their daily activities like gardening, their daily time in the sun, and their relationships with others," points out my friend Susanne Bennett, D.C., president of Wellness for Life in Santa Monica, California. Bennett advocates nutritional supplements and dietary changes rather than hormones of any kind.[1]

"We know that hormones are not a fountain of youth, nor are they as risky as they have been portrayed," writes Parker-Pope in *The Hormone Decision.* "Hormones are not good for all women, nor are they bad for all women. The question is whether they are right or wrong for you."

---

1 Bennett will occasionally use DHEA in certain cases; see page 200.

In fact, according to Parker-Pope, analysis of data from both the Nurses Health Study and the WHI found that the right lifestyle choices could have such a profound effect on health and aging that they dwarfed any protective (anti-aging) effects of hormone replacement. "The benefits of a healthy lifestyle were so powerful that they literally erased any impact of menopausal hormones," she writes. "This means that the health gains of exercise and healthful eating far exceed any potential benefit or any potential risk of hormone use."

As of this writing, we are far from knowing all the answers to balancing the risks and benefits of hormone replacement therapy for women. The best we can say for now is that the benefits and risks of estrogen (or combo estrogen/progesterone) therapy probably depend on the age of the patient, the route of administration, and individual factors best evaluated with your health professional.

At this point, the best advice seems to be to be a variation on the tired old mandate to "talk to your doctor," though I'd add that you'll want to do some due diligence in finding a specialist who's really familiar with all the issues.[2]

Progesterone: Nature's Chill Pill

Progesterone might well be thought of as the Cinderella in this hormone family. It might not get the attention of its sexy older sister, estrogen, but it is a necessary component of a normal menstrual cycle.

It is the regular rhythmic balance of these two hormones that controls menses. Most menstrual disorders are a result of imbalances in these hormones and processes. For example, as women age and approach menopause

(become perimenopausal), they frequently do not ovulate. Without ovulation, progesterone is not produced normally by the ovaries. This leads to unopposed estrogen stimulation of the uterine lining and heavy irregular bleeding, which is not at all unusual in women as they age.

Let's now address what the effects of progesterone are on your system. First, we must again make a distinction between natural progesterone and the synthetic forms of Progestins. The synthetic forms have been widely prescribed by the general medical community for many years now. Studies have indicated that the synthetic forms may actually have detrimental effects on the heart and breast tissue. They have been noted to cause fluid retention and an irritable mood.

In contrast, natural progesterone exerts a calming effect on the brain—it is a natural anti-anxiety agent and thus is best taken at bedtime. Studies have shown that it may actually inhibit breast cancer cell growth, is a natural diuretic, and may have protective effects on heart function as well. Additional studies need to be performed; however, the early evidence demonstrates just the opposite effects from the natural as opposed to the synthetic forms.

In the menopausal female with an intact uterus, it is absolutely essential to balance estrogen with progesterone. Without the progesterone component, the uterine lining would overgrow and potentially cause bleeding or theoretically a uterine cancer from unchecked overgrowth. By adding the progesterone component, it matures the lining and prevents this from occurring.

In women who have had a hysterectomy, traditionally progesterone was not given. It was generally believed that since the purpose of progesterone was to prevent the buildup of the uterine lining, that the removal of the uterus meant it was no longer necessary.

---

2 I've listed some of the best in the resource section, but you can also check the "Find a FM Practitioner" tab on the website for the Institute for Functional Medicine (www.functionalmedicine.org).

WHAT'S BEST FOR WOMEN: "CYCLICAL" OR "CONTINUOUS"?

Controversy still exists as to whether menopausal women should receive "cyclical" or "continuous" therapy. In cyclical therapy, estrogen is given during the first half of the month and progesterone is ADDED to the estrogen during the second half of the cycle. The proponents of "cyclical" regimens believe that because it mimics a woman's own natural cycle it is the safer and more natural option. Many women on the cyclical regimen continue to have menstrual periods.

Another option for menopausal females is a continuous regimen. In this type of replacement, both estrogen and progesterone are taken throughout the entire month with no breaks. The progesterone dose is lower then that of the cyclical regimen; however, because it is taken on a regular basis, it prevents the buildup or overgrowth of the uterus and still provides protection against uterine cancer. On a continuous regimen, menstrual periods normally cease.

We now know that progesterone receptors exist on other organs and exert powerful effects. We have mentioned the benefits on brain, and potentially the heart and breast, but we have not mentioned that progesterone is also an important player in maintaining bone density in women.

The type of replacement therapy you choose is between you and your physician. It is the balance of hormones and more importantly your personal response to your regimen that will provide maximal benefits in terms of both symptomatic relief and improved overall health.

THE PROS AND CONS OF USING HUMAN GROWTH HORMONE

HGH, or *human growth hormone*, is (pardon the pun) a growth industry.

Although growth hormone was around for a long time as a treatment for kids whose growth was abnormally stunted, it achieved quite a bit of media attention after *The New England Journal of Medicine* published a study in 1990 that attracted mainstream media attention.

The study looked at healthy men, aged 61 to 81, who had IGF-1 levels below those found in normal young men. (*IGF-1* is a hormone that is stimulated by growth hormone and believed to be responsible for much of growth hormone's effects. It's much easier to measure IGF-1 in the bloodstream than it is to measure growth hormone itself, so docs use IGF-1 measurements as a surrogate marker for actual growth hormone levels.) The men received growth hormone injections three times a week for six months and were compared with a group of men who received no treatment.

The treatment resulted in a decrease in fat and an increase in lean body (muscle) mass and bone density.

This study eventually gave birth to the industry that is now growth hormone replacement and ranges from highly respected anti-aging doctors doing responsible hormone testing/replacement to every scam artist on the Internet selling pills and potions that promise to "raise growth hormone naturally at a fraction of the cost!" (*Note:* As of this writing, none of them work.)

The whole growth hormone thing is somewhat (okay, a lot) controversial. Proponents swear by it. "Patients tell me they get a substantial boost in energy that's very noticeable," says Leonardi.

But it's expensive, and it requires that you inject yourself several times a week. Most important, the elephant in the growth-hormone room is the fact that anything that makes *good* stuff grow (like muscles) or makes things reproduce (like cells) might also make *bad* stuff do the same thing (like cancer). I don't think for a minute that growth hormone causes cancer, but I do think there's a disturbing possibility that if you *already have* a slow-growing cancer it might speed things along. We just don't know.

You can raise growth hormone levels (IGF-1 levels) on your own (although not nearly as much as by using the real thing). It's released during deep sleep, so anything that helps you sleep more deeply and restfully may have an effect (see melatonin, page 204). And very strenuous exercise will also raise it.

Although there are anti-aging doctors who will disagree with me on this, my personal opinion on growth hormone replacement is that it's a fairly minor weapon in the anti-aging strategy. Interestingly, when Cenegenics Medical Institute—the nation's oldest age-management and hormone replacement medical practice—opened its doors in 1998, virtually 100 percent of new patients wanted (and were put on) HGH. Now, twenty years later in 2018, only about 10 percent of Cenegenics patients are on HGH. Clearly, HGH has a place and can be very valuable for certain people, but it's no longer at the center of state-of-the-art hormone replacement therapies. If you want to try it, discuss with your age-management physician. Just don't waste your money on any of the "natural" replacements, or the so-called "HGH boosters" that you can get over-the-counter. Not a one of them is worth the price of the packaging it comes in.

IT COULD BE YOUR THYROID

Low thyroid—particularly an autoimmune condition that affects the thyroid called Hashimoto's—is a hot topic in health and hardly unknown among the general population. But back in 2007, the public consciousness about thyroid disorders was very low. That is, until Oprah Winfrey.

In October 2007, the wildly popular talk show host discussed her bout of exhaustion and weight gain that was ultimately diagnosed as a thyroid condition. She followed up with an article in her magazine, and before you could say "Dr. Phil," thyroid problems went from relative obscurity to the top of the pile on Google searches.

Hypothyroidism, a condition in which your body does not make enough thyroid hormone, is one of the most underdiagnosed diseases of the aging population. Why? One reason is that the symptoms are a bit ambiguous—weight gain, depression, fatigue. Another reason is that the symptoms are frequently written off as simply stress, overeating, menopausal, or a part of "normal" aging. Thyroid disorders are much more common in women (let's not even talk about the number of women who've been told by their doctors that the symptoms are "all in their head"). And finally, for reasons we'll talk about in a minute, the tests that many docs use are not necessarily the best ones; the results can be vague and misleading, especially for a doc who doesn't specialize in this kind of thing.

The third U.S. National Health and Nutrition Examination Survey (NHANES lll) of people aged twelve

ANTI-AGING ACTION PLAN:

Feel Better and Get Your Thyroid Checked!

"Estrogen will make thyroid hormone tests even more unreliable than they are," writes thyroid expert Richard Shames, M.D., which might explain why so many women have thyroid issues. According to a 2001 report in *The Journal of Epidemiology*, as many as 26 percent of menopausal women were hypothyroid, making their menopause years worse.

and older reports that nearly 6 percent of the U.S. population has thyroid disease. As the population ages, the proportion of people with thyroid conditions increases.

Vladimir Korenchevsky was one of the first scientists to document similarities between hypothyroidism and aging. His list of similarities shared between aging and low thyroid included the following:

- Low metabolism
- Low body temperature, (i.e., chilliness, such as cold hands and feet)
- Obesity
- Elevated cholesterol
- Poor skin elasticity with increased wrinkling
- Dry skin
- Constipation
- Brittle nails
- Poor muscle tone
- Arthritis
- Easy fatigability (physical and mental)
- Depression

Korenchevsky died in 1959, but many of his observations were prescient. The thoroughly modern *Textbook for Functional Medicine* lists as typical symptoms of low thyroid function the following: low energy, cold hands and feet, fatigue, elevated cholesterol, muscle pain, depression, and cognitive defects.

You get the idea.

Although Korenchevsky stated that thyroid hormone replacement was no "cure" for aging, he found it highly effective in reversing many of the above-listed aging and thyroid-related signs and symptoms. "Maintaining thyroid hormone function throughout the aging process may be an important hallmark of healthy aging," write Bland and Jones.

CROSS YOUR T'S WHEN IT COMES TO THYROID MEDICATION

The normal thyroid secretes way more T4 than T3. But the T4 hormone doesn't do all that much. The T3 is where the action is—it's about four times stronger than T4. This is important.

The popular thyroid medicines (Synthroid, Levo-thryoxin, Levothroid, Levoxyl) are all pure T4. It used to be thought that simply giving people T4 would correct any thyroid problem because the body converts T4 into the active form T3. But in a substantial number of people, that conversion doesn't take place very well. And, here's something your doc may not know: Converting T4 into T3 depends on the presence of a mineral called *selenium*. If you're not getting enough selenium in your diet (through food or supplements), your body is going to have an even harder time converting that T4 into T3 and you're not going to feel great, even with the standard thyroid meds.

An important study in the *Journal of Clinical Investigation* showed that merely replacing thyroid hormone with the inactive T4 hormone did not ensure normal thyroid activity in all tissues. That was followed by a landmark study in the *New England Journal of Medicine* showing that the vast majority of people felt considerably better, especially in terms of mental functioning, when they were given a combination of T4 and T3 (T3 is commonly known as *Cytomel*). *Armour Thyroid*, which is a more natural thyroid med that contains both T4 and T3, is often used by holistic doctors.

The Thyroid Mistake: Could You Have Hashimoto's?

Izabella Wentz was in the best of health and on top of the world. Originally from Poland, she had come to the United States to pursue her dreams and so far, things were going really well. She graduated from the Midwestern University Chicago College of Pharmacy with a doctorate in pharmacy at the tender age of twenty-three, became a Fellow of the American Society of Consultant Pharmacists, and met and married the man of her dreams.

Life was good.

Until the symptoms started.

She suddenly started getting really tired, sometimes sleeping up to fourteen hours in one day. She started having what's called *new onset panic attacks*, "new onset" because she'd never experienced them before. Ditto with depression, which now was a regular—and unexplainable—visitor. She'd never had allergies, but was suddenly sensitive to foods. At various times and to varying degrees she had all kinds of digestive issues with symptoms of acid reflux and irritable bowel.

Here's the maddening part. Every doctor she went to said, "it's all in your head," They offered her anti-depressants. One of them even told her "you're getting older." (She was twenty-five at the time.)

What Izabella Wentz had was a condition called Hashimoto's thyroiditis, an autoimmune disease in which your immune system goes rogue and attacks your thyroid gland. (Wentz went on to make the study of Hashimoto's her life work and she's now widely known as "the Thyroid Pharmacist".) Hashimoto's isn't a rare or exotic condition—the vast majority of hypothyroid cases are caused by it. But conventional doctors often miss Hashimoto's because they routinely treat hypothyroid with standard thyroid medication regardless of what's causing the problem.

And that's why their patients frequently don't get better. "*When doctors treat Hashimoto's, an immune disorder, with thyroid hormone medication, symptoms persist because the underlying problem—the gradual destruction of the thyroid gland—goes unchecked,*" writes Dr. Datis Kharrazian, author of *Why Do I Still Have Thyroid Symptoms*.

With Hashimoto's, your thyroid is producing less thyroid hormone because your thyroid gland is under attack—by your immune system. Your immune system wrongly perceives your thyroid tissue as a foreign invader, and it mounts an attack, ultimately leading to the destruction of thyroid tissue. The many symptoms that a person with Hashimoto's can experience—as Izabella Wentz discovered—do not disappear with a dose of Synthroid.

Because thyroid tissue is being destroyed in Hashimoto's, thyroid hormones wind up getting dumped into the bloodstream causing jitteriness, anxiety, irritability, and even mania. Later though, as your thyroid burns out, you have too *little* thyroid hormone, which can cause depression and weight gain. And because there are thyroid receptors in virtually every cell in the body, symptoms of Hashimoto's range all over the map, affecting everything from the emotions to the gut.

We don't know exactly what causes autoimmune disease but what we do know is that autoimmune diseases have triggers. And that by identifying and eliminating those triggers, some autoimmune diseases—like Hashimoto's—can go into remission, often staying in remission for very long periods of time.

So what are the triggers for Hashimoto's? Interestingly, they're pretty much the same as the triggers for all autoimmune diseases—toxins, drugs, virus, bacteria, environmental chemicals, and inflammatory foods.

The food connection is particularly interesting. Gluten molecules look suspiciously like thyroid tissue, and when gluten provokes your immune system, thyroid tissue can frequently be part of the collateral damage. If you're at all sensitive to gluten, the immune system will get riled up when you ingest it and will attack anything that resembles it (which happens to include thyroid tissue). Virtually every integrative, functional, or naturopathic doctor will advise those with Hashimoto's to avoid gluten.

There's another reason gluten can be a huge problem for anyone with an autoimmune disease. In gluten sensitive people, gluten provokes an inflammatory response in the gut. Inflammation leads to something called *leaky gut syndrome*—the normally tight junctures of the intestinal wall get looser and more porous. This allows undigested particles (peptides) to get past the intestinal barrier and enter the bloodstream where they don't belong and where they invariably trigger even more activity from the immune system. A leaky gut also makes it more likely that a microbe will get in and cause an infection, making the immune system go even crazier. The more the immune system is firing on all cylinders, the more likely thyroid tissue will get caught in the crossfire.

One of the biggest triggers for every autoimmune disease is stress. Stress does a lot of things to the immune system and to Hashimoto's in particular—none of it good. When you're under constant, chronic stress, your levels of cortisol (the main stress hormone) are always elevated. Cortisol interferes with the body's ability to convert the *inactive* thyroid hormone (T4) to the *active* kind (T3), the kind your body can actually *use*. Instead, cortisol directs some of that T4 to be converted to a different (but equally useless) kind of inactive thyroid hormone called reverse T3. The end result is that you have less active thyroid hormone in your bloodstream (and all the symptoms that go with low thyroid).

The ability to manage stress is critical for people with autoimmune diseases. Stress puts everything in your body on high alert, and the last thing someone with autoimmune disease needs is a trigger-happy immune system. (If you needed added motivation for taking stress management seriously, stress hormones are also strongly linked to weight gain.)

How do you know if you have Hashimoto's? The first step would be a test for thyroid antibodies. Any doctor trained in functional or naturopathic medicine will order that test for you and be able to determine the right course of action.

If you have low thyroid that you suspect is caused by Hashimoto's, here are seven things you can do that will really make a difference in your health.

- **See a doctor who doesn't just treat symptoms.** Physicians who are conventionally trained don't always look beyond the obvious symptoms to the root cause of the problem, especially when it comes to thyroid. Find a doctor who is more interested in looking deeper. Such a doctor is far more likely to test for thyroid antibodies and to be on the alert for Hashimoto's.

- **Lay off gluten!** It's inflammatory for many people and can provoke an immune system reaction that can wind up damaging thyroid tissue.

- **Fix your gut!** Gluten is just the first step—look for hidden food sensitivities or intolerances that could provoke inflammation. The most common food sensitivities besides wheat and gluten are dairy, corn, eggs, nuts, and soy. As Dr. Kharrizian says, "A gut ravaged by inflammation creates chronic stress and immune responses."

- **Watch your blood sugar.** The continuous surges of insulin that happen when you're insulin resistant (pre-diabetic) actually increase thyroid tissue destruction in those with autoimmune diseases. Chris Kresser, M.S., L.Ac.—who specializes in a functional medicine approach to autoimmune disease—writes, "Healthy thyroid function depends on keeping your blood sugar in a normal range and keeping your blood sugar in a normal range depends on healthy thyroid function." For most people, this means cutting way back—or eliminating—processed carbohydrates.

- **Try adrenal adaptagens.** Adaptagenic herbs like ashwaganda are like a metabolic thermostat—they help to cool you off when you're running too hot and heat you up when you're running to cold. They can be very helpful with stress.

- **Take 200 mcg of selenium.** The important mineral selenium is necessary for the conversion of inactive thyroid (T4) to active thyroid (T3). You can also get your daily selenium by eating four to eight Brazil nuts every day!

- **Take probiotics** (and/or eat fermented foods). Keeping the gut healthy is probably the number one priority with all autoimmune diseases, and the first step is to make sure there are plenty of "good guys" among the trillions of microbes that reside in your gut. Probiotics are the "good guys." You can also get them from fermented foods like whole-fat yogurt, kefir, and the Korean dish kimchi.

If you're among the minority of people with hypothyroid not caused by Hashimoto's, it's still a good idea to look at nutrition, hormones, stress, and gut health. We just saw how the nutrient selenium is needed to convert inactive thyroid hormone to active thyroid hormone. An excess of the sex hormone estrogen can have the effect of binding a lot of your thyroid hormone, making it unavailable to do its job. And high stress hormones can still interfere with your body's ability to make active thyroid, even if you don't have Hashimoto's.

Thyroid issues are one of the best examples of the fundamental difference between the approach of conventionally trained doctors—who tend to focus on the symptom—and doctors whose approach is to seek out the root cause of the problem. Conventional medicine asks "what's the symptom, and what pill will take it away." Doctors who take the "root cause" approach ask, "why is this symptom occurring in the first place?"

Asking that question can mean the difference between a lifetime of sickness and a lifetime of health.

GET YOUR THYROID LEVELS TESTED

The role of thyroid in aging has not gone unnoticed or unresearched. In 1992, Italian researchers performed a series of studies examining the importance of the thyroid during aging. They looked at thyroid function in thirty-four healthy centenarians, the youngest of whom was one hundred and the oldest of whom was—wait for it—108! They compared the results to tests for thyroid functions in a bunch of "youngsters" aged seventy to eighty-five.

One of the measures the researchers looked at was the presence of thyroid antibodies, which, as you saw above, is the key to diagnosing Hashimoto's. Remember, Hashimoto's is not a thyroid disease, it's an autoimmune disease. In some people, the immune system is overly vigilant and will mistake our own tissues for foreign invaders, mounting an attack. (This is what happens in all autoimmune diseases.) In Hashimoto's, the body creates antibodies that attack the thyroid, which is exactly what happened to Izabella Wentz. It was these antibodies, which ultimately wind up seriously compromising thyroid function, that the researchers tested for.

They found a significantly *lower* level of thyroid antibodies in the bodies of the healthy centenarians. In fact, these 100-plus-year-old folks had much lower levels of thyroid antibodies (and presumably a much better performing thyroid) than any of the seventy to eighty-five-year-olds who had varying levels of chronic diseases.

Most conventional docs do *not* routinely test for thyroid antibodies. If you're having thyroid issues—or your doc says your thyroid hormones are "low"—insist on the antibiody tests. Most conventional docs use a simple test called the TSH (*thyroid stimulating hormone*) test, which, while a useful piece of data, does not tell the whole picture on how the thyroid is performing. Indeed, for a period of time, your TSH test may be "normal" while your thyroid is under attack and well on the way to failing.

"If you've tested positive for antibodies, and have a TSH in the 'normal range' but still don't feel well, you may wish to consult with a practitioner who believes that the presence of thyroid antibodies alone is enough to warrant treatment with small amounts of thyroid hormone," advises About.com's highly regarded thyroid expert Mary Shomon, author of *Living Well with Hypothyroidism: What Your Doctor Doesn't Tell You … That You Need to Know.*

Low thyroid is one of those conditions in which how you actually feel may be as important as the lab test results. (Having all the symptoms of a low thyroid without confirmation from a lab test is often referred to as *subclinical thyroid dysfunction*.) More and more integrative medicine practitioners or holistic health care providers now treat the classic symptoms of low thyroid with thyroid meds regardless of whether the tests come back "normal."

But here's what's even more important: Low thyroid function, even in the absence of an abnormal standard test result, may be a sign that the complicated signaling processes and feedback loops in the endocrine (hormonal) systems are not working properly. In fact, it might even be the first sign you notice. (You will never "notice" high blood pressure, but it's hard to ignore feeling fatigued, cold, constipated, or depressed.) And these imbalances or dysfunctions in the hormone signaling systems in your body just might put you at risk for the conditions of aging.

THE DARK SIDE OF SOY

So why does there seem to be such an epidemic of low thyroid levels these days?

The environment we all live in clearly contributes to aging in a lot of insidious ways, some of which are obvious (stress, pollutants, toxins) and some of which aren't. One of the less obvious ways is in connection to thyroid function.

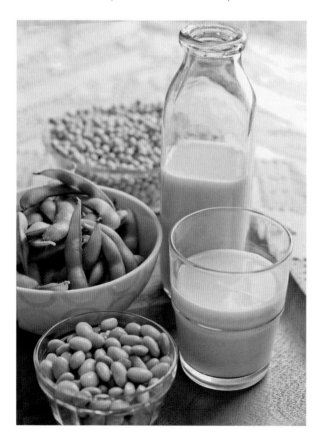

Exposure to toxic levels of heavy metals can interfere with thyroid function. "Lead and mercury invade the thyroid gland and disrupt the production of thyroid hormones," write Laura Pizzorno, M.A., and William Ferril, M.D., in the *Textbook of Functional Medicine*. Pesticides can interfere with thyroid function, as can weed killers, artificial fertilizers, and who knows what other chemicals we're exposed to on a daily basis.

"Hormone and antibiotic residues in meat and dairy products, foodborne bacteria, chemicals in cleaning products, food additives, cosmetics, and the metabolic byproducts of unfriendly gut bacteria can [interfere with] thyroid hormones," the authors point out. These things can also wreak havoc with liver function, potentially decreasing the conversion of the inactive T4 thyroid hormone into the active T3 hormone, another elegant demonstration of how "everything is related to everything" and how detoxification and a "clean" diet can have multiple beneficial effects on aging.

Another possible reason for thyroid malfunction is the fact that up until recently, practically every woman who became menopausal was put on standard hormone replacement therapy, consisting of synthetic estrogen and progesterone (Premarin and Provera). Why would this matter? Oral estrogens induce thyroid-binding globulin. Thyroid-binding globulin grabs up circulating thyroid hormones, making them unavailable for use by the tissues. Wouldn't it be ironic if the very type of hormone replacement therapy that was widely thought to be so protective for women wound up being a cause of thyroid issues for so many women?

Even foods can have a negative effect, including some that you would never suspect. The much ballyhooed health benefits of soy, for example, have come under attack by a vocal minority of holistic health practitioners who point out that soybeans contain *goitrogens*, which suppress thyroid function by interfering with iodine uptake.

"More than seventy years of studies link soy to thyroid disorders," says Kaayla Daniel, Ph.D., C.C.N., author of the book *The Whole Soy Story: The Dark Side of America's Favorite Health Food.* "The myth that soy is a healthy food has had tragic consequences, especially for women in the throes of menopause," Daniel told me, adding that *phytoestrogens* (plant chemicals that have weak estrogenic activity) found in soy products inhibit enzymes needed to produce essential thyroid hormones.

Daniel is one of a growing number of leading scientists, physicians, and toxicologists who have raised alarms about consumption of soy products high in phytoestrogens causing significant endocrine disruption and thyroid damage. "Women in midlife are already at risk for developing thyroid problems," she says. "To make matters worse, the soy industry heavily markets soymilk and other soy products to women who are menopausal as an effective and safe method of hormone replacement therapy. The truth is that it is neither effective nor safe."

Although this view remains controversial, there's pretty universal agreement, even among the "soy-hating" set, that authentic *fermented* soy products are not the problem. Tempeh, miso, and real fermented soy sauce are quite different than the hundreds of soy-based products flooding the marketplace. Fermented soy products are the kind of soy that Asians eat, and they're also the kind of soy foods eaten by some of the long-lived societies studied throughout the world. What those folks don't stock up on is soy chips, soy ice cream, soy milk, soybean oil, and other pretenders that line the shelves of the typical Western supermarket.

The United Kingdom's Committee on Toxicity of Chemicals in Food, Consumer Products, and the Environment has identified several populations at special risk for soy-induced thyroid disease: infants on soy formula, vegans who use soy as their principle meat and dairy replacement, and men and women who use isoflavone supplements to prevent or protect against cancer. And even if a certain minimum amount of soy in the diet weren't the worst thing in the world, even the "pro-soy" set no longer recommends supplementation with concentrated soy isoflavones, though these supplements remain popular and are sold everywhere. Don't take them.

Goitrogens are even found in the royalty of the vegetable kingdom—the brassica family (cabbage, broccoli, Brussels sprouts). "However, few adults and even fewer children eat these foods in excess," points out Daniel. Light cooking will neutralize most of the goitrogens in these valuable vegetables. Boiling cruciferous vegetables also reduces the goitrogens, but you'll lose a ton of important nutrients. "Patients for whom goitrogens may be problematic can be advised to briefly steam these vegetables and consume them in modest amounts," advise Pizzorno and Ferril.

Don't let the fact that cruciferous vegetables contain goitrogens stop you from eating them. Cruciferous vegetables also contain powerful plant chemicals that have a positive effect on estrogen metabolism. These plant chemicals, called *indoles*, are considered to be cancer-protective. Just be aware that if you have a thyroid problem, you might want to make sure that you steam them lightly before eating them, thus reducing the amount of thyroid disrupters while preserving the enormous nutritional benefits.

EAT YOUR WAY TO A HEALTHY THYROID

Thyroid is one of the hormones that you can definitely support with the proper diet and supplements. You may not be able to make more testosterone just by eating certain foods, but you will surely not make enough thyroid hormones if you're not providing the nutrients needed for its manufacture. Those nutrients and their best sources include the following:

- **Iodine:** Sea vegetables such as nori, arame, wakame, kombu, and kelp; sardines; eggs; haddock; shrimp; clams; oysters; and sardines
- **Zinc:** Fresh oysters, Brazil nuts, lamb chops, pecans, split peas, almonds, walnuts, and sardines
- **Vitamin E:** Mainly found in wheat germ oil (or supplements)
- **Vitamin A:** Liver, red chili peppers, collard greens, turnips, kale, Swiss chard, beet greens, apricots, winter squash, cantaloupe, papaya, and nectarines. The precursors to vitamin A, the things your body makes vitamin A from, are found in yellow and orange/green vegetables as well as some green ones.
- **Vitamin B2 (riboflavin):** Almonds, wheat germ, wild rice, mushrooms, and egg yolks

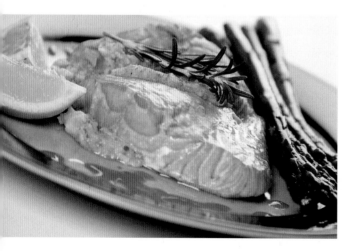

- **Vitamin B3 (niacin):** Bran, peanuts (with skin), and the light meat of turkey and chicken
- **Vitamin B6:** Sunflower seeds, tuna, liver, walnuts, salmon, trout, lentils, lima beans, navy beans, garbanzo beans, pinto beans, brown rice, and bananas

In addition, Richard Shames, M.D., recommends vitamin D (necessary for thyroid hormone production) and essential fatty acids (needed to have your thyroid hormones get to where they need to go), which I've covered extensively in this book.

DHEA: THE MOTHER HORMONE

Throughout this book, I've emphasized the interaction between the inner environment (hormones, neurotransmitters, immunity) and the external environment. As I've said before, "Genetics loads the gun, but environment pulls the trigger." Nowhere is this more evident than in the case of stress hormones.

Long-term, unremitting stress results in a loss of the ability of the adrenal glands to put out important stress hormones, a phenomenon that's becoming increasingly well known and is popularly characterized as "adrenal burnout."

The adrenal glands, two little walnut-shaped glands that sit on top of the kidneys, are responsible for secreting the stress hormones cortisol and adrenaline. But that's not all they do. They also produce an important hormone called DHEA (*dehydroepiandrosterone*) as well as a related compound called DHEA-S. And DHEA is a hormone that may have important implications for aging.

DHEA is the most prevalent hormone in the human body. And many researchers consider it a "mother hormone" because of the important role it plays in producing other hormones. The body can convert DHEA into testosterone, estrogen, progesterone, and a whole bunch of other hormones collectively called "steroid" hormones (the kind your body makes, not the kind baseball players shoot up with). Although it is considered a "minor" hormone in the scheme of things, low levels of it can result in mood changes, fatigue, and weight gain.

In normal folks, DHEA concentrations are highest around age thirty, after which they gradually decrease. By age seventy or eighty, the values are about 10–20 percent of peak values. While association doesn't mean causality, it's worth wondering if low levels of hormones are at least a partial cause of aging.

There's good reason to believe this to be true. One theory is that high circulating DHEA concentrations are actually a marker for longevity in primates. And in one study, men with low levels of DHEA had a 64 percent greater risk of death from any cause than did individuals with high DHEA levels.

Adrenal Insufficiency

Folks with a condition known as adrenal *insufficiency* don't produce enough of the important adrenal hormones, of which DHEA is one. Studies of people with this condition provide some of the strongest evidence for a beneficial effect of DHEA replacement.

The most well known of the adrenal insufficiency conditions is Addison's disease, from which President John F. Kennedy famously suffered. When women with adrenal insufficiency received 50 milligrams of DHEA daily, they experienced improved overall well-being, mood, and sexual activity. In another study of fifteen women and twenty-four men with Addison's disease, three months

of 50 milligrams a day of DHEA corrected the hormonal deficiency and improved self-esteem, while it also tended to enhance overall well-being, mood, and energy.

So now, of course, the question is: Will it benefit people without adrenal insufficiency? Although there isn't a definitive answer yet, emerging evidence suggests that it might.

Epidemiological studies suggest an association between decreasing levels of DHEA (and DHEA-S) and the adverse effects of aging. One large observational study showed a small but meaningful relationship between low DHEA levels and the risk of cardiovascular mortality in men. Another study of more than two thousand people (men and women) younger than sixty-five found that both "all-cause" and cardiovascular mortality were highest in men with the lowest levels of DHEA (though there was no significant relationship for women). Other studies have associated low DHEA levels with depressed mood and bone loss in women.

Then, there was the study published in the Proceedings of the National Academy of Science that followed 622 adults with an average age of seventy-four upon study entry. The researchers followed DHEA levels and tracked them with total mortality risk, functional status, psychological state, and mental status over a period of four years. In women, DHEA levels were directly related to scores of well-being, cognitive function, and functional status. And in men, DHEA levels were inversely related to total mortality risk.

The decline in circulating DHEA levels parallels many age-related changes such as loss of bone density and muscle mass. DHEA is believed to both decrease the bone loss that occurs with aging and enhance the formation of new bone. And it increases estrogen, which is known to build healthy bone matrixes.

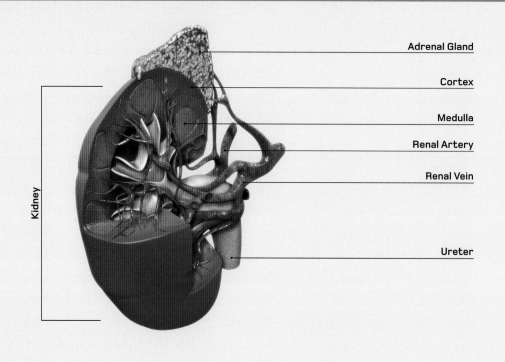

DHEA levels seem to be a marker for good things. One famous study of aging—The Massachusetts Male Aging Study—confirmed that men with higher DHEA levels were less likely to have heart disease. Several studies have demonstrated improved mood and sense of well-being with DHEA supplementation. Some research validates the notion that higher levels of DHEA are associated with higher levels of sexual satisfaction in women. Even low doses of DHEA may improve quality of life, sexual interest, and libido in females. Also, as a precursor to testosterone, it will increase sexual interest and response in both men and women. Low levels of DHEA in men have been associated with erectile dysfunction.

So is low DHEA simply a biomarker of aging, or is it causally related to mortality in the elderly? Hard to say. One research study investigated the effect of giving 50 milligrams of DHEA a day to men and women forty to seventy years old and found that they improved in measures of both physical and psychological well-being. Another study used 100 milligrams daily (a very large dose) for men and women fifty to sixty-five years of age and found that the men had decreased fat mass and enhanced muscle strength. And in a study of 280 men and women sixty to seventy-nine years old, 50 milligrams of DHEA a day increased the women's libido and sexual function (as well as slightly increased their bone mineral density).

As mentioned previously, the adrenals produce both cortisol and DHEA, but here's the thing: The relationship is like that of sharks and dolphins. Where you see a lot of sharks in the water, you won't see Flipper and his crew, and when you see a lot of dolphins, Jaws is nowhere to be found. Cortisol and DHEA have a kind of seesaw relationship; when one is up, the other tends to be down. Unfortunately, in modern life, it's cortisol that's usually elevated and DHEA that's down. An increased cortisol/DHEA ratio seems to be a contributing factor to an aging immune system, according to the *Physician's Desk Reference for Nutritional Supplements*. In general terms, cortisol tends to suppress immunity while DHEA enhances it. DHEA is a powerful immune-system stimulant that can improve your metabolism, energy levels, mood, memory, and sexual function, according to Linda Ojeda, Ph.D., of the Institute for Functional Medicine. Studies show that seniors who maintain a higher level of DHEA do, in fact, experience a longer and healthier life.

DHEA is available over-the-counter and I almost wish it weren't. When all is said, it's still a hormone, and though replacement of some hormones can be a powerful anti-aging strategy, it should still be done under the supervision of health practitioners who know what they are doing. You wouldn't fill up the gas tank in your car with a set amount of gas; you'd let the amount you put in be determined by how full (or empty) the tank was in the first place. So why would you replace hormones in your body without measuring them first, so you can know how much you need?

"It's very important to precede the administration of DHEA with salivary or serum tests for DHEA and DHEA-S, as well as testosterone and estradiol," write Bland and Jones. "A baseline hormone analysis is critical to establish the overall influence of DHEA on [hormone] balance." Most anti-aging docs use DHEA regularly as part of an overall anti-aging strategy that involves monitoring various hormones and replacing as needed to levels that make sense. Anything else is throwing darts at a dartboard blindfolded.

Because DHEA is a slight mood elevator, it could potentially—I repeat, potentially—clash with antidepressants, according to Michael Lam, M.D., M.P.H. Theoretically, the dose of antidepressants might be lowered if you took DHEA, but check with your health care practitioner.

Worth noting: In a laboratory, test-tube situation, DHEA can be synthesized from substances in wild yams, which has led to a persistent myth that if you buy an over-the-counter product made from wild yams, the body will naturally convert this into DHEA. Most health food store clerks will tell you that. This is precisely why you should not get your nutrition information from health food store clerks. Your body can't synthesize DHEA from natural wild yams. Save your money, and if you decide DHEA is worth a try, go to an anti-aging doc and get the real thing. Getting a hormone panel done by a doctor versed in age-management medicine makes a lot of sense, and it's likely that DHEA will be on the list of hormones the doc recommends. The evidence is pretty strong that DHEA can help, and it appears to elicit few short-term side effects when used in the recommended doses.

MELATONIN: BUSTING THE AGE-ROBBERS

Chances are good that you've heard of melatonin. You may even be taking it. It's famous for its ability to fight jet lag. But it's true role in human health is far more nuanced and complex.

Melatonin is a substance secreted in the evening by the pineal gland that is involved in the control of circadian rhythm. Darkness in the eye tells the brain to make melatonin so the body can prepare for sleep.

As we grow older, the pineal gland—big surprise—produces less melatonin. Also, light from night lights, TVs, and other electronic devices can literally reduce the production of melatonin by the brain. In addition, there are a multitude of other factors that may reduce melatonin, all leading to poorer sleep quality.

So yes, melatonin is great for helping you fall asleep and great for jet lag. But it has a much more impressive resume than just that. It's also been shown to do the following:

- Stimulate the immune system
- Relieve certain types of depression (i.e. seasonal affective disorder)
- Reduce migranes
- Reduce stress hormones (cortisol)
- Protect the heart and have a mild beneficial effect on blood pressure
- Support growth hormone production
- Alleviate glaucoma
- Reduce the side effects of chemotherapy and enhance the death of cancer cells during chemo while at the same time protecting healthy cells

Melatonin is a potent antioxidant and may therefore help protect the brain against one of the Four Horsemen of Aging: oxidative damage. It protects cell membranes even more than vitamin E does and is more effective than glutathione (an important antioxidant in the body) at neutralizing a deadly free radical that causes oxidative damage, *hydroxyl radicals*. Melatonin also supports immune function in a number of ways and may even play a role in protecting against cancer, as mentioned above. (One reason scientists believe that blind women have significantly less breast cancer risk is because blind women, with their reduced exposure to light, presumably make a greater amount of melatonin.) So although melatonin is not by itself a miracle anti-aging supplement, it helps protect against a number of age-robbers.

Take sleep, for example. During sleep, a great deal of cellular damage that occurs during the day is repaired, and that repair process is initiated by secretions of melatonin. And because disturbed sleep so often accompanies aging, anything that can help us sleep better (with ancillary benefits to boot and no side effects) might be something to take note of. Melatonin definitely fits the bill.

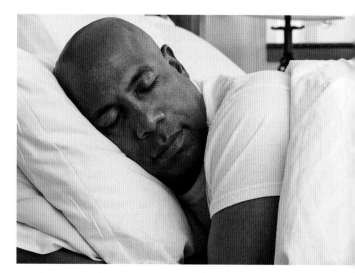

Poor sleep quality reduces the growth hormone, an important (though minor) hormone that helps us keep muscle and lose fat. It may also raise levels of stress hormones such as cortisol. "This may argue strongly for sleep therapy and/or melatonin being of primary importance in the management of some symptoms associated with … aging," write Bland and Jones.

And because melatonin plays an important role in setting our "biological clock," it influences metabolism. Just as this was being written, researchers at the University of California, Irvine discovered that proteins involved with circadian rhythms and metabolism are in fact intrinsically linked with and dependent upon each other. "Our circadian rhythms and metabolism are closely partnered to ensure that cells function properly and remain healthy," said researcher Paolo Sassone-Corsi, distinguished professor and chair of pharmacology.

Circadian rhythms are twenty-four-hour cycles that govern fundamental processes in the body. They operate like an inner clock, respond to light and darkness, and anticipate environmental changes. When these rhythms are disturbed, serious health consequences can result. In fact, disruption of these internal rhythms has been linked to diabetes, depression, heart disease, and cancer.

According to Sassone-Corsi, when the balance between circadian rhythms and metabolism is upset it can ultimately lead to illness and disease. Lack of rest or disruption of normal sleep patterns can increase hunger, leading to obesity-related illnesses and accelerated aging. Because melatonin is so helpful in getting a good night's sleep, the use of melatonin as a supplement may have far-reaching consequences for many of the conditions that interfere with healthy aging.

And if all of this weren't enough, melatonin may also be good for the heart. Researchers tested melatonin supplements on women aged forty-seven to sixty-three and found that supplementation improved the "day-night" rhythm of blood pressure, significantly decreasing nighttime blood pressure. "Melatonin, in addition to being an incredibly powerful antioxidant, may well turn out to be cardio-protective," says Traylor.

Melatonin is available over-the-counter. You might think after all I said that I wouldn't be hugely happy about its over-the-counter status.

Actually, I think it's fine and here's why: Melatonin is a hugely important hormone with many overlapping benefits. Virtually everyone over the age of forty doesn't make enough, and taking extra doesn't seem to have any negative side effects. So, I'm comfortable with people trying it on their own.

Melatonin has been used successfully as a supplement for sleep in doses from as low as 0.1 milligram to as much as 10 milligrams (which, if you're curious, is what I take nightly).

CHAPTER 12

What Do I Do Next?

At this point, you might well be wondering: What do I do next?

Glad you asked!

This final chapter is my best answer to that question. It's a distillation of everything I've learned studying health and longevity, in a convenient, easy-to-follow "how-to" guide that I hope will serve you well as you look to develop habits that will keep you active and healthy for decades.

If I had one chance to leave my loved ones with a blueprint for how to live a life as rich, and full, and vibrant as mine has been (and I hope will continue to be!) this would be it.

Can I "prove" every one of these suggestions will result in your life being extended by a specific amount of months or years? Of course not. But I'm known for having a pretty good BS detector. And in a field crowded with contradictory advice and misinformation, the following principles are ones that I believe will stand the test of time. These are the ones I practice. I hope they will serve you as well as they have served me.

But first, a warning.

Many of the recommendations you'll see below are based on what I call "connect the dots" knowledge. We know, for example, that inflammation is a major promoter of every degenerative disease on the planet. We also know that omega-3s are anti-inflammatory. My reading of the massive research on this question has led me to believe that omega-3 supplements are a really smart idea. But again— that's my opinion.

And really, that's all this chapter is about: The conclusions I've personally reached after twenty-eight years as a health professional. These are the things that matter. These are the things that make a difference. I hope you'll try them out and find they make as much a difference in your life as they do in mine.

FOOD

Do not eat a low-fat diet. Quite the contrary. Consume a fair amount of healthy fat—such as coconut oil, Malaysian palm oil, olive oil, avocado oil, macademia nut oil, grass-fed butter, and ghee. Include lots of vegetables and fruits and a moderate amount of clean protein (i.e. grass-fed meat, wild salmon, cage-free eggs) every day (about 80 to 120 grams will do it for most people). Add beans, nuts, green tea, pomegranate juice and berries. Drink lots of water. Throw in some dark chocolate a few times a week. Don't worry about how many servings a week or any of that stuff. Just put those foods and beverages in your refrigerator and pantry, keep them in heavy rotation, and eat them regularly and often. Avoid: bread, pasta, cereal, cakes, crackers, chips, donuts, and sodas.

Practice hara hatchi bu. Hara hatchi bu is a Confucian saying that roughly translated means "push away from the table when you're 80 percent full." With all the hundreds of books' worth of information on what to eat, what tends to get lost is this simple truth: Eating less extends life. Don't wait till you're stuffed to leave the table.

Consider intermittent fasting. Intermittent fasting is "trending" big-time and has been for the last couple of years prior to this writing (2018). I suspect it will continue. Unlike many trends and fads, this one has excellent science behind it. There's a lot of ways to do it, and it's not difficult at all. And the health benefits are quite real. (Best resource: *The Complete Book of Fasting* by Jason Fung, M.D., and Jimmy Moore)

SUPPLEMENTS

Take these five supplements every day: Omega-3 fish oil (I recommend Barlean's), magnesium, a high-quality multiple, vitamin D (at least 2,000 IUs daily depending on your vitamin D blood test results), and probiotics. For probiotics, look for a formula that contains these five species: *Lactobaccilus plantarum*; *Lactobaccilus acidophilus*; *Lactobaccilus brevia*; *Bifidobacterium lactis* (also called *B. animalis*); and *Bifidobacterium longum*.

If you want to go further, consider curcumin, trans resveratrol, and sulforaphane (extract of broccoli), all of which are part of my daily supplement routine. I'm also a fan of collagen supplements—collagen is the most abundant protein in the body. We stop making it when we're forty, and when it goes, it causes skin wrinkling, other signs of aging, and joint pain. Collagen supplements make sense to me.

EXERCISE

Walk every day. Try to get thirty (or more) minutes. Vary your intensity—i.e. a minute fast, a minute slow, or variations on that theme (it's called interval training). Strength train twice a week for fifteen to twenty minutes. And don't sit for more than an hour at a time without getting up to stretch or walk to the water cooler. The last ten years of research has shown pretty conclusively that extended periods of sitting are almost as bad for you as smoking.

MEDITATE

Tim Ferris has one of the most interesting podcasts on the planet and routinely interviews high performers like Bill Gates, Tony Robbins, Peter Thiele. One thing that over 80 percent of the incredibly successful people he's interviewed have in common is that they do some kind of meditation. There's a ton of research on the benefits of meditation, going back over forty years to Herbert Benson, M.D., and the Mind-Body Institute at Massachussets General Hospital. For years, I thought meditation was something I could not do, even though I knew how good for you it was. Then, at age seventy, I began a practice of transcendental meditation and I've never looked back. If I can meditate, so can you. It's probably one of the healthiest habits—for mind and body—that you can develop. There's a million ways to do it—find one that works for you and make it a habit.

GET SOME SUN

We've become so sun phobic that we slather on 55 SPF just to go to the mailbox. And we have an epidemic of low vitamin D levels, with as high as 70 to 75 percent of the population having levels way below optimal. Ten minutes of unprotected exposure a few times a week is all it really takes to up your vitamin D levels (and even so, I still recommend vitamin D as a supplement). And if you get outdoors and can be around greenery, so much the better. There's a whole science called ecotherapy that demonstrates how exposure to nature—particularly greenery—actually changes mood, reduces depression scores by 71 percent, improves mental health, and even lowers blood pressure.

LEARN TO SLEEP RIGHT!

Sleep is so important to our health that I called it one of the Pillars of Longevity and gave it its own section in the book. Let me sum that section up for you now: During sleep, you replace important biochemicals. You release important hormones. You parse and "clean up" circuits in the brain (which is why we're always told to "sleep on it" when we have a problem). But in order to get all these benefits, you have to have relatively uninterrupted, restful sleep, enough hours to make you feel good during the day. (If you're constantly dragging and fatigued, you're not getting enough. Period.) So, read the sleep section and follow the suggestions. Not sleeping long enough or soundly enough has serious hormonal consequences including raising a hormone that puts on belly fat. Turn the lights off, turn the temperature down, and don't fall asleep with the TV on.

MAKE A GRATITUDE LIST

Anyone who's ever watched TV knows that when someone is about to explode in anger, the first thing you tell him is to take a deep breath. That's because deep breathing is basically incompatible with anger. Well, it's the same thing with gratitude. It's really hard to be pissed off at the world when you're counting (and thinking about) your blessings. When you put some psychic energy on the things you're grateful for—I frequently make a list of the first ten that come to mind—it literally changes your physiology. You can feel it. Your brain relaxes. Your breathing calms. And now, there's actual research showing that practicing gratitude in one way or another has significant health benefits. Plus it feels good. Try it. It's an important practice.

SOCIALIZE

Finally—and perhaps most important of all—connect with other people. A social network—and I'm not just talking about Facebook friends—is one of the best predictors of long (and healthy) life. Remember, every long-lived society on earth has several things in common. They eat a diet absent of processed foods. They stay active every day. And they have strong ties to their community, neighbors, friends, and relatives.

SECTION III

The Secrets of Emotional Intelligence: Underrated and Ignored—Until Now

I want to start by telling a little story about fish.[1] Two young fish are swimming along and they happen upon an older fish swimming the other way. The older fish nods hello and says, "Morning boys, how's the water?" The two young fish keep swimming on for a bit, and eventually one of them turns to the other and says, "What the hell is water?"

To some extent, every one of us is like those young fish, swimming in a milieu, inside a perspective that we take so for granted we can't actually reflect upon it. In popular parlance, it's where we're coming from. It's our way of being, and it's so much a part of us that we don't even notice it. Our "water" is our personal perspective—it's the self-evident fact that we see everything through the view of "me."

---

1 This story comes from the writer David Foster Wallace's 2005 commencement address at Kenyon College in Ohio. If you haven't read this legendary gem, I highly recommend it; simply Google "David Foster Wallace commencement speech." *The Wall Street Journal* published an excellent adaptation on September 19, 2008, which you can find online as well.

And when you think about it, how could we not? Every single thing that happens to you is experienced through the filter of your own brain, eyes, experience, and history. From the news you watch on television to the color of a flower you notice in a garden to the relationships that form the fabric of your life, all are filtered through your eyes and your experience of them. When we begin to look beyond that view, then we begin to see (and hopefully appreciate) how others view things. And that ability is a cornerstone of anti-aging.

If you have kids, you have a living, breathing laboratory to observe how this works. One of the stages of infant development is when babies begin to realize that there's another person in the room. Slowly, over time, they begin to anticipate another person's perspective. When that perspective expands, you can actually see how others might see something, what it's like to live in their shoes, what it's like to see things from their perspective. We call that being well adjusted. You've adjusted your natural, personal "me" perspective to one that incorporates other people and other things.

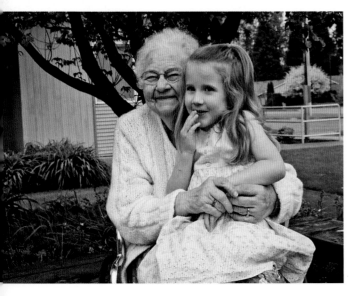

The fish story is a good starting point for what I want to talk about in this section of the book, and the term I've chosen to use for what I'm going to talk about is *emotional intelligence*. Emotional intelligence is what happens when you adjust and expand that "me" perspective—when you're able to take on another person's perspective and, ultimately, the community's perspective. With that achievement comes empathy, sympathy, altruism, the reduction of stress, and a kind of wisdom that in many ways is far more important than IQ. That "adjustment and expansion," or emotional intelligence, is the key (perhaps the most important key) to aging well and living long.

Now, that might seem like a radical concept. But consider this: The longest-lived societies in the world (and we're going to talk about a few of those) don't take supplements. They don't have "designer genes." They're not the beneficiaries of stem cell treatments. They don't have *nanobots* (microscopic electronic devices envisioned by the pioneers of anti-aging medicine) circulating in their bloodstream. They don't go to the gym. Yet, in many of these societies it's not uncommon to see ninety-four-year-olds out tilling the fields, or shepherds in their late eighties climbing mountains with their sheep, or people in their late nineties milking cows before dawn.

How do they do it?

ANOTHER KIND OF STRENGTH

One thing every one of them has is this ambiguous, hard-to-define, amorphous set of qualities that, for want of a better term, I call emotional intelligence. For the purpose of this book, I'm defining emotional intelligence as everything that comes under the heading of relationships, community, and contribution. That includes relationships with self (being at peace, contented, and satisfied) and relationships with others. In fact, a fast definition of emotional intelligence is the ability to deal with people effectively from a place of integrity and self-awareness.

We can trace the most distant roots of the whole concept of emotional intelligence to Darwin, who discovered that there was an evolutionary purpose in having a developed emotional intelligence, even though he didn't call it that. Why? Because you needed to be able to read cues from other people to survive. You needed to know right away: Is this guy friendly? Is he dangerous? Is this wildebeest staring me down on the African Serengeti wanting to be petted or is he about to make me lunch? Life-and-death decisions hinged on the ability to read others' signals. Am I food for this creature or is he food for me? Is this tribesman friend or foe? This kind of intelligence is not the sort that lets you win a chess game or perform brain surgery, but it's an intelligence that's necessary for survival, and as we'll see, it's vital for living well and living long.

Around the 1920s, a psychologist named E. L. Thorndike started to use the term *social intelligence* to describe the skill of understanding and managing other people. Decades later, in 1983, a psychologist named Howard Gardner put forth a theory of multiple intelligences. He defined *interpersonal* intelligence as the capacity to understand the intentions and motivations of other people, whereas *intrapersonal* intelligence was the capacity to understand ourselves; it was the ability to look inward and appreciate our own feelings, fears, and motivations.

In 1990, psychologists Peter Salovey and John Mayer published their landmark article "Emotional Intelligence" in the journal *Imagination, Cognition and Personality*. They basically defined the term as a part of social intelligence that involves "the ability to monitor one's own and others'

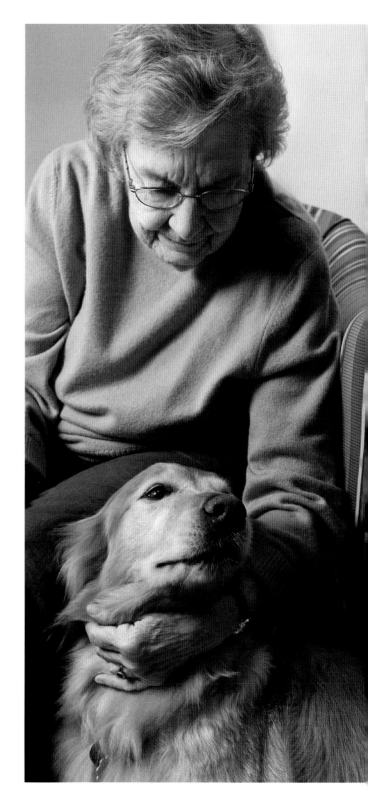

feelings and emotions," and to discriminate among them and use this information as a guide to our own feelings and actions. Emotional intelligence involves the perception of emotion, the ability to reason using emotions, the ability to understand emotion, and the ability to manage emotion, according to Salovey and Mayer. (The term emotional intelligence burst through into the popular consciousness with the 1995 release of psychologist and *New York Times* science writer Daniel Goleman's seminal book *Emotional Intelligence: Why It Matters More Than IQ*, which currently has more than 5 million copies in print worldwide in thirty languages!)

What's important to remember is that despite differences in approach, all of the writers on emotional intelligence talk about the same thing: how you relate; how you adapt; how you handle your own feelings; and how you manage your relationships with others, the wider community, and in fact, the whole planet.

THE FABRIC OF LIFE

Remember those long-lived societies? These are the healthy civilizations that we keep going back to in order to get the secrets of a long and healthy life. These folks have never heard of this peculiarly academic and Western concept of emotional intelligence. If we went and asked them about this they'd look at us like we were crazy. Emotional intelligence is just something that they live with. They don't have a word for it, or books about it, or even a definition of it. It's part of their lives—like exercise, healthy food, and sleep—there for us to observe (and hopefully emulate, or at least adapt to our own circumstances).

If you asked them about emotional intelligence, they'd respond just like those two young fish: "What the heck is emotional intelligence?" It's so much a fabric of their lives that to question or label it would be like asking a fish about water or a person about air.

So, if you look at every one of the longest-lived and healthiest people on the planet, what would you see? What patterns would emerge from their daily activities? What could you say about their relationships to themselves, each other, and their community?

As it turns out, quite a lot.

First and foremost, every one of them has firm family and community connections. Every single study of healthy centenarians shows that the number one thing about them is that they're connected. There is no such thing as a healthy one-hundred-year-old who is isolated. Scientists would be happy to study any such person or people, but the problem is they just don't exist. There are people who defy every other "rule" of long living; those who, for whatever strange reason, are able to smoke, not exercise, take lousy care of their bodies, and somehow, by some miracle of the genetic lottery, live long and seem to be healthy.

But there's not a single person on the planet who has been able to do that in isolation, sans connections to family, community, social group, religious institution, or some other entity that gives their life meaning and purpose.

Not one.

THE ROSETO EFFECT

To give you an idea of the true power of community and connectedness, you need to look no further than Roseto, a close-knit little town of Italian immigrants in Pennsylvania.

The study of the Roseto effect began quite by accident in the 1960s. A local doctor was having a couple of beers with the head of medicine at the University of Oklahoma

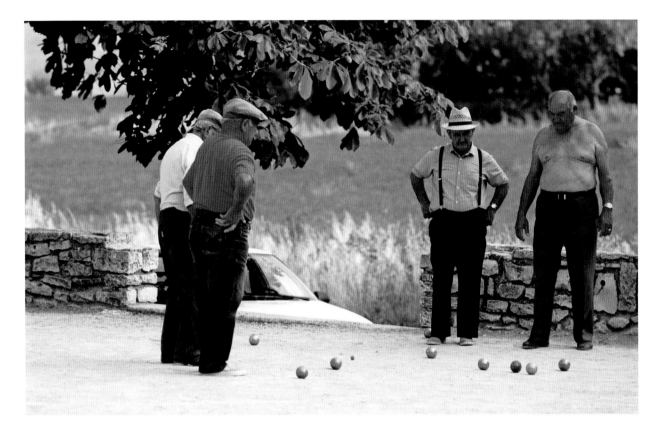

and casually mentioned something he'd noticed: that heart disease in Roseto seemed to be far less prevalent than in the adjoining towns. Word of this spread among the doctor rumor mill and eventually captured the attention of some scientists, who began to seriously study cardiac mortality in Roseto. And what they found was astonishing.

It's well known that the frequency of death from heart disease rises with age, but in Roseto, the rate of death from heart disease was near zero for men aged fifty-five to sixty-four. And for men over sixty-five, the rate of death from heart disease was about half of the national average. Scientists quickly began poking around, extensively interviewing the Rosetans, but this simply deepened the mystery. All the data ruled out any genetic or physical cause of the apparent resistance to heart disease among the people of Roseto.

To make matters worse, or shall we say, more maddening to the conventional medical thinkers, these people had the worst lifestyle imaginable. They smoked like chimneys. They drank. They spent their days in what has been described as "backbreaking, hazardous labor," working underground in the slate mines. Their traditional Italian food was modified and Americanized in a way that would drive a dietitian nuts. Not able to afford the traditional olive oil, for example, they simply fried everything in lard.

So why weren't they dropping like flies from heart disease?

Subsequent research uncovered some very interesting facts. Number one, nearly all the houses in Roseto contained three—count 'em, three—generations of the family. Rosetans didn't put their elderly out to pasture; they incorporated them into community life, treating them as the wise village elders. Those enormous lard-ridden dinner tables offered nourishment and nurturing for the human spirit. The villagers took evening strolls, belonged to numerous social clubs, and participated in church festivals in which the whole community was engaged. And, by the way, both the crime rate in Roseto and the applications for public assistance were zero.

The Roseto effect seemed to be caused by something that escaped traditional investigations.

In their book, *The Power of Clan*, Stewart Wolf, M.D., and sociologist John Bruhn speak about the phenomena seen in Roseto (and elsewhere). They talk of the mutual respect and cooperation that contribute to the health and welfare of a community and also note that lack of concern for others and self-indulgence in general seem to exert the exact opposite influence.

"People are nourished by other people," says Wolf, adding that the characteristics of tight-knit communities predict heart health better than cholesterol or even tobacco use. According to Wolf, an isolated and unconnected person is far more likely to be overwhelmed by the problems of everyday life than someone who is connected in the way the Rosetans are connected. Being overwhelmed then turns into stress, which, as we've seen in this book, is arguably the most destructive of the Four Horsemen of Aging.

"We looked at the social structure of healthy communities," Wolf said, "and found that they are characterized by stability and predictability. In those communities, each person has a clearly defined role in the social scheme."

Now, there are things about life in Roseto in the 1960s that most people reading this book might find suffocating.

It was a town based on predictability and conformity (characteristics it seemed to share with many of the modern long-lived societies like those in Okinawa, Sardinia, and Loma Linda, California). Display of wealth was taboo. People knew from early on what they would be doing. If you were a boy and your father worked in the mine, so would you, and if you were a girl and your mother worked in one of the small blouse factories found in the village, that was likely to be where you'd wind up as well.

Even meals were somewhat ritualized. "Monday," recalled sixty-six-year-old Angie Martocci, "almost everyone in town ate *spezzati* (a spinach and egg soup). Tuesdays, it was spaghetti and gravy (tomato sauce). Wednesday was roast chicken and potatoes. Thursday, spaghetti again. Fish on Fridays, of course. Veal and peppers on Saturday; and antipasto, meatballs, and spaghetti on Sunday."

And always, there was the work ethic. Virtually everyone worked, and they worked toward the shared communal goal of creating a better life for their children. This work ethic and shared goal was part of the fabric of Roseto life, virtually from the town's beginnings. The very first priest in Roseto, Father Pasquale de Nisco, who arrived in 1896, took up a pick and shovel and started breaking ground next to the church to build a graveyard.

TOO MUCH TO CHOOSE FROM

The absence of choice and the emphasis on conformity and the social order is anathema to today's generation, where choices are limitless (and overwhelming) and attention is limited. (It's interesting that until recently, such emphasis on conformity and community was deeply embedded in Japanese life, where people smoke like chimneys and live longer than we do!) But that enormous buffet of choices that we enjoy, in everything from jeans to colleges to mates, comes with a price.

There's a great deal of stress involved in choosing among hundreds of options, a phenomena that has been noted time and again, notably in Barry Schwartz's brilliant book, *The Paradox of Choice: Why More Is Less.*[2] And although none of us would probably be willing to go back to a time when everything was static and predictable, it's worth considering some of the positive aspects of communities where regularity and predictability are the norm and seeing whether we can adapt some of those good things to a more modern life. Especially because whatever those folks are doing seems to be life-extending.

First, let me give you the executive summary on the above-mentioned good things (and then we'll get into the details). Every long-lived society on earth has several things in common: sleep, friends, community, exercise, and a diet absent of processed foods.

Sure, their career and lifestyle choices might be limited. They might not be able to access the Internet or buy any of the two hundred styles of jeans available in any mall. They might not have Facebook and Twitter, or endless channels of digital cable. In fact, life in these places might even seem downright boring compared to what we're used to in modern Western societies. But let's face it—we're not doing so great when it comes to living long and well, and they are. Maybe we can dig a little deeper to find out exactly what works so well for these people and then find a way to graft some of our modern amenities onto those basics that seem to produce such robust health for people in several hidden corners of the globe. Maybe there's a way to have

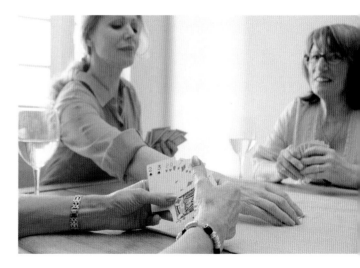

our organic whole-grain cake—and eat it, too. (Hopefully, you'll agree after finishing this book.)

GREEK PARADISE

One of those places where people live longer, healthier lives is the Greek island of Ikaria. Ikaria is the ultimate Mediterranean paradise. It's ninety-nine square miles of mountainous terrain, filled with gorgeous green valleys and eye-popping beaches. (The more I read about Ikaria while researching this book, the harder it was to resist booking a vacation there immediately!) The people of Ikaria routinely live into their nineties and beyond. In fact, they reach the age of ninety at four times the rate that we do in the United States! More important, they have far fewer years of disease and poor health (remember "rectangularizing the curve"?). As Anderson Cooper put it on his CNN special on Ikaria, "I'm guessing [that] living on a Greek island doesn't exactly lead to depression, but for those of us who can't pack up and move to a Mediterranean paradise, we can reap the benefits of Ikarian culture at home."

My sentiments exactly.

---

2 You can watch the twenty-minute video of Schwartz's entertaining presentation on choice all over the Internet, notably on the www.TED.com site or on YouTube. Or you can Google "Schwartz video paradox of choice." Highly recommended!

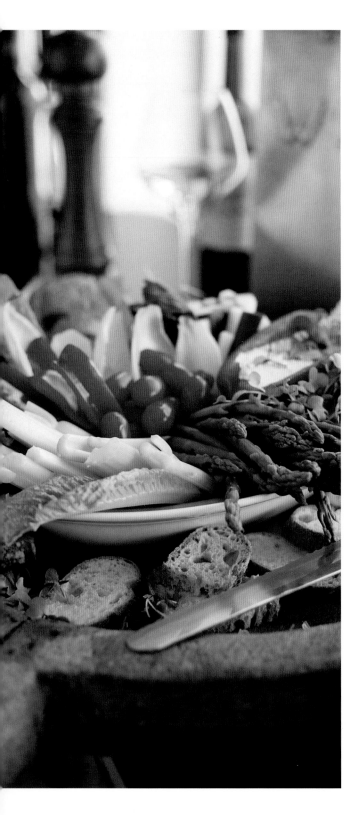

One person who knows firsthand what it looks like to "transport" the best of Ikarian culture to America is chef and author Diane Kochilas. Kochilas's Ikarian mom (and aunt on her dad's side) lived to age ninety-five, and her husband's paternal Ikarian grandmother lived to age ninety-eight! Diane herself grew up in an Ikarian home in Queens, New York. Here's how she describes growing up:

"We always had a stream of guests dropping in and our kitchen table was always ready to accommodate them. The foods were usually simple: a salad, boiled greens (picked in the New York of the 1960s during countless Sunday outings to Long Island), some cheese, bread, olives, some bean dish or other that was my father's specialty. Maybe a savory pie filled with more greens, usually spinach. Olive oil was part of every dish, even many of the sweets we ate, even then, before the Mediterranean Diet was discovered. But most of all, it was the conviviality of it all I remember, the open hospitality, the de rigueur offering of food and wine to anyone who came through our door."

We've covered foods for longevity elsewhere in this book, so let's concentrate on those other aspects of how Ikarians live. As we'll see, the lifestyle of the Ikarians has a lot in common with the lifestyle of the other longest-lived peoples in the world. And that isn't an accident.

Take, for example, Okinawa.

This little Pacific archipelago is about a thousand miles from Tokyo and has been described by explorer and researcher Dan Buettner as a "Japanese Hawaii" with a "warm, temperate climate, palm trees, and sugar-sand beaches hemming a turquoise sea." Okinawans have one of the highest life expectancies on the planet and one of highest centenarian rates (about 5 per 10,000 people). Compared to the United States, they have one-fifth the rate of cardiovascular disease, one-fourth the rate of breast and prostate cancer, and one-third of the rate of dementia.

One Okinawa senior, Fumiyasu Yamakawa, cycles to the beach every morning at 4:30, swims for a half hour, runs for a half hour, does yoga, and then meets with a group of other seniors. They stand in a circle and laugh.

"Why is that?" asked Buettner.

"It's vitamin S," replied Yamakawa. "You smile in the morning and it fortifies you all day."

No kidding.

There's something in Okinawan life called a *moai*, which, according to Buettner, means "meeting for a common purpose." It could be a group of lifelong friends or it could be a social support network. Doesn't matter. It's the fabric of social connection that's important here, and it appears to be central to Okinawan longevity. It might not be the single cause of long life—after all, Okinawans also eat in a healthy way and exercise regularly—but it sure is a big part of the secret of living longer and better.

And it's not just the Okinawans. In every area of the globe where people live long, robust lives, social connections are essential. In Sardinia, for example, Buettner tells us that men gather in the street each afternoon to laugh with and at each other. (There aren't too many better ways to reduce stress than that.) The Adventists in Loma Linda, California, are encouraged to volunteer through their church and consistently told Buettner that they found a sense of purpose doing just that, often staving off depression by focusing on helping other people. And in the Nicoya Peninsula off Costa Rica, the fourth of Buettner's "Blue Zones," where people live the longest and maintain their health into their ninth and tenth decades, the oldest people live with their families, not by themselves or in assisted living homes. Their children and grandchildren

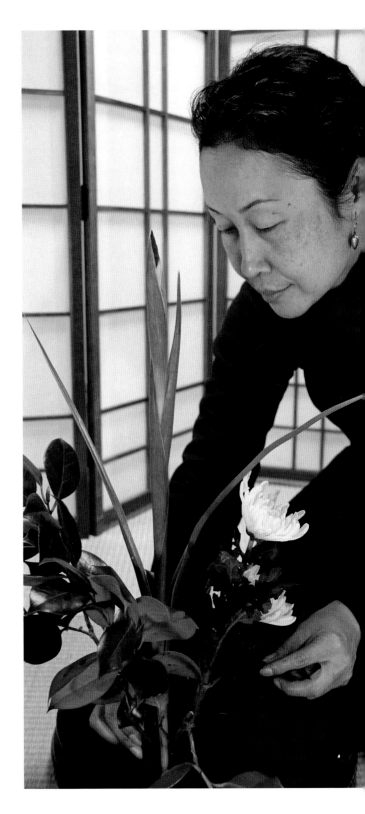

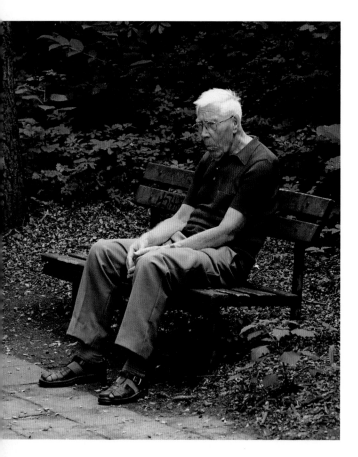

YOU'VE GOT TO HAVE FRIENDS

Closer to home, one of the most famous studies of successful aging is the MacArthur Foundation Study, which is widely believed to be the most comprehensive and extensive study on aging in America. Many of the healthy, long-lived people in the MacArthur Foundation Study report that they thrive because of social bonds with family and friends. Many credit friendship with being the single most important factor in keeping their lives active and emotionally stable.

Geriatrician John Rowe, M.D., of Mount Sinai Medical Center, is the chair of the MacArthur Foundation Research Network on Successful Aging. Here's what he had to say about social connections:

"We know four important things about the connection between social relations and health, and all apply to older people. First, isolation, a lack of social ties however measured, is a powerful risk factor for poor health. Second, social support in its many forms—emotional, actual physical assistance, and so on—has direct positive effects on health. Equally important, but less widely known, social support can buffer or reduce some of the health-related effects of aging. Finally, and perhaps most important, no single type of support is uniformly effective for all people and all situations."

As the song famously says, "You've got to have friends."

"Human beings are not meant to live solitary lives," adds Rowe. "Talking, touch, and relating to others are essential to our well-being."

Caring for others extends to the nonhuman universe as well. In a classic experiment in 1977, researchers gave each resident of a nursing home a plant. Half the residents were told the plant would be cared for by the staff while the other half were told that the plant was their responsibility.

provide support and a sense of belonging and purpose. Their neighbors visit frequently. They find joy in the physical chores of everyday life. "They know how to listen, laugh, and appreciate what they have," says Buettner.

What all these folks have in common is emotional intelligence. It's their "water." It's their way of being. It's what keeps them "young" even when, as so many of them have, they reach the age of one hundred.

If there's any one take-away message that stands out in the studies of all these robust and healthy older people it's this—social connections matter. Social connections are life-extending and health promoting. This has been demonstrated in virtually every study of centenarians or of long-lived societies like the ones in Okinawa and Ikaria.

THE RIGHT OF KIND OF EMOTIONAL SUPPORT

Nearly all the research on robust aging has found an interesting distinction between emotional support and direct assistance. And the best way to illustrate that distinction is to remind you of when you learned to ride a bike.

Most of us can remember the exact moment when we were able to remove those training wheels and feel the exhilaration of being able to balance on the two-wheeler. I know I do. It was a Sunday night in front of our apartment in Jackson Heights, Queens, New York. I was about eight years old and my father took off the training wheels and began to run alongside the bike, helping to balance it from behind as I pedaled with some uncertainty and wobbliness, slowly picking up speed, until he was finally able to let go as I shrieked, "I can do it!"

That moment of autonomy, which most of us have experienced, at least those of us who learned to ride a two-wheeler, is significant. And it has a lot to teach us about aging well. My father provided emotional support, but he also knew when to let go and let me do it myself. In research on aging, it's been shown time and again that emotional support fosters autonomy and well-being, but the kind of direct assistance (helping someone with a task or doing it for him) is associated with the exact opposite.

"Even if that assistance were given with the best intentions, providing *more assistance than people really need* can reduce their belief in themselves, as well as their ability to function," says geriatrician John Rowe, M.D. "Giving direct assistance in excess of what people need or perhaps want is a frequent, well-meant, but mistaken form of support" (italics mine).

"The current slogan of 'use it or lose it' applies not only to exercise and athletic ability, but to basic physical and cognitive function as well," says Rowe. Or as Tennyson put it in his classic poem *Ulysses*, "Shine in use!"

People feel best when they're self-sufficient and making a contribution to others, when they're participating in life, and we don't really need a scientific study to prove that (although we have plenty of them). Nothing extends life and well-being like the feeling of competence, and nothing destroys it like a lack of autonomy. Support is one thing; dependence is another.

The people who took care of their plant had better medical outcomes, better blood tests, fewer visits to the doctor, and higher scores on virtually every measure of well-being that the researchers could come up with. Just caring for a plant improved their health measurably and significantly! And that's a plant!

One of the participants in the MacArthur Foundation Study was eighty-two-year-old Stanley, who told the researchers that, besides his many human connections, his nonhuman social bonds were also vitally important in keeping him healthy and happy. Gardening, for example. "If you're involved in the garden, you're involved in living things that depend on you, and you're in a sense in a spiritual relationship with them—you do for them and they do for you," he told them. "I have a dog, too, and the same can be said for her, even more so. The joy is rather like friendship, and keeps you young, because you keep concerned and healthy."

Rowe sums it up perfectly: "Loneliness breeds both illness and early death," he says. "As a rule, people whose connections with others are relatively strong—through family (including marriage), friendships, and organizational memberships—live longer."

In fact, for people who have few relationships, or whose relationships with others are weak, the risk of death is between two and four times greater than it is for those who have strong social bonds. This is regardless of age, race, socioeconomic status, physical health, smoking, alcohol use, physical activity, or even obesity. "The bottom line is we do not outgrow our need for others," Rowe says. "The life-giving effect of close social relationships holds throughout the life course."

Having friends, community, and social relationships even protects your brain and helps preserve your memory. Harvard researchers looked at data from 16,000 study participants from the Health and Retirement Study. The researchers checked for marital status, volunteer activity, and frequency of contact with children, neighbors, and parents. Based on this information, they assigned each participant a "social integration" score. (Those with the most contact with others received the highest scores, and those with the least contact received the lowest.)

Then, the researchers gave the participants a standard battery of memory tests. Those with the lowest "social integration" scores had much greater loss of memory than those with the highest scores. In fact, their memory declined at twice the rate as those who had the most social connections! "Our study provides evidence that social integration delays memory loss among elderly Americans," the researchers concluded.

The protective effects of social relationships aren't just limited to the brain. In a classic 1979 study of the residents of Alameda County, California, researchers found that people who lacked social and community ties were far more likely to die during a nine-year follow-up period than those who had more extensive and meaningful contact with others, regardless of any other health practices, including smoking.

David Snowdon, Ph.D., author of *Aging with Grace*, puts it quite well: "It has now been convincingly demonstrated," he writes, "that marriage, membership in churches, clubs or other social groups, and regular contact with family and friends all reduce the risk of death from the major killers, coronary heart disease and stroke."

John Rowe (of the MacArthur Foundation Study) agrees: "The more [that] older people participate in social relationships, the better their overall health," he says. Rowe points out that there are all kinds of venues for social contact and support that promote healthy and successful aging, such as phone conversations, visits from family, neighbors, and friends, participation in religious groups, and attendance at meetings of organizations. In fact, the two strongest predictors of well-being, according to Rowe's research, are frequency of visits with friends and frequency of attending meetings of organizations. "All these interactions [predict] robust aging," Rowe writes, "an index of overall well-being that includes involvement in productive activity, emotional and mental status and functional level." "Interestingly," he adds, "the more meaningful the contribution in a given activity, the greater its impact on health."

So if there is something you care about passionately and that has deep personal meaning to you—volunteering at an animal shelter or participating in Habit for Humanity, for example—you get double the life-extending benefit!

The bottom line: Get involved. It's a good bet it will extend your life.

A WORD FROM THE WISE

At this point, we've come full circle. We've discussed the goal of longevity that is to "square the curve," making old age so healthy and robust that it no longer seems like anything we need to dread and doesn't even look like anything our parents would recognize as old age. Not only that, but the goal is to keep it that way right up to the very end. We've discussed the major systems of the body, how they (typically) break down, and how they can be protected, even enhanced! And finally, in this section, we've discussed the personal and social aspects of living well and long: emotional intelligence, social connectedness, and the inevitable wisdom and peace that come with both.

And here's a little secret: It's all pretty simple.

Dan Buettner interviewed many extraordinary people for his research on healthy aging, but one of the wonderful folks he spoke to stands out: Kamada.

Kamada is 102 years old, healthy, active, serene, and beautiful. Surely, she knows something about living long and well. Not surprisingly, Buettner asked her what the secret was to living to 102. Here's what she said:

"Eat your vegetables, have a positive outlook, be kind to people, and smile."

As a simple prescription for a long life, and, as a bonus, for wisdom, it doesn't get much better than that.

The take-home message of this chapter is pretty simple: Live life well, reduce stress by simplifying your life, keep your friends and families close, and contribute to others.

It's hard to come up with a scientifically accurate prescription that dictates how you might accomplish all that, but I'm going to give you my own personal take on how to develop a program for emotional intelligence. Think of it as a personal training program for developing both inner peace and social connectedness. I can't claim that this list of suggestions is either perfect or complete, but it's what I would personally suggest if you were my client and I were your personal trainer in the field of longevity and robust living.

Developing Emotional Intelligence: Your Personal Training Program for Extending Life

Shakespeare's famous words "know thyself" were never more appropriate, because emotional intelligence begins with self-awareness. (Self-awareness morphs easily into empathy and from there into compassion, caring, and contribution.) By developing an inner sense of peace and contentment, you will not only reduce stress and increase well-being, but you will also develop precisely the kinds of social connections that have been found to extend life in virtually every study of healthy robust aging that's ever been done.

This is my personal training program for developing both. My Emotional Intelligence Workbook on page 244 may help you get the ball rolling.

1. Acknowledge Someone

An acknowldgement is a simple statement of another's value. It's a small act that can contribute enormously to the well-being of another and will also make you feel good at the same time (trust me on this one). You can acknowledge the most significant person in your life, or you can acknowledge a stranger, or both. Just tell them what they mean to you.

How about thanking a waiter for excellent service and for making your dinner a pleasant experience? Or telling your partner how much his or her smile lights up the room? Approach the world with new eyes and look for an opportunity where you can express even a small amount of thanks to someone every single day. Look for opportunities where you can acknowledge somebody's worth, especially when there are no strings attached. Think about how you feel when somebody tells you what a great job you're doing or what a difference you make in that person's life. We don't get acknowledged enough, and more important, we don't give enough acknowledgments. Acknowledge somebody on a daily basis. It takes virtually no time or effort and repays in dividends that would make Wall Street blush.

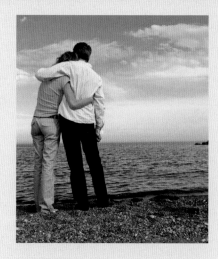

2. Practice Forgiveness

Full disclosure: I actually think that forgiveness (together with the next item I'm going to talk about, gratitude) is the key to happiness and longevity.

In my very, very first book, *Shape Up* (it's out of print, you'll never find it), I told the story of a young New York City cop named Terry McDonald. McDonald was on patrol in New York City during the early 1990s, when crime was at an all-time high in the city. He got shot in a gunfight during a robbery attempt and was paralyzed. The bullet went into his spine and he never was able to walk again.

I remember this story when it happened. I lived in New York at the time and it was headline news, particularly in the *New York Post* and the *New York Daily News* for several days. People were outraged and angry about the injustice of it all, and there was an outpouring of sympathy for McDonald and his family.

McDonald had every reason to be bitter and hateful. He was cut down in the prime of his life by a heartless young punk, confined to a wheelchair in his thirties, and unable to live a normal life with his wife and two kids (with a third on the way, thank you very much). Who would blame him for being bitter and angry? McDonald, however, didn't quite see it that way.

He decided to forgive.

It wasn't easy. But he did it. Somehow, over time, he decided to forgive the person who shot him and release the anger he felt. He decided to find the opportunity in his tragedy and he wound up taking his experience and turning it into a career about bringing people together. When last heard from, he was leading peace marches in Ireland between the two warring factions there—in his wheelchair.

Here's what forgiveness is not: It's not about making it be "okay" that someone did something really horrible and unforgivable. It is about releasing something that is poisoning you. If you think of anger as a little ball of fire that you're holding on to in your hand, consider who's getting burned. Who does anger and resentment ultimately hurt?

Exactly.

Anger takes up psychic space and it drives your stress hormones through the roof. Stress, as we've seen throughout this book, shortens

your life. On a more metaphysical level, anger and resentment poison and pollute your soul. Who needs them? And one thing can be said clearly and unequivocally about the long-lived people mentioned throughout this book: They are not angry. Not even a little.

Forgiveness is an art, and like any art, it needs practice. It's also a muscle, and like a muscle, it needs training. A good way to start is by making a list of everyone for whom you feel any anger or resentment.

Then, forgive someone on the list.

As an exercise, put yourself in that person's place and try to see the world through his eyes. What would it have been like to be that person while he was doing whatever he was doing that made you feel angry? Maybe whatever he did to you was born of his own fear or frustration or ignorance. Whatever. Remember this is not about "excusing" him or making him "right"; it's about you letting go of the disappointment, rage, frustration, or anger that you're left with.

I don't recommend that you start practicing your forgiveness muscle by trying to forgive the worst offender on your list. (That would be like a beginning golfer taking on Tiger Woods!) So you may not be able to forgive the stepdad who abused you, but you may be able to forgive the person who cut in front of you in line at the cafeteria, or the waitress who brought the wrong dish, or the coworker who didn't thank you

for the work you did that saved his butt. The important thing is to start practicing with something you can actually manage. Remember, it's a muscle. It needs practice. You don't start doing bicep curls with fifty-pound (23 kg) weights; you start with little hand weights. And it's the same with forgiveness.

Forgiveness is an amazing "muscle." If you develop it, it will extend your life and your well-being and those of everybody around you as well.

3. Volunteer

"Volunteering makes the heart grow stronger," says David Eisner, CEO of the Corporation for National and Community Service.

He's absolutely right. A boatload of research has found a significant connection between volunteering and good health. Volunteers have lower mortality rates, greater functional ability, and lower rates of depression later in life than those who do not volunteer, according to a comprehensive 2007 report. Here are a few of the findings from the report, titled *Health Benefits of Volunteering: A Review of Recent Research*:

→ Older volunteers are most likely to receive the most health benefits from volunteering. These benefits include improved physical and mental health.

→ Volunteering leads to greater life satisfaction and lower rates of depression.

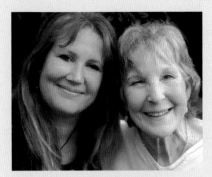

→ Volunteering and physical well-being are part of a positive reinforcing cycle.

→ Individuals who volunteer live longer.

It's more than a little interesting that the rate of volunteering in any given state in the United States is strongly correlated with the physical health of that state's population!

And no wonder. A study of longitudinal data from the Americans' Changing Lives survey found that those who volunteered reported higher levels of happiness, life satisfaction, self-esteem, sense of control over life, and general physical health.

Not a bad group of benefits just for helping other people.

If you've spent any time at all around what is unfortunately called *the self-help movement* (what I would prefer to call the *personal growth movement*), you may have attended a weekend seminar by one of the great motivational leaders, such as my friends Mark Victor Hansen, Jack Canfield, or T. Harv Eker. At any one of these seminars, you can find dozens of volunteers who do all these amazing things for the participants. These guys arrive early and stay late, working insanely long hours for . . . let's see now . . . no pay. Zero. Nada. Zilch.

Why do they do it?

Well, it may have started back in the 1970s with the brilliant teacher and innovator Werner Erhard. (Sharp-eyed readers may have noted that Werner is thanked in every book that I've ever written and will continue to be for as long as I'm writing.) When Werner had a weekend seminar called *EST training* (which later evolved into what is now *The Forum*), he began the concept of assisting at seminars, and he did it with a very simple rule: He told volunteers at his centers that the value they created for the organization by assisting had to be bettered by the value they created for themselves by doing it. He demanded that the situation be not only a win-win for the assistant volunteers but also that the assistants win even more!

This philosophy has permeated every personal growth organization I've ever seen in action, and the energetic volunteers who "work the room" at all those weekend events will be the first to tell you what a gift and a privilege it is to do so.

Why?

Because contributing to the world feels good.

Remember those long-lived societies we keep coming back to? They don't have personal growth seminars, nor do they have formal organizations for volunteering, and many of them don't even know how to spell the word charity, let alone what it means.

But every one of them volunteers on a regular basis. They may not call it volunteering, preferring to consider it just the part of life when you help out where needed. But help out they do, whether through their church, community, *maoi*, or circle of friends or just by bringing a dish to the village potluck dinner. "Volunteering" is simply a way of life for them; it's their "water."

Volunteering lets you focus on something other than yourself, at least for a while, providing a kind of therapeutic "time-out" from self-involvement. And that's something from which most of us who grew up as part of the "me" generation could well benefit.

It allows us to feel we're contributing and that we're productive, and that is one of the most life-extending, life-enhancing feelings on the planet. It produces feelings of accomplishment, it engages our compassion and empathy circuits, and—although this hasn't been tested—I'm absolutely sure it produces beneficial biochemical changes in our brain.

And of course, it reduces our stress hormones.

4. Make a Gratitude List

Gratitude is the other side of forgiveness, and together they are the cornerstones of any youthful, energetic, happy life.

Most of us don't spend nearly enough time actually focusing on what we have and what we're grateful for.

Years ago, Steven Sills recorded a song called "Love the One You're With" that spoke to a generation of baby boomers. Maybe it's time to recall the metaphysical sentiment of that song, which was that we would all be better off celebrating what we have instead of always questing after something that we don't have.

We live in a very acquisitive, materialistic society, and it's easy to get caught up in aspiring to "something better." Although there's nothing wrong with wanting more out of life, what often happens is that we focus so intensely on what we want (and what, by definition, we don't have) that we forget what we do have.

Gratitude is the enemy of stress. It's hard to be angry, frustrated, or resentful—all emotions that produce bucketfuls of stress hormones— when you're taking a deep breath and thanking the universe for the gifts you've been given.

The thing of it is, when people begin the exercise of making a gratitude list, something profoundly changes for them. I've seen it countless times. You can even try it for yourself (and I hope you do). Simply make a list of any ten things you're grateful for. They can range from the seemingly insignificant (like your new wide-screen TV) to the profoundly important (your relationship with your son).

You can be grateful for the ability to see or hear, for the ability to smell a rose outside your dining room window, for your new computer, for the good health of your loyal ferret. Doesn't matter. Just focusing on gratitude and satisfaction will reduce your stress hormones, brighten your day, and increase your well-being.

Studies on gratitude suggest that subjects who were instructed to keep gratitude journals actually showed higher levels of positive emotions, more life satisfaction, more vitality, lower levels of depression, and lower levels of stress. You get better quality sleep. You have less pain. You're more likely to exercise, and you're more likely to actually make progress toward important personal goals. That sure sounds to me like the beginnings of a prescription for longevity.

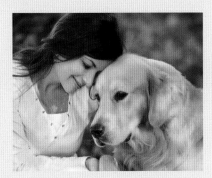

I can't prove it, but my guess from reading interviews with dozens of folks in the long-lived "Blue Zones" of the planet is that gratitude is a deep and persistent part of their lives and that they feel it profoundly on a daily basis. Innkeeper Ishikichi Tanaka, for example, ninety-nine years young, summed it up wonderfully:

"I never pray for a long life, but I just express my gratitude for another day. It reminds me that every day is important."

Make that list and then read it every single morning for thirty days.

CONCLUSION

A Plan for You: The 7 × 3 Matrix of Healthy Aging

Thank goodness for the vision of three young guys named Steve Chen, Chad Hurley, and Jawed Karim working out of a garage in Menlo Park, California, in 2005. Because without them, we wouldn't have YouTube, and I wouldn't be able to start this chapter with the following request:

1. Go to your computer.
2. Go to either Google or YouTube and type in: "Never Underestimate an Old Gal."
3. Watch.
4. Return to this book.

Okay, on the off-chance that you might not have followed my directions to the T or would prefer to watch the video another time, let me give you the summary of what happens on that clip, which, as of this writing, is sweeping the Internet.

The video was made during the finals of a salsa dance test in a big auditorium somewhere in South America. A handsome, fit Latin man in a white suit enters from one side of the stage while his female partner, dressed in sequins, enters from the other. Over the course of the next 4 minutes and 45 seconds they put on a dazzling display of classic salsa. There's attitude, sexiness, athleticism, and dazzling technique, some of which includes leg extensions, lifts, spins, and dips that produce jaw-dropping amazement in the audience and result in a tumultuous standing ovation at the end of the routine. It is, to be blunt, awe-inspiring.

Oh, I forgot to mention: The female partner in this duo is eighty-seven years old.

Now, let's be clear: Following every piece of advice in this book doesn't guarantee you'll be performing world-class salsa routines in your ninth decade. Or that you'll be conducting grueling workouts in Malibu like our friend Don Wildman. Or still teaching and training jujitsu like ninety-year old Helio Gracie, or choreographing until her death at age ninety-six like the great modern dancer Martha Graham, or painting "Young Bather with Sand Shovel" at the age of ninety like Pablo Picasso, or even shepherding flocks in the mountains like many of the ninety-plus-year-old citizens in Sardinia. Fact is, we don't completely understand why some people are vital and robust and still having fun forty years after some of their contemporaries can barely drag themselves off their recliners.

But, we've got some ideas.

This concluding chapter is, in some ways, the most personal chapter in the book because the opinions expressed here are solely my own. These are the core strategies that seem to me, after reading as much research as I could get my hands on about living long and well, to be the most important things you can do to increase the odds of a long and healthy life.

Remember, we don't have any multi-decade studies that examine the precise effect of each one of these strategies, and we probably never will. (We also don't have any double-blind studies that "prove" water puts out fire, but the fire department of every major city acts on the assumption that it's true!) So here, for what it's worth, is my own "water puts out fire" theory, boiled down into a matrix I call the "7 × 3 Matrix of Healthy Aging." These are the strategies I try to follow, and although I can't prove it to the satisfaction of the most hard-nosed scientists in the world of academia, it's a good bet that these strategies will increase the odds that you'll be among those left standing, jogging, shepherding, painting, dancing the salsa, or just plain having fun long after many of your contemporaries have sadly departed this universe.

And one more thing, a footnote, if you will: If you happen to be reading this book and your age has any number less than four as the first digit, congratulations. Here's what I've discovered about anti-aging strategies and life: They parallel what happens with a car.

Let me explain.

I drive a really nifty little two-seater car that never breaks down. But it only has 30,000 miles on it. When a car has low mileage, you will not usually see the result of poor car maintenance. You can lease a car and totally neglect it for the first three years of its life (and the length of the typical lease) and nothing will happen. Ignore the oil changes, drive it into the ground, don't rotate the tires—it doesn't much matter because the car's youth will ensure that it can weather the damage (which is, after all, cumulative). By the time you trade in the car, it will still perform pretty much the way it was when you drove it off the lot. You won't notice a difference in performance at all.

But the next owner will.

Most damage, to cars and to the human body, is cumulative. So the person who takes up smoking a pack of cigarettes a day doesn't notice a change in his health for the first year, maybe even the first twenty, except perhaps an annoying hacking cough when he wakes up that usually goes away by midday. His first wakeup call is when he gets that X-ray with a suspicious spot on it, and that might well be twenty years down the road. The first "symptom" of heart disease is often death, and high blood pressure, which seriously increases the risk, usually has no symptoms at all. The same with diabetes.

But back to the car.

So my lovely little convertible performs great at 30,000 miles, and you would expect that it would no matter how it was taken care of. But the fact is, I take great care of it. It never misses a service or an oil change. It's garaged. The tires are changed regularly and even rotated pretty much on schedule. So why do I do that?

Because when the car has 75,000 miles, or 175,000 miles, I expect it will still run great.

I have good reason to suspect that. Because my *other* car, a fifteen-year-old version of the new one, has nearly 180,000 miles and I've taken care of it in the same way as I take care of the newer car, and guess what—it never breaks down. It runs like a dream, and except for a little aging of the mechanical parts, it's almost as good as new. Sure, it creaks a bit here and there, but it's certainly as good as cars half its age, and it still elicits smiles and waves when I drive it with the top down on the Pacific Coast Highway.

I was thinking about that this morning as I got off the tennis court. I feel the way I felt when I was in my thirties, maybe better. Of the major complaints that are a daily occurrence in people my age—constipation, low back pain, joint aches, inflexibility, low energy—I have none. (The sound you hear is me knocking wood—I never said I wasn't suspicious or grateful!)

When I fill out those medical questionnaires (e.g., "have you ever had . . ."), I draw a big circle around all the "no's" on the page. And I'm 100 percent convinced that the reason that is so is because I do most of what I've talked about in this book. I started at age thirty-eight, but I know people who've started a lot later than that. (Friends of mine, like the fit and muscular Jeff Life, M.D., the "poster boy" for the anti-aging clinic Cenegenics in Las Vegas, started at fifty-seven.) The point is, start now. Even if you don't notice the results while you're young, look around you in your decades that start with five, six, and seven and beyond, and wonder why everyone else looks and sounds and feels old and you don't.

And trust me with one more thing—it's worth it.

TWENTY-ONE STRATEGIES FOR AGING WELL

So here's the 7 × 3 Matrix of Healthy Aging. The "7 × 3" comes from the fact that there are three categories—food, supplements, and lifestyle—each of which contains seven simple strategies. It's the program I try to follow on a daily basis and I hope you will, too.

1. Food: Age Well with the Right Foods

Hippocrates, the father of modern medicine, said, "Let food be thy medicine and medicine be thy food." How right he was. Remember, heart disease isn't a Lipitor deficiency. If you give the body what it needs in the way of fuel, it will make everything it needs to keep you healthy, glowing, and robust for decades. And though there are probably hundreds of different diets (or eating styles), there are a few standout foods and beverages that seem to be found in the diets of the healthiest people on earth. These are the ones that form the core seven strategies below.

Green tea: Arguably the healthiest beverage in the world, or at least one of the top five, green tea contains compounds that have been found to reduce the risk of esophageal cancer, breast cancer, and heart disease. Mayo Clinic scientists found that components in green tea kill human prostate cancer cells in test tubes. Green tea may also help you lose weight. Emerging research suggests that the chemicals found in green tea may also protect the brain against Alzheimer's and Parkinson's diseases. I recommend a minimum of two cups a day and think that if you can drink five you're golden!

Nuts: Some of the largest and most important long-term studies of diet and health have shown a consistent 30 to 50 percent lower risk of heart attacks or heart disease associated with eating nuts several times each week. Nuts are a regular part of the daily menu in virtually every one of the Blue Zones. "We don't know if it's the omega-3s in the nuts or the fact that by eating nuts they're not eating salty chips, but we do know that people who eat a handful of nuts four times a week live on average two years longer than those who don't," *The Blue Zones* author Dan Buettner told Diane Sawyer on *Good Morning America*.

The magic number from the research seems to be one ounce (28 g) four to five times a week. Enjoy! (And it doesn't much matter which kinds of nuts you choose.)

Beans: Beans are the cornerstone of every one of the diets in the Blue Zones. They reduce the risk of cancer, heart disease, and diabetes. One study found that women who eat the most beans had a 38 percent reduction in the risk for diabetes, not surprising because beans are one of the greatest sources of fiber on the planet and fiber helps stabilize blood sugar. (A high-fiber intake is also associated with a lower risk of colon cancer.) When it comes to antioxidants, beans are among the richest sources, with red beans, red kidney beans, and pinto beans being particularly outstanding. And in one major research study, four or more one-cup servings of cooked legumes per week was enough to decrease the risk of heart disease by 22 percent. I recommend four servings per week.

Grass-fed meat: As of this writing, the controversies and misunderstandings about meat and health continue to rage. (We won't resolve the debate here.) It's worth noting, however, that even in the Blue Zones, people eat meat. They just don't eat it that often and they don't eat the processed, factory-farmed junk that we routinely consume in Western societies. Grass-fed meat is absent of steroids, antibiotics, and growth hormones, and the fat is

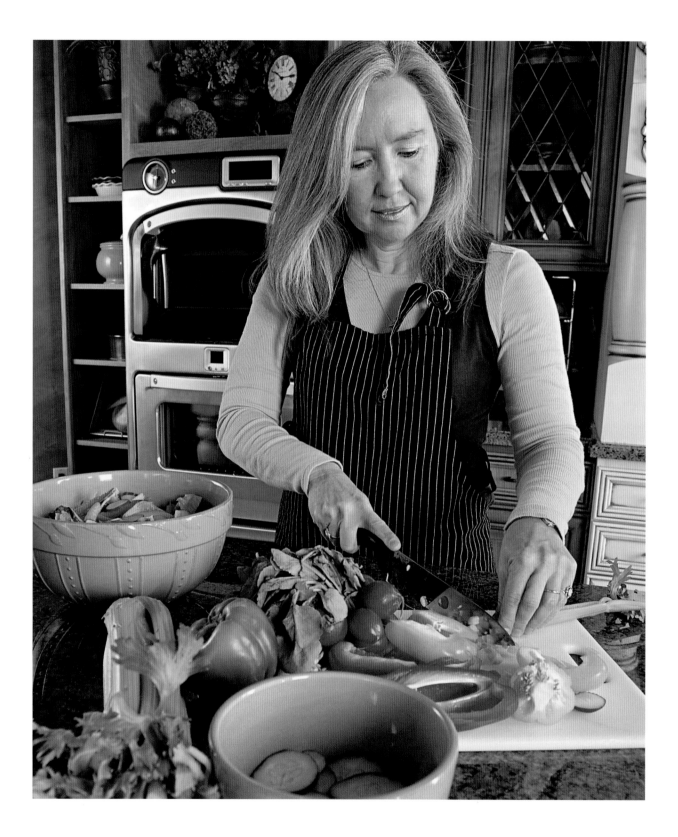

rich in omega-3 properties and cancer-fighting conjugated linolenic acid (CLA). And meat remains one of the best sources of protein and vitamin B12. My recommendation: Eat grass-fed red meat once a week.

Fish: Fish is a major component in the diet of virtually every long-lived society. Fish is the ultimate anti-aging food. High in protein, low in calories, it's a nutritional bonanza. Cold-water fatty fish like (wild) salmon, sardines, mackerel, and herring contain omega-3 fats that protect the brain and the heart, improve mood, and lower blood pressure and triglycerides. I recommend a minimum of two servings per week, but there's no problem with eating it more often than that!

Berries (and other fruits): I can't say enough good things about berries, but I'll mention just a few, starting with my favorite, blueberries. In a series of remarkable experiments, James Joseph, Ph.D., of the U.S. Department of Agriculture Human Nutrition Center on Aging at Tufts University found that when you feed animals blueberries, they behave like young stud muffins. Motor function, memory, and performance on assorted tests for muscle coordination and strength all improve. Cranberries are high in *phenolic acids*, plant chemicals known to protect against a wide range of health conditions. Raspberries are loaded with fiber, calcium, magnesium, phosphorus, potassium, vitamin C … should I go on? And they're also one of the best sources in the world of a plant chemical known as *ellagic acid* (also found in strawberries), which has been shown to inhibit the growth of tumors. I recommend a cup of berries every day or at least five days a week. But don't neglect other great anti-aging fruits like apples, grapefruit, and cherries. A twenty-six-year prospective study of men

in Sweden provided evidence that fruit intake in general is associated with greater longevity.

Vegetables: You can't find a Blue Zone where vegetables aren't a big part of every meal. The vegetable kingdom is rich in antioxidants and anti-inflammatories, not to mention cancer-fighting plant compounds like indoles (found in the cabbage family), carotenoids, fiber, vitamins, minerals, and phytochemicals, all of which have substantial health benefits and can reasonably be assumed to keep you alive and disease-free for a long time. Data from two of the longest running studies of diet and health ever done—the Nurses Health Study and the Health Professionals Follow-Up Study—showed that men and women who ate the most vegetables (nine or ten servings a day) had a 20 percent lower risk of coronary artery disease compared to those who ate the least (only two or three servings a day). Other studies have shown an even greater reduction in risk of heart attacks (38 percent), and still others have shown decreased risk for stroke, diabetes, and a variety of cancers.

You don't have to be vegetarian to get the benefits of a high-vegetable intake—just eat them at every single meal. There's no maximum recommendation, but at minimum try for seven servings a day (nine is even better). It's not as much as you might think considering that one serving is only a half a cup.

So there you have it, and it winds up being pretty simple: green tea, nuts, beans, grass-fed meat, fish, berries and fruits, and vegetables. A glass of wine here and there wouldn't hurt either, nor would a square or two of dark chocolate. With minor variations, those foods seem to be part of the diet of just about every place on earth where folks live a long time in good health.

2. Get Nutritional Insurance with the Right Supplements

Okay, I can easily imagine the obvious question—if most of the people who live long and healthy lives don't even know what a supplement is, why would nutritional supplements be on the short list of strategies for a life-extension program? Can't you manage perfectly well without them?

Well, yes, you can. Especially if you live in the lush paradise of a Greek Isle and walk ten miles (16 km) a day and eat only organic, locally grown food, breathe clean air, and enjoy low levels of stress.

Unfortunately, most of us don't.

I look at supplements as a high-tech delivery system for the nutrients that, in the best of all possible worlds, we would get from food. But most of us don't get anything like the optimal doses of certain nutrients from our food, even when we're eating really, really well.

There are two major reasons for this—besides the fact that most of us don't eat all that terrifically in the first place. One, nutrient levels in food have fallen over the years, due in large part to the way food is grown, processed, and prepared. Important nutrients have declined between 5 and 40 percent, according to comprehensive research by professor Donald Davis, Ph.D. Other researchers have shown even greater losses. David Thomas, D.C., analyzed and compared government tables for food composition in 1940 and 2002 and found losses of 55 to 60 percent in iron and 60 percent in copper just in meat alone, largely due to intensive farming methods.

Two, optimal doses are far from adequate doses. It's hard to get 400 IUs of vitamin E from food, for example, and next to impossible to get any meaningful dose of such important nutrients as alpha-lipoic acid or coenzyme Q10. But it's easy to get them through supplements.

So even if you followed the above dietary recommendations to the letter, you might still benefit from additional quantities of certain nutrients. In previous chapters, we've discussed how certain supplements can provide added protection for specific organs or systems in the body (the brain, heart, and bones), and you can certainly expand the following list of supplements with any of the ones mentioned in those chapters. But here, for what it's worth, is my list of seven supplements that seem to have demonstrated the most bang for the buck when it comes to protecting your body, brain, and heart and which have the strongest likelihood of ensuring a longer life.[1]

Omega-3 fatty acids (fish oil): Throughout this book you've heard references to omega-3s, those fatty acids found in fish and flax. They protect the heart and brain and improve mood. They keep you young. They are arguably the most important supplement you should take for a long and healthy life.

The ratio of omega-6s (vegetable oils) to omega-3s (fish oil, flax) is thought by most people who know what they're talking about to have a tremendous influence on human health. The ideal ratio is about 1:1; we typically consume about 16:1 or more in favor of the pro-inflammatory omega-6s. Omega-3s lower inflammation, blood pressure, and triglycerides.

Omega-3s are the one supplement I wouldn't be without no matter what. I recommend at least 1 gram a day of DHA and EPA, the two important fatty acids found in fish oil. (I personally take 2 grams a day.) If for some reason you can't or won't take fish oil or fish oil capsules, you can take flax oil instead but you'll need to take substantially more to

---

1   Especially if taken as part of an overall plan like the one described in this chapter.

get enough EPA and DHA in your system—at least 2 to 4 tablespoons (30 to 60 ml) a day. Only a relatively small portion of the omega-3 fatty acid in flaxseed converts in the body to the two omega-3 fatty acids, EPA and DHA, which are most important for human health.

Selenium: Selenium might just be the most important mineral you've never heard of. It's absolutely essential for your immune system, and without a healthy immune system, you are at a big disadvantage when it comes to healthy aging. When animals are deficient in selenium and exposed to a flu virus, the virus mutates into a much worse (and more life-threatening) form, which is then passed on to other animals, research has found. A decline in selenium levels is a hallmark of AIDS progression, but studies have found that selenium supplementation can suppress HIV-1.

But bolstering your immune system is hardly the only thing selenium does (although if it was, it would be reason enough to take it!). Mortality rates are significantly higher in individuals with low selenium levels. And, according to a study in the journal *Epidemiology*, selenium may help slow cognitive decline. "Selenium status decreases with age and may contribute to declines in neuropsychologic[al] functions among aging people," concluded the researchers.

Finally, selenium has a clear anticancer effect. In one classic study published in the *Journal of the American Medical Association*, 1,312 patients with a history of skin cancer were treated for an average of four and a half years with either 200 micrograms of selenium or a placebo. The total cancer incidence was reduced by 37 percent in the selenium group, which also had 63 percent less prostate cancer, 58 percent less colorectal cancer, and 46 percent less lung cancer.

There's a lot of hoopla about selenium toxicity, but most of it is nonsense. The "toxic symptoms" (garlic breath, brittle fingernails) occur at huge doses. Studies in China have found that nail and hair problems occur at the level of 4,990 micrograms a day (about twenty-four to forty-eight selenium capsules daily). I recommend 200 to 400 micrograms of selenium every day.

When the first edition of this book came out, there was a phase 3 study of 32,500 men, funded by the National Cancer Institute, testing the benefits of selenium and vitamin E on preventing prostate cancer. I wrote then that the results would be released after the 2013 completion date of the study, but I also warned readers not to expect much. Why? Because the U.S. Food and Drug Administration chose a ridiculously low dose of selenium, 55 micrograms per day, to test in the study. It's difficult to imagine that 55 micrograms of selenium a day will do very much to prevent cancer. (It remains *very* possible that selenium, together with other nutrients we don't get much of, has a synergistic effect!)

Well, my prediction was correct. Not surprisingly, no benefit was found in taking 55 micrograms of selenium. What's more, a follow-up study showed that men who took 400 IUs of vitamin E (without selenium) had a very slightly *increased* risk for prostate cancer. The form of vitamin E they used—dl-alpha-tocopherol—might have had something to do with it (it's the least effective and possibly most harmful kind of vitamin E, one which no nutritionist ever recommends). Or it's possible the increased risk was found because of some other factor—or combination of factors—not taken into account.

Here's Dr. Andrew Weil commenting on a different study that showed vitamin E supplements in a bad light: "My feeling is that the health status of the study participants could be the problem here—perhaps the vitamin E had some unpredictable bad effect on their pre-existing conditions or didn't mix well with certain medications. The researchers also may have overlooked controlling for the form of vitamin E used in the various studies. Natural vitamin E in the form of mixed tocopherols can possibly provide different benefits than synthetic versions limited to alpha tocopherol."

The point is that studies can be all over the map when it comes to supplements, drugs, foods, and various other things we study. No one study "proves" anything, it just "suggests" evidence for a hypothesis. In my opinion, looking at *all* the evidence, 200 to 400 micrograms of selenium a day as part of your supplement regime (or as an ingredient in your multiple vitamin) continues to make good.

Vitamin D: If you had to pick one vitamin that achieved superstar status in the decade from 2000 to 2010, it would have to be vitamin D. The résumé of health and potentially life-extending (and quality-of-life-improving) benefits of this long underappreciated vitamin is simply stunning. The conservative *Physicians' Desk Reference for Nutritional Supplements* summed it up best: "Over the past several years, studies have indicated that vitamin D may play beneficial roles in a wide range of disease and disorders, including osteoporosis, cancer, multiple sclerosis, heart disease, psoriasis, and Alzheimer's disease."

A 2008 study showed that people with low levels of vitamin D are significantly more likely to die for *any* reason than are people with higher levels. A diet lacking in adequate vitamin D may increase the risk for cancer. And the definition of "adequate" intake is rapidly changing,

especially because clinical experience shows that far more people than you might imagine have much lower than optimal levels of this vitamin.

"We found a marked increase in vitamin D deficiency over the past two decades," said vitamin D researcher Adit Ginde, M.D., assistant professor of surgery at the University of Colorado Denver School of Medicine. "Over three out of four Americans now have vitamin D levels below what we believe is necessary for optimal health. African-Americans and Hispanics are at particularly high risk—nearly all have suboptimal levels."

Indeed. Vitamin D may help prevent diabetes and heart attacks, and people with higher levels of vitamin D have a significantly lower risk of cognitive impairment when they get older. Vitamin D also improves physical performance in older adults. It's also absolutely essential for strong bones, an important concern as we get older. For goodness sake, it may even help prevent colds.

There are few food sources of vitamin D, which is one reason I strongly recommend this vitamin in your 7 × 3 strategy for robust aging. In 2008, several health organizations, including the American Pediatrics Association, recommended doubling the recommended daily allowance for vitamin D, but they're being conservative. I recommend 2,000 IUs of vitamin D on a daily basis. If you're in the sun, a source of vitamin D, for hours on end, you could reduce that to 1,000 IUs, but you're probably not in the sun for that long anyway.

Don't worry about toxicity. Your body makes many times that amount when you're in the sun all day, and studies have shown that up to 2,000 IUs a day is perfectly safe. Noted researcher Michael F. Holick, M.D., director of the Vitamin D Laboratory at Boston University, says, "We are in desperate need to have a marked increase in the adequate intake recommendation, and hopefully that will be 1,000 to 2,000 IUs per day—and raise the safe upper limit to at least 10,000 IUs a day."

Folic acid: Here's a prediction: Folic acid is poised to become the "next" vitamin D, in the sense that researchers are still discovering the huge benefits of this nutrient and that we have woefully underestimated the optimal daily intake of this member of the B vitamin family.

We don't get enough folic acid in our diet or at least not nearly the optimal amount. To make matters worse, the body doesn't absorb folate, the form of folic acid found in food, all that well. Folic acid, the form used in supplements, is actually much better absorbed. But none of this would make much difference if it weren't for what's been learned about low folate (folic acid) status and its impact on human health and longevity.

Low concentrations of folate in the blood have been associated with poor cognitive function, dementia, and Alzheimer's disease, not to mention a higher risk for colorectal, lung, esophageal, brain, cervical, and breast cancers. The *Encyclopedia of Dietary Supplements*, which was written by a blue-ribbon panel of scientists from the National Institutes of Health, says, "Observational studies continue to indicate an inverse relationship between folate (folic acid) intake . . . and the risk of developing certain common cancers." Low intake has also been associated with depression and other psychiatric symptoms. And let's not forget about homocysteine (see page 102), a risk factor for both heart disease and stroke. Folic acid is a key player in lowering this toxic compound in the blood.

But the main thing that convinced me to put folic acid on the short list of essential supplements for a long and healthy life was the Nun Study.

The Nun Study is a longitudinal study of aging and Alzheimer's disease funded by the National Institute on Aging. The participants are members of the School Sisters of Notre Dame and are between 75 and 106(!) years old. The idea was to look at this homogenous population of women, all of whom pretty much lead the same lifestyle, eat the same food, and have similar patterns of alcohol and cigarette use (which would be zero), and to determine which factors might account for the fact that some of them develop Alzheimer's and some don't. Good idea, right?

Here's what David Snowdon, Ph.D., the lead researcher in the Nun Study, had to say: "Nine years into the Nun Study, we finally found a nutrient that appeared to stave off the brain-damaging effects of Alzheimer's disease in the sisters."

That nutrient? Folic acid.

I recommend taking 800 to 1,000 micrograms (1 mg) of folic acid daily.

Worth knowing: The current recommended dietary intake is 400 micrograms (about ½ gram), which is very low. The National Academy of Sciences' Food and Nutrition Board recommends 1,000 micrograms as a safe upper limit, but what's important to know is that number is not related to any possible toxicity of folic acid. Folic acid is not toxic or dangerous; doses of up to 15,000 micrograms (15 grams) in healthy adults have not produced any reported serious adverse effects.

In my opinion, the only reason the recommendations for folic acid haven't been higher is that the people who make these recommendations are concerned about the fact that folic acid can mask vitamin B12 deficiency, which is something you definitely *don't* want. My solution to that is simple: Just make sure you get adequate levels of B12 (which you will get from grass-fed meat and many kinds of fish). Taking a multiple vitamin or a B complex should clear up any concerns about getting enough B12.

Probiotics: When you think about it, all the food and supplement recommendations we've made so far are only beneficial to you if you are able to digest and absorb them. Probiotics, the "good" bacteria that live in your gut, help make digestion and absorption possible.

Your gut is teeming with bacteria, some of it good (probiotics), some of it not so good (*Candida albicans*, or "yeast"). There's a constant turf battle going on, and you want the good guys to win. Not only does a good balance of "good" to "bad" bacteria in the gut help with digestion and absorption, but growing evidence suggests that it may support the immune system as well. And emerging research is showing that probiotic benefits, including lowering inflammation, may extend to the whole body.

"If I could only get people to take one supplement a day, it would be a probiotic," says my friend and nutritionist Allison Tannis, M.Sc., R.H.N., author of *Probiotic Rescue: How You Can Use Probiotics to Fight Cholesterol, Cancer, Superbugs, Digestive Complaints, and More.* "The benefits of probiotics are so far-reaching it's mind-boggling."

Many people in countries where fermented food is routinely consumed get plenty of probiotics in their diet. Traditionally fermented sauerkraut, for example, or olives, or the Korean dish kimchi are all wonderful sources of these beneficial bacteria. But unless you're eating fermented food or a ton of yogurt that contains active cultures, you probably could use some extra help. Many health professionals are beginning to put probiotics on their short list of the most important supplements for general health. I agree.

Get a good brand that mixes various "families" of probiotics (like *lactobacillus* and *bifidobacterial*) and take it daily, with food or just after a meal. (*Note:* The dose per enteric-coated capsule is given in billions of organisms—remember, these bacteria are really, really tiny!) You can also get probiotics in a powder, which is both convenient and effective. Sprinkle it on yogurt, fruit, or any cold dish. And unless the package says it's "shelf stable," remember to refrigerate it; the bacteria are alive and you want to keep them that way for as long as possible—until they hit your gut, where they can do some good!

Resveratrol: The fact that red wine is good for you is hardly news. For years, we've heard about wine, which contains hundreds of chemical compounds that fall into the family of polyphenols. And the polyphenol that's gotten the lion's share of attention, at least when it comes to wine and grapes, is resveratrol.

Resveratrol is found in the skin of dark grapes. In every species studied, from yeast cells to fruit flies to mice, resveratrol seems to extend life. Research by Harvard Medical School professor of pathology David Sinclair, M.D., has shown that resveratrol extends the life span of mice by up to 24 percent and the life span of other animals by as much as 59 percent.

It's believed that resveratrol exerts its magic by turning on the SIRT genes, which are involved in longevity. (Some SIRT genes are turned on by caloric restriction, another well-known age-extending strategy, albeit a difficult one to follow.) Scientists are hard at work to develop a drug that turns on the SIRT genes, which, if successful, may be the pharmaceutical equivalent of the Fountain of Youth.

And many are counting on resveratrol to be the main ingredient. (You can be sure that just as soon as the pharmaceutical companies come up with a way to work it into a patented medicine, they'll not only do so, but they'll also make a killing.)

Resveratrol is also a powerful antioxidant. And it's been found to inhibit the growth of several cancer cell lines and tumors, "suggesting," according to the *Physicians' Desk Reference for Nutritional Supplements*, "that it has an inhibitory effect on cancer promotion [and] progression."

You'd have to drink an enormous amount of wine to get the amount of resveratrol available in a single supplement pill. I recommend you take at least 250 milligrams a day, although many of the experts I spoke to take a lot more.

Worth noting: The only form of resveratrol shown to be effective so far is the *trans*-resveratrol form. The label on the bottle will tell you exactly how much trans-resveratrol you're getting. If, for example, you have a 500 milligram capsule of resveratrol "standardized for 20 percent trans-resveratrol," that means it contains 100 milligrams of tran-resveratrol (20 percent of 500 milligrams). Calculate your dose based on the trans-resveratrol each pill provides, not on the total amount of resveratrol per pill.

Coenzyme Q10: A healthy heart is a great thing to have if you want to live long and well, and coenzyme Q10 is one of the greatest nutrients for the heart on the planet.

Coenzyme Q10, or CoQ10 for short, is a vitally important nutrient for energy. It literally recharges the energy production furnaces in the cells (called the *mitochondria*). The heart cells produce more energy than any other organ, so CoQ10 and the heart are a natural fit. Indeed, CoQ10 is given as a prescription drug for congestive heart failure in Japan—it's that effective at helping the heart produce energy.

Our bodies make CoQ10, but as we age, we produce substantially less. And don't think you're going to make up the difference with food—CoQ10 is found mainly in organ meats (heart, liver, and kidney). Other foods that have it, like sardines and beef, contain paltry amounts, and you'd need a ton of them to get even 30 milligrams a day,

the absolute minimum dose for healthy folks looking for general protection.

Emerging evidence suggests that CoQ10 may be helpful in preventing certain neurodegenerative diseases. It also helps prevent migraines and lowers blood pressure. And if that weren't enough, it's also a powerful antioxidant. I recommend at least 60 to 100 milligrams of CoQ10 daily for anyone over forty.

3. Adopt the Age-Management Lifestyle

The best foods in the world and the most potent supplements will not make you happy. They will give your body everything it needs in the way of fuel, but that's not enough. You could put the highest quality gas in a Ferrari, but to get the fun from a Ferrari, you still have to take it out of the garage and drive it! (Well, I assume you do. I personally never have, but you get the point.)

The following strategies are drawn from themes I've discussed in these pages. They're the same themes that come up in every single piece of research I've seen on successful aging, whether it's the MacArthur Foundation Study, the Nun Study, the Baltimore Longitudinal Study of Aging, the Adventist Study, or in Dan Buettner's book, *The Blue Zones*. I've taken what I think to be the most important common denominators and put them together in seven basic strategies. Obviously, you can argue that not every healthy centenarian does every one of these things. But if I were a betting man, I'd bet the family farm that the following strategies represent an effective program for aging well that is bound to keep you active and happy for a long time.

Walk thirty minutes every day. I'm not saying you'll lose a ton of weight with this strategy, but that's not why it's on the list. Walking at a moderate clip has been shown to grow new brain cells in both animals and humans. It's the perfect natural antidepressant and mood elevator. Duke University researchers found that over sixteen weeks, walking (or jogging) for thirty minutes (plus warming up and cooling down) worked as well as antidepressant medications in improving mood. And the American Cancer Society's cancer prevention guidelines state that at least thirty minutes a day of dedicated exercise (like brisk walking) is needed to reduce cancer risk. Walking is good for the heart, the lungs, the brain, and, especially if you do it outside amid greenery and beauty, the soul.

Weight train twice a week. Walking is great, but you also need muscular strength if you're going to navigate through life effortlessly. I'm not necessarily talking about bench-pressing four hundred pounds (91 kg) here; I'm talking about keeping your muscles strong and useful so that you can do the daily tasks of life without any great problem. And muscles are the truest example of the old adage "use it or lose it." You lose about half a pound (225 g) of muscle a year if you don't do anything to stop the loss. And it's not just muscle you lose. Because calories are burned primarily in the muscle cells, losing muscle means you lose calorie-burning ability and gain fat much more easily.

Weight training can significantly slow that loss of muscle to a negligible amount. You may not win the Mr. Universe contest at eighty, but you'll be strong as an ox and look pretty darn good to boot. And don't believe for a second that you're too old to start. Noted strength researcher Wayne Wescott, Ph.D., has done a number of studies on weight training with elderly people, some of whom were in wheelchairs, and nearly all of them improved in strength and autonomy. Ronald Reagan started using weights when he was eighty-two and even he gained some muscle!

The good news is that you don't have to train all that hard or all that frequently. Twice a week for a half hour or so is all you need to make sure those muscles don't atrophy.

Breathe—deeply! You can substitute mediation for this if you like, or stick with the basics of deep breathing (see below). Breathing deeply gets oxygen to the brain, calms the mind and the soul, lowers stress hormones, and is incompatible with anger and other destructive emotions. In case you don't want to look it up, here's how to do it in the simplest possible way:

1. Sit comfortably with your eyes closed.
2. Pay attention to your breathing and repeat a word, phrase, or prayer silently to yourself as you exhale.
3. Slowly fill your lungs up deeply and exhale fully.
4. When you notice your mind wandering, which it most definitely will, passively bring your attention back to your breathing.
5. Practice for approximately twenty minutes every day (or at least three or four times a week).

Although sitting quietly and meditating (or breathing deeply) is one way to reduce stress and calm the brain, don't rule out a more structured approach like gentle yoga, tai chi, or qi gong. They all accomplish the same thing. It's probably no accident that most of the healthy people you see in parks doing tai chi are over seventy!

Get out in the sun for at least ten minutes a day. Not only does it give you some vitamin D the natural way, but sunshine is also a great mood enhancer. It's no accident that seasonal affective disorder (SAD) hits people most in winter or in the darker, colder months. It's also no accident that the tropics are frequently called paradises; you don't see too many people enjoying carefree vacations in Antarctica.

Remember that deeply etched into our DNA is a whole cascade of hormonal and biochemical responses that are regulated by light and dark. We ignore these at our peril. The sun is our original source of light, and it's no accident that so many of the longest-lived people in the world spend a lot of time outdoors and are probably much more in tune with the natural rhythms of light and dark produced by the cycle of night and day.

The importance of these rhythms was underscored recently in a surprising study of suicide in Greenland. Greenland has one of the highest suicide rates in the world, and researchers have found that suicides are far more pronounced during the periods in which the sun never sets—the months known as "constant day." In the north of the country, 82 percent of the suicides occurred during these months, and these suicides were almost exclusively violent. The researchers speculate that light-generated imbalances in the brain chemical serotonin may be responsible.

The point is that light and darkness form an exquisite balance that has profound effects on our well-being. To paraphrase Goldilocks, when it comes to sun we need "not too much, not too little, but just enough." Don't be sun phobic. The sun is your friend, but so (as we'll see below) is darkness. Embrace both.

Sleep well! Prior to the invention of electricity, our sleep patterns were pretty stable. After all, we had no options to override the natural rhythm of light and dark. We went to bed in darkness when the sun set and woke up with the light, when the sun rose. There's a deep and abiding wisdom in this, one we would do well to copy in our modern life, especially if we want to live long and feel good!

How well you sleep has an enormous and sometimes underappreciated relationship to how good you feel.

Undersleeping elevates stress hormones, increasing blood pressure, inflammation, irritability, and weight gain and decreasing energy. (Point of interest: People who sleep fewer than seven or eight hours a night are more likely to be overweight or obese, possibly because undersleeping disrupts hormones like leptin and ghrelin, which have a significant effect on appetite.)

Recent research has linked sleep and longevity. In 2007, researchers from the University College London Medical School studied 10,308 British civil servants to try to find out whether there was any link between the number of hours slept per night and what is technically called "all-cause mortality"—the likelihood of dying for any reason. They looked at the civil servants at two points in their lives: 1985 to 1988 and those still alive in 1992 and 1993. The researchers statistically adjusted for all the important factors, such as age, sex, smoking, alcohol use, weight, and physical illness, and were then able to isolate the effect that changes in sleep patterns over five years had on mortality rates eleven to seventeen years later.

The results were eye-opening. Those who had cut their sleeping from seven hours to five hours or fewer had a 1.7-fold increase in the risk of dying from any cause and twice the likelihood of dying from a cardiovascular problem.

"In terms of prevention, our findings indicate that consistently sleeping around seven hours per night is optimal for health and a sustained reduction may predispose to ill health," said the researchers.

During sleep, important biochemicals are replaced, hormones are released, and the body is rejuvenated and refreshed. Sleeping well and soundly makes you feel energized, increases well-being, and helps you maintain your weight at a healthy level. It also bolsters your memory.

Make getting a good night's sleep—every night of the year—a priority. It's one of the cornerstones of living well and living long. Although there are definitely individual variations, all indications point to seven hours a night as being the magic number needed for optimal health. (Full disclosure: I sleep six hours a night, but I'd worry if it were consistently less than that.)

Practice *hara hatchi bu.* With all the hundreds of books' worth of information on what to eat, what tends to get lost is this simple truth: Eating less extends life.

Clearly what you eat matters greatly—I wouldn't have written several books on the subject if I didn't think it was important. But what's also important is how you eat (relaxed, without stress, and mindfully) and how much you eat.

In every species studied so far, calorie restriction extends life. Seriously. But don't let the term *restriction* scare you. You don't have to join one of those calorie-restriction societies and count every single calorie every day of your life. Just eat about one-third to one-fourth less than you normally would. The benefits are enormous. (Though no authoritative figures are available, most estimates put the "average" daily caloric intake of Americans in the 3,600 range, with many people eating far more than that.)

The long-lived folks on Okinawa eat up to 40 percent fewer calories than Americans do and 17 percent less than the Japanese average. It seems to be working. Not only do they have one of the highest life spans of any group ever studied, but, compared to Americans, Okinawa elders are 75 percent more likely to retain their cognitive ability, develop 80 percent fewer breast and prostate cancers, have 50 percent fewer ovarian and colon cancers, experience 50 percent fewer hip fractures, and suffer 80 percent fewer heart attacks.

The Confucian saying "*Hara hatchi bu*" sums it up best—"Eat until you are 80 percent full." The folks in the Okinawa peninsula live by this mantra.

You and I should do the same.

Connect. I've saved the best and most important part for last. Connect—that simple word sums up the most important message in this entire book. More than food, more than supplements, more than exercise, more than virtually any other strategy I can think of to extend both the length and the quality of life, connecting with others is the most important thing you can possibly do if you want to live long and well.

I've said it before, but it bears repeating. People have lived a very long time with some very unhealthy habits. I don't think it makes a lot of sense to risk the odds on this, but still, it's worth noting that every family has an Uncle Jack who smoked two packs a day and drank a fifth of Jack Daniels and lived to a hundred.

But no family has an Uncle Jack who lived to a hundred in isolation.

Whether it's friends, family, or extended family, whether it's church, temple, mosque, or charity, connection to something or someone outside of you is a prerequisite for living well and seems to be a prerequisite for living long.

Every society studied has intricate social networks where people offer help, assistance, companionship, friendship, and outreach. As we've seen in this book, even taking care of a houseplant improves medical outcomes substantially. If taking care of a plant and paying attention to something outside yourself improves medical outcomes that much, imagine what taking care of—or contributing to—people, animals, and causes can do. People who volunteer live longer and healthier lives. People who are connected to others thrive; people who don't, wither away.

IKAGI

On a personal note: I've spent most of my life studying human beings and health—first as a psychologist and then as a nutritionist—and the more I learn, the more I profoundly understand how little I know. I've changed what I believe about food and exercise (or at least modified it) many times over the two decades I've been in the health and wellness field. But one belief I've never changed is this: People want to contribute.

Many people on this planet want nothing more than to contribute, be heard, make a difference, and have a meaningful life. No matter whether we are conscious of it or not, and regardless of whether we express it or not, the desire to contribute and make a difference is at the core of what every human being truly wants. It is what makes us human. It is what makes life both beautiful and fulfilling.

The Japanese have a word for that—*ikagai*. It means "purpose"—what you value in life, what gives your life meaning, what lights you up and fulfills you. With a purpose, an "ikagi," as the Okinawans say, you have a reason for staying alive. if you didn't have a purpose, all the anti-aging strategies in the world won't mean much. So if I had but one "anti-aging" strategy to leave you with it would be this: Find your purpose.

And then live in accordance with it. Every single day.

With a purpose, you have a reason for staying alive.

I hope this book has given you the tools to do exactly that.

Enjoy the journey.

My Emotional Intelligence Workbook

Emotional intelligence is the ability to be both personal and interpersonal, to have relationships, community, and contribution, and deal with people from a place of integrity and self-awareness.

Working through the steps in this workbook will increase your awareness of yourself and your relationship to others. Copy these questions onto another piece of paper or other journal format of your choice.

Emotional intelligence encompasses most areas of our connection to other people (and our ability to be at peace with ourselves). Remember that one of the defining characteristics of the longest-lived and healthiest people on the planet—a characteristic that consistently shows up in every study of people around the globe who live extremely long and healthy lives—is connection to others. This includes friendships, marriages, relatives, community, and church or spiritual groups.

In this workbook, I've broken down the components of emotional intelligence into specific categories that allow you to focus on the little steps you could take to increase the enormous sense of well-being that comes with reaching out to other people and taking attention off yourself. Use this as a way to take inventory of where you are in your relationships, and where you would like to go. Consider it a working, breathing document, always subject to revision, and notice the effect taking these (sometimes small) actions have on your overall well-being, vitality, and longevity!

ACKNOWLEDGMENT (STATEMENT OF ANOTHER'S VALUE)

You can acknowledge the most significant person in your life or share with an acquaintance. You can even make a difference to a stranger. How about thanking a waiter for excellent service and for making your dinner a pleasant experience? Approach the world and look at where you can thank someone, where can you acknowledge somebody's worth. Bonus points if you acknowledge someone and expect nothing in return.

- Who did I acknowledge?
- How did that make me feel?
- Who could I acknowledge?
- Who will I acknowledge?

PRACTICE FORGIVENESS

Forgiveness is an emotional muscle. It needs practice. You may not be able to forgive the stepdad who abused you. You want to start with the person who cut you off on the highway. Start with something small that you can manage. Practice this idea of letting go of anger and forgiving.

- Who did I forgive?
- Who *could* I forgive?
- Who *will* I forgive? (And by when?)

VOLUNTEERING YOUR SERVICES

Helping other people *actually* makes you healthier and happier. You will get more satisfaction out of life and experience better health and less depression. Volunteering is an enormous thing that you can do, not only for the world, but also for yourself, and there are many ways to do it.

- Where did I volunteer?
- How did it make me feel?
- Where *could* I volunteer?
- Where *will* I volunteer? (And by when?)

MAKE A GRATITUDE LIST

Make a list of some of the things you're grateful for in life. It can be your relationship, it can be the dogs that you're lucky enough to share space with, it can be your home or the vegetables you grow in your garden. It can be *anything*.

- What am I grateful for?
- Expand your list … What else am I grateful for?

Read this list *and the expanded list* every day for thirty days. This keeps your mental focus on things that are actually peaceful and happy. You will focus on things that you care about and things that you're grateful for rather than on things you don't have. It's a powerful healing technique.

PERFORM A RANDOM ACT OF KINDNESS

Perform a random act of kindness. *Bonus points if the act of kindness is completely anonymous.* Put a quarter in somebody's meter. Go on the Internet and make a donation to something. Giving back is rewarding to the person doing the giving, as well as the person receiving it.

- Where did I perform a random act of kindness?
- How did that make *me* feel?

- How could I perform a random act of kindness? *Get creative!*
- How *will* I manifest a random act of kindness?

PRACTICE MINDFULNESS

Mindfulness is the key to everything from relationships to safety. Practice *noticing*. Practice being mindful. Be present for your life and present in the moment.

- In what areas of my life did I stay present and mindful?
- What did I notice that was different about this experience?
- In what areas of my life *could* I stay present and mindful?
- In what areas of my life *will* I stay present and mindful?

STAY CONNECTED

Stay connected. *Face-to-face connection.* Nurture your social ties. These can be religious or spiritual affiliations, social groups, family, friends, and animals. It's all about connections.

- Who did I connect with?
- Who *could* I connect with?
- Who *will* I connect with? (And by when?)

Remember to use this workbook as a living, breathing document. It's a work in progress, just like our lives! Use it to monitor what you're doing for yourself (and others) and notice how these steps, taken or intended, can benefit your well-being, energy, vitality, and longevity!

My Longevity Journal

Use these prompts to keep track of the changes you're making in your life in your journal.

Sometimes, we're actually taking steps to being healthier without giving ourselves full credit for it. Writing down each thing you're doing helps make it more concrete and real for you. Acknowledge how far you've come—and use this journal as a springboard to go even further, one step at a time.

You can also use this journal to plan future steps you might take in each of the seven key areas of longevity. You may find that small actions might occur to you that would be worth jotting down as goals, such as a one-day fast. Even if you haven't done it yet, put it down in the *future goals* section, and make a game of moving items from the "to-do in the future" list to the "actions accomplished" list!

FIRST PILLAR OF LONGEVITY: FOOD

What things have I done today (or this week) to improve my diet and increase my longevity? These items could be foods that you've added to your diet, changes you've made to your protein intake or calorie consumption, foods that you've eliminated, or any other dietary improvements.

What things might I do in the *near future* that would make a difference in my diet and would increase my energy, vitality, and longevity? (This could be foods you're planning to eat more of, fast food meals you're planning to eliminate, or any other dietary strategy that would represent a step forward.)

SECOND PILLAR OF LONGEVITY: SUPPLEMENTS

What supplements am I taking now on a regular basis? Include everything, even if you're only taking a simple one-a-day formula.

What supplements might I add in the *near future* that would make a difference in my health and overall longevity on a long-term basis? Consider the basic ones discussed in this book, especially in section II, and others that seem like they make sense. Think about any supplements you may have taken in the past and whether they made you feel better. If so, in what way? Include those as well.

THIRD PILLAR OF LONGEVITY: DETOXIFICATION

What things have I done today (or this week) to reduce my exposure to toxins? This could include switching to a "green" laundry detergent or organic strawberries, for example. Think about the various toxins you are exposed to on a daily basis—food, water, air, even relationships!—and see what steps you've already taken to reduce their effects.

What things might I do in the *near future* that would further reduce my exposure to toxins or that would support detoxification pathways in my own body? This could include things like dry skin brushing, an infrared sauna, or going on a one-week detox diet. It could also include taking liver support supplements such as milk thistle or alpha-lipoic acid. What might I do that could increase my energy, vitality, and longevity?

FOURTH PILLAR OF LONGEVITY: EXERCISE

What things have I done today (or this week) for exercise? You can include any activity at all; remember, it all starts with small steps. If you walked from the bus stop, put it in. If you gardened today, put it in. Or, if you're already a "gym rat," put down what you've done. Be specific. How many minutes did you walk/jog? Did you lift weights? What exercises? How many reps? Did you play tennis? You may find that you actually spend more time away from your desk than you thought. Use this part of the journal to acknowledge that.

What things might I do in the *near future* that would make a difference in my exercise or activity level and would increase my energy, vitality, and longevity? This could be anything from "park farther from the office and walk across the parking lot" to "run a marathon." It could be an extra ten pounds (4.6 kg) on your bench press or an extra fifteen minutes of gardening. Anything that adds to the total load of activity could be used in this section as a future goal. Have fun!

FIFTH PILLAR OF LONGEVITY: SLEEP

What things have I done today (or this week) to improve the quality of my sleep? This can include going to bed an hour earlier, banning the computer from the bedroom, or any other strategy to increase the quality (and quantity) of your sleep.

What things might I do in the *near future* that would improve my sleep? This could include anything from buying a new mattress to banning the television from the bedroom or any other strategy to increase the quantity and quality of your sleep and increase your energy, vitality, and longevity.

SIXTH PILLAR OF LONGEVITY: STRESS REDUCTION

What things have I done today (or this week) to reduce my stress? This can include anything from organizing your inbox to taking a five-minute deep breathing break. It can also include bigger things such as removing a toxic relationship from your life or setting boundaries on one that's causing you stress.

What things might I do in the *near future* that would reduce my stress and increase my energy, vitality, and longevity?

SEVENTH PILLAR OF LONGEVITY: EMOTIONAL INTELLIGENCE

What things have I done today (or this week) that have the potential to improve the quality of my relationships—with people, my community, and the world around me—and ultimately improve my well-being?

What things might I do in the near future that would improve my relationships with others, myself, my community, and the world around me? This could include anything from donating time (or money) to volunteering. It can also include any increased efforts to reach out to other people in your life—be they family, friends, strangers, or animals!

Remember to use this workbook as a living, breathing document. It's a work in progress, just like our lives! Use it to monitor what you're doing for yourself or, in some cases, others, and notice how these steps, taken or intended, can benefit your well-being, energy, vitality, and longevity!

Resources

BRAIN

Amen, Daniel. *Change Your Brain, Change Your Life*. New York: Three Rivers Press, 1999.

Amen, Daniel. *Magnificent Mind at Any Age*. New York: Harmony, 2008.

Khalsa, M.D., Dharma Singh, and Cameron Stauth. *Brain Longevity*. New York: Grand Central Publishing, 1999.

McCleary, Larry. *The Brain Trust Program*. New York: Perigee Trade, 2007.

Perlmutter, David, and Carol Colman. *The Better Brain Book*. New York: Riverhead, 2005.

EMOTIONAL INTELLIGENCE

Buettner, Dan. *The Blue Zones*. National Geographic, 2009. www.bluezone.com

HEART

Houston, M.D., Mark, with Barry Fox, Ph.D., and Nadine Taylor, M.S., R.D. *What Your Doctor May Not Tell You About Hypertension*. New York: Warner Books, 2003.

Sinatra, M.D., Stephen, and James Roberts, M.D. *Reverse Heart Disease Now*. Hoboken, NJ: Wiley and Sons, 2007.

Stoll, M.D., Andrew L. *The Omega-3 Connection*. New York: Fireside, 2001.

Oz, M.D., Mehmet C., and Dean Ornish. *Healing from the Heart*. New York: Plume, 1999.

HORMONES

Bowden, Jonny. *Living Low Carb*. New York: Sterling, 2010.

Brownstein, David. *Overcoming Thyroid Disorders*. West Bloomfield, MI: Medical Alternatives Press, 2002.

Daniel, Kaayla T. *The Whole Soy Story*. Winona Lake, IN: New Trends, 2005.

Gittleman, Ann Louise. *Before the Change*. Harper Collins, 1998

Northrup, Christiane. *The Wisdom of Menopause*. New York: Bantam, 2001.

Parker-Pope, Tara. *The Hormone Decision*. Emmaus, PA: Rodale, 2007.

Reiss, Uzzi. *Natural Hormone Balance for Women*. New York: Atria, 2002.

Sarrel, Philip. "Women's Health Initiative Study on HRT Stopped: What the News Means to You." He@lthLINK, Yale-New Haven Hospital.

Schwartz, Erika. *The 30-Day Natural Hormone Plan*. New York: Grand Central Publishing, 2005.

Schwartz, Erika. *The Hormone Solution*. New York: Grand Central Publishing, 2002.

Shames, Richard, and Karilee H. Shames. *Thyroid Power*. New York: Collins Living, 2002.

Sholomon, Mary. *Living Well with Hypothyroidism*. New York: HarperCollins, 2000.

INFLAMMATION

Cannon, Christopher P. and Elizabeth Vierck. *The Complete Idiot's Guide to the Anti-Inflammation Diet*. New York: Alpha, 2014.

Sears, Barry. *The Anti-Inflammation Zone*. Harper Paperbacks, 2005.

THE MEDITERRANEAN DIET

Acquista, Angelo. *The Mediterranean Prescription*. New York: Ballantine, 2006.

Schulman, Martha Rose. *Mediterranean Light*. New York: William Morrow, 2000.

Simopoulos, Artemis P., and Jo Robinson. *The Omega Diet*. New York: Collins Living, 1999.

MUSCLES, BONES, AND JOINTS

Knopf, Karl. *Stretching for 50+*. Berkeley, CA: Ulysses Press, 2005.

Knopf, Karl. *Weights for 50+*. Berkeley, CA: Ulysses Press, 2005.

Lanou, Ph.D., Amy, and Michael Castleman. *Building Bone Vitality*. McGraw-Hill, 2009.

McCormick, R. Keith. *The Whole-Body Approach to Osteoporosis*. Oakland, CA: New Harbinger, 2009.

Nelson, Miriam. *Strong Women, Strong Bones, updated edition*. New York: Perigee, 2006.

Neporent, Liz, Suzanne Schlosberg, and Shirley Archer. *Weight Training for Dummies*. Indianapolis, IN: Wiley, 2006.

Sanson, Gillian. *The Myth of Osteoporosis*. Ann Arbor, MI: MCD Century Publications, 2003.

Schlosberg, Suzanne, and Liz Neporent. *Fitness for Dummies*. Hoboken, NJ: Wiley, 2005.

Weatherby, Craig, and Leonid Gordin. *The Arthritis Bible*. Rochester, VT: Healing Arts Press, 1999.

Westcott, Wayne, and Thomas R. Baechle. *Strength Training Past 50*. Champaign, IL: Human Kinetics, 1997.

DOCTORS AND CLINICS SPECIALIZING IN HORMONE REPLACEMENT AND ANTI-AGING

Ann Louise Gittleman, Ph.D., C.N.S
UniKey Health Systems, Inc.
181 West Commerce Drive
Hayden, ID 83835
800-888-4353, www.unikeyhealth.com

David Leonardi, M.D.
Leonardi Institute
225 Union Boulevard, Suite 400
Lakewood, CO 80228
303-462-5344, www.leonardiinstitute.com

Prudence Hall, M.D.
The Hall Center
406 Wilshire Boulevard
Santa Monica, CA 90401
301-566-6688, www.thehallcenter.com

Preventative Medical Center of Marin
Elson M. Haas, M.D.
4340 Redwood Highway, Suite A-22
San Rafael, CA 94903
415-472-2343, www.pmcmarin.com, www.elsonhaas.com
(This is an Integrative Medicine Clinic that accepts multiple insurances, including Medicare.)

Erika Schwartz, M.D.
724 5th Avenue, 10th floor
New York City, NY 10019
212-873-3420, www.eshealth.com

Beth Traylor, M.D.
Cenegenics Medical Institute
851 South Rampart Boulevard, Suite 100
Las Vegas, NV 89145
702-953-1560
www.cenegenics.com

For more recommendations, go to the Institute for Functional Medicine (ww.ifm.org) and click "find a practitioner."

References

SECTION I: REIN IN THE FOUR HORSEMEN OF AGING

Campion, E.W. Aging better. *N Eng J Med* 338, no. 15 (1998): 1064–66.

"Cancer Prevention Tied to Diet and Way of Life." *New York Times*, Nov. 20, 1996.

"Diet and Cancer Research," The Cancer Project. www.cancerproject.org/diet_cancer/facts/major_killers.php.

Doll, R. and R. Peto. The causes of cancer: quantitative estimates of avoidable risks of cancer in the United States today. *J Natl Cancer Inst* 66, no. 6 (1981): 1191–1308.

"Heart Disease and Stroke," Canadian Diabetes Association. www.diabetes.ca/diabetes-and-you/complications/heart-disease-stroke.

Jones, David S., ed. *Textbook of Functional Medicine*. Gig Harbor, WA: Institute for Functional Medicine. 2005.

Stampfer, M., F. Hu, J. E. Manson, E. B. Rimm, and W. C. Willett. Primary prevention of coronary heart disease in women through diet and lifestyle. *N Eng J Med* 343, no. 1 (July 6, 2000): 16–22.

U.S. Centers for Disease Control and Prevention. *National Vital Statistics Reports* 54, no. 13 (April 19, 2006).

Vita, A. J., R. B. Terry, H. B. Hubert, and J. F. Fries. Aging, health risks, and cumulative disability. *N Eng J Med* 338, no. 15 (1998): 1035–41.

Yusuf, S., S. Hawken, S. Ounpuu, et al. on behalf of the INTERHEART Study Investigators. Effect of potentially modifiable risk factors associated with myocardial infarction in 52 countries (the INTERHEART study): case-control study. *Lancet* 364 (2004): 937–952.

Chapter 1: Fight the First Horseman of Aging—Free Radicals

Aslan, M., and T. Ozben. Reactive oxygen and nitrogen species in Alzheimer's disease. *Curr Alzheimer Res.* 1 (2004): 111–119.

Aubrey, Allison. "The Full-Fat Paradox: Dairy Fat Linked to Lower Diabetes Risk." April 18, 2016. https://www.npr.org/sections/thesalt/2016/04/18/474403311/the-full-fat-paradox-dairy-fat-linked-to-lower-diabetes-risk.

Blatt, Harvey. *America's Food: What You Don't Know About What You Eat*. Cambridge, MA: MIT Press, 2008

De Alzaa, F, et al. "Evaluation of Chemical and Physical Changes in Different Commercial Oils during Heating." Acta Scientific Nutritional Health, 2018. actascientific.com/ASNH/pdf/ASNH-02-0083.pdf.

Halliwell, B. Oxygen and nitrogen are pro-carcinogens. Damage to DNA by reactive oxygen, chlorine and nitrogen species: measurement, mechanism and effects of nutrition. *Mutat Res* 443 (1999): 37–52.

Harman, D. Nutritional implications of the free-radical theory of aging. *J Am Coll Nutr* 1 (1982): 27–34.

Johnson, S. The multifaceted and widespread pathology of magnesium deficiency. *Medical Hypotheses*, 2001: 163-170.

Knight, J. A. The biochemistry of aging. *Adv Clin Chem* 35 (2000): 1–62.

Knutson K.L., K. Spiegel, P. Penev, E. Van Cauter. The Metabolic Consequences of Sleep Deprivation. *Sleep medicine reviews*. 2007;11(3):163-178. doi:10.1016/j.smrv.2007.01.002.

"Leading Causes of Death," Centers for Disease Control and Prevention. 2016. https://www.cdc.gov/nchs/fastats/leading-causes-of-death.htm.

Maroon, Joseph C., and Jeffrey Bost. *Fish Oil: The Natural Anti-Inflammatory*. Laguna Beach, CA: Basic Health Publications, Inc., 2006.

McCall, M. R., and B. Frei. Can antioxidant vitamins materially reduce oxidative damage in humans? *Free Radic Biol Med* 26, no. 7-8 (1999): 1034–53.

Mishra, B.N. Secret of Eternal Youth; Teaching from the Centenarian Hot Spots ("Blue Zones"). *Indian Journal of Community Medicine : Official Publication of Indian Association of Preventive & Social Medicine*. 2009;34(4):273-275. doi:10.4103/0970-0218.58380.

Moore, Jimmy. "Tim Russert's Fatal Heart Attack Was Preventable, He Followed Antiquated Advice." Jimmy Moore's Livin La Vida Low-Carb. June 18, 2008. http://livinlavidalowcarb.com/blog/tim-russerts-fatal-heart-attack-was-preventable-he-followed-antiquated-advice/2403.

Nago, N., S. Ishikawa, T. Goto, and K. Kayaba. "Low cholesterol is associated with mortality from stroke, heart disease, and cancer: the Jichi Medical School Cohort Study." *Journal of Epidemiology*, 2011: 67-74.

"National Report on Human Exposure to Environmental Chemicals," Centers for Disease Control and Prevention, http://www.cdc.gov/exposurereport.

Neighmond, Patti. "Sitting All Day: Worse for You Than You Might Think." April 25, 2011. https://www.npr.org/2011/04/25/135575490/sitting-all-day-worse-for-you-than-you-might-think.

Pesticide Data Program, Annual Summary: Calendar Year 2005. United States Department of Agriculture. 2006.

Prior, R.L., L. Gu, et al. Plasma antioxidant capacity changes following a meal as a measure of the ability to alter in vivo antioxidant status. *J Am Coll Nutr* 26 (2): 170–181.

Ryan-Harshman, M., and W. Aldoori. The relevance of selenium to immunity, cancer, and infectious/inflammatory diseases. *Can J Diet Prac Res* 66 (2005): 98–102.

Sachdeva, A., et al. "Lipid levels in patients hospitalized with coronary artery disease: an analysis of 136,905 hospitalizations in Get With The Guidelines." *American Heart Journal*, 2009: 111-117.

Shoppers Guide to Pesticides in Produce. Environmental Working Group. 2018. https://www.ewg.org/foodnews/.

Valko M., M. Izakovic, M. Mazur, C. J. Rhodes, and J. Telser. Role of oxygen radicals in DNA damage and cancer incidence. *Mol Cell Biochem* 266 (2004): 37–56.

Wu, S., Y. Ding, F. Wu, G. Xie, J. Hou, P. Mao. Serum lipid levels and suicidality: a meta-analysis of 65 epidemiological studies. *Journal of Psychiatry & Neuroscience*. 2016;41(1):56-69. doi:10.1503/jpn.150079.

Chapter 2: Put out the Fire of the Second Horseman of Aging—Inflammation

Brod, S.A. Unregulated inflammation shortens human functional longevity. *Inflamm Res* 49, no. 11 (November 2000): 561–70.

"Inflammation, Heart Disease and Stroke: The Role of C-Reactive Protein." American Heart Association.

Knight, J.A. The biochemistry of aging. *Adv Clin Chem* 35 (2000): 1–62.

Mora, S., and P.M. Ridker. Justification for the use of statins in primary prevention. *Am J Cardiol* 97, no. 2A (2006): 33A–41A.

Simopoulos, A.P. Evolutionary aspects of diet, the omega-6/omega-3 ratio and genetic variation: Nutritional implications for chronic diseases. *Biomed Pharmacother* 60, no. 9 (November 2006): 502–07.

Stanner, Sara, Keith N. Frayn, and British Nutrition Foundation. *Cardiovascular Disease: Diet Nutrition and Emerging Risk Factors: The Report of a British Nutrition Foundation Task Force.* London: Blackwell, 2005.

Chapter 3: Avoid the Damage of the Third Horseman of Aging—Glycation

Vlassara, H., W. Cai, J. Crandall, et al. Inflammatory mediators are induced by dietary glycotoxins, a major risk factor for diabetic angiopathy. *Proc Natl Acad Sci USA* 99, no. 24 (Nov. 26, 2002): 15596–601.

Chapter 5: How Much Influence Do Genes Have on the Four Horsemen of Aging?

Hursting, S.D., J.A. Lavigne, D. Berrigan, et al. Calorie restriction, aging, and cancer prevention: mechanisms of action and applicability to humans. *Annu Rev Med* 54 (2003): 131–152.

Yu, B.P., E.J. Masoro, I. Murata, et al. Life span study of SPF Fischer 344 male rats fed ad libitum or restricted diets: Longevity, growth, lean body mass and disease. *J Gerontol* 37, no. 2 (March 1982): 130–41.

Zhang, J., J. Asin-Cayuela, J. Fish, et al. Strikingly higher frequency in centenarians and twins of mtDNA mutation causing remodeling of replication origin in leukocytes. *Proc Natl Acad Sci USA* 100, no. 3 (Feb 4, 2003): 1116–1121.

SECTION II: HOW TO KEEP THE KEY PLAYERS IN YOUR BODY FIT

Carey, Benedict. "At the Bridge Table, Clues to a Lucid Old Age," *New York Times*, May 22, 2009.

Chapter 6: Start with the Eight Pillars of Living Young

Bartholomew, J. B., D. Morrison, and J. T. Ciccolo. Effects of acute exercise on mood and well-being in patients with major depressive disorder. *Med Sci Sports Exer* 37, no. 12 (December 2005): 2032–7.

Chandalia, M. Beneficial effects of high dietary fiber intake in patients with type 2 diabetes mellitus. *New England Journal of Medicine*, 2000; 342(19): 1392-8

Demet, W. C. and C. C. Vaughan. *The Promise of Sleep.* New York: Delacorte Press, 1999: 274.

"Diet, Nutrition and the Prevention of Chronic Diseases." Report of a Joint FAO/WHO Expert Consultation. Geneva World Health Organization. 2003. (WHO Technical Report Series No. 916).

Dunstan, D.W., et al. Television Viewing Time and Mortality. The Australian Diabetes, Obesity and Lifestyle Study, 2010: 384-391.

Erickson, K. I., R. S. Prakash, M. W. Voss, et al. Aerobic fitness is associated with hippocampal volume in elderly humans. *Hippocampus*, Jan 2, 2009.

Jiamton, S., J. Pepin, R. Suttent, et al. A randomized trial of the impact of multiple micronutrient supplementation on mortality among HIV-infected individuals living in Bangkok. *AIDS* 17, no. 17 (2003): 2461–9.

Ludwig, D.S., et al., Dietary Fiber, Weight Gain, and Cardiovascular Disease Risk Factors in Young Adults. *Journal of the American Medical Association* 282 (1999): 1539-1546.

New Hampshire Department of Health and Human Service. How Much Sugar Do You Eat? You May Be Surprised! https://www.dhhs.nh.gov/dphs/nhp/documents/sugar.pdf.

Pereira, A. C., D. E. Huddleston, A. M. Brickman, et al. An in vivo correlate of exercise-induced neurogenesis in the adult dentate gyrus. *Proc Natl Acad Sci USA* 104, no. 13 (March 27, 2007): 5638–5643.

Rezende L.F.M., Sa T.H., Mielke G.I., et al. All-Cause Mortality Attributable to Sitting Time: Analysis of 54 Countries Worldwide. *American Journal of Preventive Medicine*, 51 (2016): 2, pp. 253-263.

Shankle, W. R. and D. G. Amen. *Preventing Alzheimer's: Ways to Help Prevent, Delay, Detect, and Even Halt Alzheimer's Disease and Other Forms of Memory Loss.* New York: G. P. Putnam's Sons, 2004.

Spiegel, K., R. Leproult, and E. Van Cauter. Impact of sleep debt on metabolic and endocrine function. *Lancet* 354, no. 9188 (1999): 1425–9.

Spiegel, K., J. F. Sheridan, and E. Van Cauter. Effect of sleep deprivation on response to immunization. *JAMA* 288 (2002): 1471–2.

Stamatakis, E., M. Hamer, and D.W. Dunstan. Screen-based entertainment time, all-cause mortality, and cardiovascular events: population-based study with ongoing mortality and hospital events follow-up. *Journal of the American College of Cardiology*, 2011: 292-299.

Taheri, S., L. Lin, D. Austin, et al. Short sleep duration is associated with reduced leptin, elevated ghrelin, and increased body mass index. *PLoS Med* 1, no. 3 (December 2004): e62.

The $11 Trillion Reward. Union of Concerned Scientists. https://www.ucsusa.org/sites/default/files/legacy/assets/documents/food_and_agriculture/11-trillion-reward.pdf

The World Health Report 2002: Reducing Risks, Promoting Healthy Life. Geneva: World Health Organization. 2002.

Chapter 7: Keep Your Heart in Shape

Addison, *Can Med Assoc J, 18: 281–285, 1928, cited in Modern Nutrition in Health and Disease*, vol 2, 8th ed. Shils, Olson, Shike, eds. Philadelphia, PA: Lea & Febiger, 1994, p 1290.

Houston, et al. *What Your Doctor May Not Tell You About Hypertension.* New York: Warner Books, 2004.

Kalea, A., F. Lamari, A. Theocharis, et al. Wild blueberry (*Vaccinium angustifolium*) consumption affects the composition and structure of glycosaminoglycans in Sprague-Dawley rat aorta. *J. Nutritional Biochemistry* 17, no. 2 (Feb 17, 2006): 109–116.

Krikorian, R., M. Shidler, T. Nash, et al. Blueberry supplementation improves memory in older adults. *J Agric Food Chem*, 2010 58 (7), 3996-4000 DOI: 10.1021/jf9029332.

Kuriyama, S., T Shimazu, K. Ohmori, et al. Green tea consumption and mortality due to cardiovascular disease, cancer, and all causes in Japan: The Ohsaki Study. *JAMA* 296, no. 10 (Sep. 13, 2006): 1255–65.

"Leading Causes of Death," Centers for Disease Control and Prevention, 2005.

Lyon, Chris. "Blueberries: Colorful Protection for a Healthier Heart, Sharper Brain, and Cancer Defense." *Life Extension Magazine.* Feb 2009.

Medicinal Food, Spring 2005; 8(1):8–13.

Sinatra, S. *Reverse Heart Disease Now.* Hoboken, NJ: Wiley and Sons, 2007.

"Top 10 Causes of Death," WHO (World Health Organization), 2005.

Chapter 8: How to Keep Your Brain Sharp

Ames, B. N. and J. Liu. Delaying the mitochondrial decay of aging with acety-l-carnitine. *Ann N Y Acad Sci* 1033 (2004): 108–116.

Ammon, H. P., H. Safayhi, T. Mack, et al. Mechanism of anti-inflammatory actions of curcumine and boswellic acids. *J Ethnopharmacol* 38, no. 2-3 (1993): 113–119.

Balestreri, R., L. Fontana, and F. Astengo. A double-blind placebo controlled evaluation of the safety and efficacy of vinpocetine in the treatment of patients with chronic vascular senile cerebral dysfunction. *J Am Geriatr Soc* 35, no. 5 (May 1987): 425–430.

Bone, Kerry. "Amazing New Uses for an Old Herbal Standby." *Nutrition and Healing.* November 2008. www.wrightnewsletter.com.

Carmel, R. Megaloblastic anemias. *Current Opinion in Hematology* 1 (1994): 107–12.

Chandra, V., R. Pandav, H. H. Dodge, et al. Incidence of Alzheimer's disease in a rural community in India: The Indo-U.S. study. *Neurology* 57, no. 6 (2001): 985–989.

Colcombe, S. J., K. I. Erickson, P. E. Scalf, et al. Aerobic exercise training increases brain volume in aging humans. *J Gerontol A Biol Sci Med Sci* 61, (2006): 1166–1170.

de Quervain, D. J., B. Roozendaal, R. M. Nitsch, et al. Acute cortisone administration impairs retrieval of long-term declarative memory in humans. *Nature Neuroscience* 3 (2000): 313-314.

"Dietary Supplement Fact Sheet: Vitamin B12," Office of Dietary Supplements, National Institutes of Health, https://ods.od.nih.gov/factsheets/Vitaminb12-HealthProfessional/.

Esch, T., G. B. Stefano, G. L. Fricchione, et al. The role of stress in neurodegenerative diseases and mental disorders. *Neuoro Endocrinology Letters* 23, no. 3 (June 2002): 199–208.

Greendale, G., D. Kritz-Silverstein, T. Seeman, et al. Higher basal cortisol predicts verbal memory loss in postmenopausal women: Rancho Bernardo Study. *Journal of the American Geriatrics Society* 48 (2000): 1655–1658.

"Healthy glucose levels the key to a healthy ageing brain." Australian National University. 2017. https://medicalxpress.com/news/2017-08-healthy-glucose-key-ageing-brain.html.

The Hospital for Sick Children, press release. "Canadian kids don't get enough vitamin D." May 4, 2009.

Kedar, N. P. Can we prevent Parkinson's and Alzheimer's disease? *Journal of Postgraduate Medicine* 49, no. 3 (July–September 2003): 236–245.

Lupien, S., M. de Leon, S. de Santi, et al. Cortisol levels during human aging predict hippocampal atrophy and memory deficits. *Nature Neuroscience* May 1998.

"Mayo Clinic research shows that improving brain processing speed helps memory," *Life Extension Daily,* Feb. 11, 2009.

"Omega-3 fatty acids," University of Maryland Medical Center. https://www.umms.org/ummc/patients-visitors/health-library/medical-encyclopedia/images/omega3-fatty-acids.

Ono, K., K. Hasegawa, H. Naiki, et al. Curcumin has potent anti-amyloidogenic effects for Alzheimer's beta-amyloid fibrils in vitro. *J Neurosci Res* 75 (2004): 742–50.

Perlmutter, David, and Carol Colman. *The Better Brain Book.* New York: Berkley Publishing Group, 2004.

"Salk study links diabetes and Alzheimer's disease," Salk Institute. May 15, 2008. https://www.salk.edu/news-release/salk-study-links-diabetes-and-alzheimers-disease/.

Scarmeas, N., Y. Stern, R. Mayeux, et al. Mediterranean diet and mild cognitive impairment. *Arch Neurol* 66, no. 2 (2009): 216–225.

Shukla, P. K., V. Khanna, M. Khan, et al. Protective effect of curcumin against lead neurotoxicity in rats. *Human & Experimental Toxicology* 22 (2003): 653–58.

"Vitamin D and your Health: Deficiency," Vitamin D Council, www.vitamindcouncil.org/health/deficiency/am-i-vitamin-d-deficient.shtml.

Walsh, E.I., M. Shaw, P. Sachdev, K.J. Anstety, and N. Cherbuin. Brain atrophy in ageing: Estimating effects of blood glucose levels vs. other type 2 diabetes effects. *Diabetes & Metabolism* 44, no. 1 (Feb. 2018): 80-83

Witte, A.V., M. Fobker, R. Gellner, et al. Caloric restriction improves memory in elderly humans. *Proc Natl Acad Sci USA* 106, no. 4 (Jan. 27, 2009): 1255-60.

Xu, W., C. Qiu, B. Winblad, et al. The effect of borderline diabetes on the risk of dementia and Alzheimer's disease. *Diabetes* 56 (2007): 211–216.

Yang, F., G. P. Lim, A. N. Begum, et al. Curcumin inhibits formation of amyloid {beta}oligomers and fibrils, binds plaques, and reduces amyloid in vivo. *J Biol Chem* 280 (2005): 5892–5901.

Chapter 9: How to Protect and Maintain Strong Bones, Muscles, and Joints

"Baseball's Money Business on the Upswing." *USA Today.* Nov. 11, 2006.

Centers for Disease Control and Prevention. National and state medical expenditures and lost earnings attributable to arthritis and other rheumatoid conditions—United States, 2003. *Morbidity and Mortality Weekly Report* 56, no.01 (2007): 4–7.

Coates, Paul, ed. *Encyclopedia of Dietary Supplements.* New York: National Institute of Health, Marcel Dekker, 2005.

"Cox-2 Inhibitors," MedicineNet.com. www.medicinenet.com/cox-2_inhibitors/article.htm.

"D-bunking the role of vitamin d in bone health," American Medical Women's Association, www.amwa-doc.org/index.cfm?objectid=97141F72-D567-0B25-5E6E71C12C78F497.

Felson, D., Y. Zhang, J. M. Anthony, et al. Weight loss reduces the risk for symptomatic knee osteoarthritis in women. The Framingham Study. *Ann Intern Med* 116 (1992): 535–539.

Green, C.J., K. Bassett, V. Foerster, et al. Bone mineral density testing: Does the evidence support its selective use in well women? British Columbia Office of Health Technology Assessment, Sep. 1998, *www.chspr.ubc.ca.*

Janssen, I., D. S. Shephard, P. T. Katzmarzyk, et al. The healthcare costs of sarcopenia in the United States. *J Am Geriatr Soc* 52, no. 1 (2004): 80–85.

Maetzel A., L. C. Li, J. Pencharz, et al. The economic burden associated with osteoarthritis, rheumatoid arthritis, and hypertension: A comparative study. *Ann Rheum Dis* 63, no. 4 (2004): 395–401.

McAlindon, T., M. LaValley, J. Gulin, et al. Glucosamine and chondroitin for treatment of osteoarthritis: A systematic quality assessment and meta-analysis. *JAMA* 283, no. 11 (2000): 1469–1475.

Messier, S., D. J. Gutekunst, C. Davis, et al. Weight loss reduces knee-joint loads in overweight and obese older adults with knee osteoarthritis. *Arthritis & Rheum* 52, no. 7 (July 2005): 2026-32.

"Orthopaedic Surgery: Hip Fracture," University of Virginia Health System, www.healthsystem.virginia.edu/uvahealth/adult_orthopaedics/hipfract.cfm.

Pavelká, K., J. Gatterová, M. Olejarová, et al. Glucosamine sulfate use and delay of progression of knee osteoarthritis: A three-year, randomized, placebo-controlled, double-blind study. *Arch Intern Med* 162, no. 18 (2002): 2113–2123.

Reginster, J. Y., R. Deroisy, L. C. Rovati, et al. Long-term effects of glucosamine sulfate on osteoarthritis progression: A randomised, placebo-controlled clinical trial. *Lancet* 357, no. 9252 (2001): 251–256.

Stenlake, Richard. "How Do Glucosamine and Chondroitin Work." The Arthritis & Glucosamine Information Center.

Chapter 10: Boost Your Immune System

Bogden, J. D., A. Bendich, F. W. Kemp, et al. Daily micronutrient supplements enhance delayed-hypersensitivity skin test responses in older people. *Am J Clin Nutr* 60 (1994): 437–447.

Burns, E. "Aging and the Immune System," Healthlink.

Chandra, R. K. Nutrition, immunity and outcome: Past, present and future. 11th Gopalan Gold Medal Oration. *Nutr Res* 8 (1988): 225–237.

David Servan-Schreiber, *Anticancer: A New Way of Life*. New York: Viking Penguin, 2008.

"Diet, Exercise, Stress and the Immune System." Cleveland Clinic website, accessed March 15, 2009.

Foote, J., A. Giuliano, and R. Harris. Older adults need guidance to meet nutritional recommendations. *J Am Coll Nutr* 19 (2000): 628–640.

Giammanco, M., E. Tripoli, G. Tabacchi, et al. The phenolic compounds of olive oil: structure, biological activity and beneficial effects on human health. *Nutrition Research Reviews* 18, no. 1 (June 2005): 98–112.

Haaland, D. A., T. F. Sabljic, D. A. Baribeau, et al. Is regular exercise a friend or foe of the aging immune system? A systematic review. Clin J Sport Med 18, no. 6 (Nov 2008): 539–548.

Head, J. F., F. Wang, R. L. Elliott, et al. *Ann N Y Acad Sci* 690 (1993): 340–342.

Institute of Medicine, P.O.M. *Dietary Reference Intakes*. Washington, DC: National Academy Press, 2006.

Isolauri, E., Y. Sütas, P. Kankaanpää, et al. Probiotics: Effects on immunity. *Am J Clin Nutrition* 73, no. 2 (Feb 2001): 444S–450S.

Levy, S. M., R. B. Herberman, M. Lippman, et al. Immunological and psychosocial predictors of disease recurrence in patients with early-stage breast cancer. *Behav Med* 17, no 2 (1991): 67–75.

Life Extension Foundation Interview with Simin Meydani. "Vitamin E: Revitalizing Your Immune System." *Life Extension Magazine*. February 1999.

Meydani, S. N., M. Meydani, J. B. Blumberg, et al. Vitamin E supplementation and in vivo immune response in healthy elderly subjects: A randomized controlled trial. *JAMA* 277 (May 7, 1997): 1380–1386.

Rountree, Robert, and Carol Colman. *Immunotics*. New York: G T Putnam's Sons, 2000.

Sano, J., S. Inami, K. Seimiya, et al. Effects of green tea intake on the development of coronary artery disease. *Circ J* 68, no. 7 (Jul 2004): 665–70.

Segerstrom, S., S. Taylor, M. Kemeny, et al. Optimism is associated with mood, coping, and immune change in response to stress. *J of Personality and Soc Psychology* 74, no. 6 (June 1998): 1646–1655.

"Theraputic Benefits of Laughter," Holisticonline. www.holistic-online.com/Humor_Therapy/humor_therapy_benefits.htm.

Wachi, M., M. Koyama, M. Utsuyama, et al. Recreational music-making modulates natural killer cell activity, cytokines, and mood states in corporate employees. *Med Sci Monit* 13, no. 2 (Feb 2007): CR57–70.

Wintergerst, E. S., S. Maggini, and D. H. Hornig. Contribution of selected vitamins and trace elements to immune function. *Ann Nutr Metab* 51 (2007): 303–23.

Yan, Y. S. Effect of Chinese tea extract on the immune function of mice bearing tumor and their antitumor activity. *Zhonghua Yu Fang Yi Xue Za Zhi* 26, no. 1 (Jan 1, 1992): 5–7.

Chapter 11: What You Should Know about Hormones

Allen, B.G., S.K. Bhatia, C.M. Anderson, et al. Ketogenic diets as an adjuvant cancer therapy: History and potential mechanism. *Redox Biol.* 2014; 2: 963–970.

Araujo, Andre B. et al. Clinical Review: Endogenous Testosterone and Mortality in Men: A Systematic Review and Meta-Analysis. *The Journal of Clinical Endocrinology and Metabolism* 96.10 (2011): 3007–3019.

Arlt, W., F. Callies, J. van Vlijmen, et al. Dehydroepiandrosterone replacement in women with adrenal insufficiency. *NEJM* 341, no. 14 (1999): 1013–1020.

Barrett-Connor, E., and D. Goodman-Gruen. The epidemiology of DHEA-S and cardiovascular disease. *Ann NY Acad Si* 774 (1995): 259–270.

Baulieu, E. E., G. Thomas, S. Legrain, et al. Dehydroepiandrosterone (DHEA), DHEA sulfate, and aging: contribution of the DHEAge Study to a sociobiomedical issue. *Proc Natl Acad Sci U S A* 97, no. 8 (2000): 4279-4284.

Berr, Claudine Berr et al. Relationships of dehydroepiandrosterone sulfate in the elderly with functional, psychological, and mental status, and short-term mortality: A French community-based study. *Proceedings of the National Academy of Sciences of the United States of America* Nov 1996, 93 (23) 13410-13415; DOI: 10.1073/pnas.93.23.13410

Bland, Jeffrey S., and David S. Jones, "Clinical Approaches to Hormonal and Neuroendocrine Imbalances." *Textbook of Functional Medicine*, Institute for Functional Medicine, 2005.

"Body clock regulates metabolism, finds UCI study," NewsRx.com, March 26, 2009, www.lef.org/news/LefDailyNews.htm?NewsID=8058&Section=Aging.

Bunevicius, R., G. Kažanavičius, R. Žalinkevičius, et al. Effects of thyroxine as compared with thyroxine plus triiodothyronine in patients with hypothyroidism. *NEJM* 340, no. 6 (February 11, 1999): 424-429.

Cagnacci, A., M. Cannoletta, A. Renzi, et al. Prolonged melatonin administration decreases nocturnal blood pressure in women. *Am J Hypertens* 18, no. 12 (December 2005): 1614-1618.

Canonico, M., E. Oger, G. Plu-Bureau, et al. Estrogen and Thromboembolism Risk (ESTHER) Study Group. Hormone therapy and venous thromboembolism among postmenopausal women: impact of the route of estrogen administration and progestogens: the ESTHER study. *Circulation* 115 (2007): 840–845.

Edwards, Kim. "Older Men May Not Live As Long If They Have Low Testosterone." June 5, 2007. http://ucsdnews.ucsd.edu/archive/newsrel/health/06-07LowTestosteroneKE-.asp.

Escobar-Morreale, H. F., M. J. Obregón, F. Escobar del Rey, et al. *J Clinical Invest* 96, no. 6 (Dec 1995): 2828–38.

Gnagnarella, P., S. Gandini, C. La Vecchia, et al. Glycemic index, glycemic load and cancer risk: A meta-analysis. *Am J Clin Nutr* 87, no. 6 (June 2008): 1793–1801.

Greendale, G. A., S. Edelstein, and E. Barrett-Connor. Endogenous sex steroids and bone mineral density in older women and men: The Rancho Bernado Study. *J Bone Miner Res* 12, no. 11 (1997): 1833–1843.

Greenspan, F.S., et al. "Chapter 7: The Thyroid Gland," *Basic and Clinical Endocrinology*, 5th edition. New York: Appleton and Lange; 1997.

Harding, Anne. "Men's testosterone levels declined in last 20 years." January 19, 2007. https://uk.reuters.com/article/health-testosterone-levels-dc-idUKKIM16976320061101.

Hunt, P. J., E. M. Gurnell, F. A. Huppert, et al. Improvement in mood and fatigue after DHEA replacement in Addison's disease in a randomized double-blind trial. *J Clin Endocrinol Metab* 85, no. 12 (2000): 4650–4656.

Institute for Functional Medicine, *Textbook of Functional Medicine*, 2005.

Korenchevsky, V. *Physiological and Pathological Aging*. Basel, Switzerland: S. Karger, 1961.

Maggio, Marcello et al. "Relationship Between Low Levels of Anabolic Hormones and 6-Year Mortality in Older Men: The Aging in the Chianti Area (InCHIANTI) Study." *Archives of Internal Medicine* 167.20 (2007): 2249–2254.

Marigliano, V., C. Bauco, F. Campana, et al. Normal values in extreme old age. *Ann N Y Acad Sci* 673 (December 6, 1992): 23–28.

Mariotti, S., P. Sansoni, G. Barbesino, et al. Thyroid and other organ-specific autoantibodies in healthy centenarians. *Lancet* 339 (1992): 1506–8.

Michigan Medicine–University of Michigan. "Low total testosterone in men widespread, linked to chronic disease." *ScienceDaily*. April 19, 2018.

Morales, A. J., J. J. Nolan, J. C. Nelson, et al. Effects of replacement dose of dehydroepiandrosterone (DHEA) in men and women of advancing age. *J Clin Endocrinol Metab* 78, no. 6 (1994): 1360–1367.

Morales, A. J., R. H. Haubrich, J. Y. Hwang, et al. The effect of six months treatment with a 100 mg daily dose of DHEA on circulating sex steroids, body composition and muscle strength in age-advanced men and women. *Clin Endocrinol (Oxf)* 49, no. 4 (1998): 421-433.

Nakahata, Y., S. Sahar, G. Astarita, et al. Circadian control of the NAD+ salvage pathway by CLOCK-SIRT1. *Science* 324, no. 5927 (March 12, 2009): 654-657.

Pizzorno, Lara, and William Ferril. "Thyroid." *Textbook of Functional Medicine*, edited by David S. Jones. Gig Harbor, WA: Institute for Functional Medicine, 2005.

Poff, A.M., C. Ari, P. Arnold, T.N. Seyfried, and D.P. D'Agostino. Ketone supplementation decreases tumor cell viability and prolongs survival of mice with metastatic cancer. *Int J Cancer*. 2014 Oct 1; 135(7): 1711–1720.

Roth, George S., et al. Biomarkers of Caloric Restriction May Predict Longevity in Humans. *Science* 02 Aug 2002 : 811.

Trivedi, D.P., and K.T. Khaw. DHEA-S and mortality in elderly men and women. *J Clin Endocrinol Metab* 86, no. 9 (2001): 4171–4177.

Vann, Madeline. "1 in 4 Men Over 30 Has Low Testosterone." September 13, 2007. https://abcnews.go.com/Health/Healthday/story?id=4508669&page=1.

CHAPTER 12: What Do I Do Next?

Bushak, Lecia. Benefits of Ecotherapy: Being in Nature Fights Depression, Improves Mental Health and Well-Being. October 26, 2013. https://www.medicaldaily.com/benefits-ecotherapy-being-nature-fights-depression-improves-mental-health-and-well-being-261075.

Emmons, Robert A. *The Little Book of Gratitude: Create a life of happiness and wellbeing by giving thanks*. London, England: Gaia, 2016.

"Probiotics: Five Core Specifics." drperlmutter.com. https://www.drperlmutter.com/learn/resources/probiotics-five-core-species.

SECTION III: THE SECRETS OF EMOTIONAL INTELLIGENCE: UNDERRATED AND IGNORED— UNTIL NOW

AM SURV: House, James. Americans' Changing Lives: Waves I, II, III, and IV, 1986, 1989, 1994, and 2002. Inter-University Consortium for Political and Social Research (2008).

Berkman, L.F., and S.L. Syme. Social networks, host resistance and mortality: A nine-year follow-up study of Alameda county residents. *Am Journal of Epidemiology* 109, no. 2: 186-204.

Buettner, Dan. *The Blue Zones*. Washington, DC: National Geographic, 2008.

Ertel, K. A., M. M. Glymour, and L. F. Berkman. Effects of social integration on preserving memory function in a nationally representative US elderly population. *Am J Public Health* 98, no.7 (2008): 1215-20.

Harrington, Ann. *The Cure Within*. New York: W.W. Norton, 2008.

Kochilas, Diane. "Ikarian Diet a Key to Health and Longevity," Anderson Cooper 360°. ac360.blogs.cnn.

Langer, E. and Rodin, J. The effects of choice and enhanced personal responsibility for the aged: A field experiment in an institutional setting. *J Pers Soc Psychol* 34, no. 2 (1976): 191-198.

Rowe, John and Robert Kahn. *Successful Aging*. New York: Dell Publishing, 1998.

Snowdon, David. *Aging with Grace: What the Nun Study Teaches Us about Leading Longer, Healthier and More Meaningful Lives*. New York: Bantam, 2001.

"Volunteering Produces Health Benefits," press release, AmeriCorps / Corporation for National and Community Service, www.americorps.gov/about/newsroom/releases_detail.asp?tbl_pr_id=687 .

Wolf, Stewart and John Bruhn. *The Power of Clan*. New Brunswick, NJ: Transaction Publishers, 1992.

Conclusion: A Plan for You: The 7 x 3 Matrix of Healthy Aging

Akbaraly, T. N., I. Hininger-Favier, I. Carrière, et al. Plasma selenium over time and cognitive decline in the elderly. Epidemiology 18, no. 1 (Jan. 2007): 52-58.

Akbaraly, T. N., J. Arnaud, I. Hininger-Favier, et al. Selenium and mortality in the elderly: Results from the EVA Study. *Clinical Chemistry* 51 (2005): 2117-2123.

Alexopoulos, N., C. Vlachopoulos, K. Aznaouridis, et al. The acute effect of green tea consumption on endothelial function in healthy individuals. *Eur J Cardiovasc Prev Rehabil* 15 (2008): 300-305.

Bazzano, L. A., J. He, L. G. Ogden, et al. Legume consumption and risk of coronary heart disease in US men and women. *Arch Intern Med* 161 (Nov. 26, 2001): 2573-2578.

Blumenthal, J. A., M. A. Babyak, K. A. Moore, et al. Effects of exercise training on older patients with major depression. *Arch Intern Med* 159 (1999): 2349-2356.

Clark, L. C., G. F. Combs Jr., B. W. Turnbull, et al. Effects of selenium supplementation for cancer prevention in patients with carcinoma of the skin: A randomized controlled trial. *JAMA* 276 (Dec. 25, 1996): 1957-1963.

Coates, Paul, ed. *Encyclopedia of Dietary Supplements*. New York: Marcel Dekker, 2005.

Colcombe, S. J., K. I. Erickson, P. E. Scalf, et al. Aerobic exercise training increases brain volume in aging humans. *J Gerontol A Biol Sci Med Sci* 61 (2006): 1166-1170.

Davis, D. Declining fruit and vegetable nutrient composition: What is the evidence? *J HortScience* 44 (2009): 15-19.

Ehrnhoefer, D. E., J. Bieschke, A. Boeddrich, et al. EGCG redirects amyloidogenic polypeptides into unstructured, off-pathway oligomers. *Nature Structural and Molecular Biology* 15 (May 30, 2008): 558-566.

Ferrie, J. E., M. J. Shipley, F. P. Cappuccio, et al. A prospective study of change in sleep duration: Associations with mortality in the Whitehall II cohort. *Sleep* 30, no. 12 (2007): 1659-66.

Galpern, W. R., and M. E. Cudkowicz. Coenzyme Q10 treatment of neurodegenerative disease of aging. *Mitochondrion* 7, supp.1 (2007): S146-153.

Gao, Y. T., J. K. McLaughlin, W. J. Blot, et al. Reduced risk of esophageal cancer associated with green tea consumption. *J Natl Cancer Inst* 86, no. 11 (June 1,1994): 855-858.

Ginde, A.A., J. M. Mansbach, and C. A. Camargo. Association between serum 25-hydroxyvitamin d level and upper respiratory tract infection in the third National Health and Nutrition Examination Survey. *Arch Intern Med* 169, no. 4 (Feb. 23, 2009): 384-90.

Giovannucci, E., Y. Liu, B. W. Hollis, et al. 25-hydroxyvitamin D and risk of myocardial infarction in men: a prospective study. *Arch Intern Med* 168, no. 11 (June 9, 2008): 1174-80.

"Greenland's Constant Summer Sunlight Linked to Summer Suicide Spike," Science Daily. May 10, 2009.

Heller, L. "Scientist concerned at plummeting nutrient levels," Food Navigator, foodnavigator-usa.com, 2006.

Hendler, Sheldon and David Rorvik. *Physicans' Desk Reference for Nutritional Supplements*, 2nd edition. Montvale, NJ: Physicians' Desk Reference, Inc., 2008.

Hirano, R., Y. Momiyama, R. Takahashi, et al. Comparison of green tea intake in Japanese patients with and without angiographic coronary artery disease. *Am J Cardiol* 90, no. 10 (2002): 1150-1153.

Hoffman, P. R. and M. J Berry. The influence of selenium on immune responses. *Mol Nutr Food Res* 52, no. 11 (Nov. 2008): 1273-80.

Houston, D. K., M. Cesari, L. Ferrucci, et al. Association between vitamin D status and physical performance: The InCHIANTI study. *J Gerontol A Biol Sci Med Sci* 62, no. 4 (April 2007): 440-446.

Hurwitz, B. E., J. R. Klaus, M. M. Llabre, et al. Suppression of human immunodeficiency virus type 1 viral load with selenium supplementation: A randomized controlled trial. *Arch Intern Med* 167, no. 2 (Jan. 22, 2007): 148-54.

Joshipura, K. J., F. B. Hu, J. E. Manson, et al. The effect of fruit and vegetable intake on risk for coronary heart disease. *Ann Int Med* 134 (2001): 1106-1114.

Kagawa, Y. Impact of Westernization on the nutrition of Japanese: Changes in physique, cancer, longevity and centenarians. *Preventive Medicine* 7, no. 2 (June, 1978): 205-17.

Kelly Jr., J. H. and J. Sabaté. Nuts and coronary heart disease: An epidemiological perspective. *Br J Nutr* 96, Suppl 2 (Nov. 2006): S61-7.

Knekt, P., M. Laaksonen, C. Mattila, et al. Serum vitamin D and subsequent occurrence of type 2 diabetes. *Epidemiology* 19, no. 5 (Sep. 2008): 666-71.

Lappe, J. M., D. Travers-Gustafson, K. M. Davies, et al. Vitamin D and calcium supplementation reduces cancer risk: results of a randomized trial. *Am J Clin Nutr* 85, no. 6 (Jun 2007): 1586-91.

Lawrence, Felicity. "Mineral Levels in Meat and Milk Plummet Over 60 Years," The Guardian, Feb 2, 2006.

Liu, S., J. E. Manson, I. M. Lee, et al. Fruit and vegetable intake and risk of cardiovascular disease: The Women's Health Study. *Am J Clini Nutri* 79 (2000): 922-928.

Llewellyn, D. J., K. M. Langa, and I. A. Lang. Serum 25-hydroxyvitamin D concentration and cognitive impairment. *J Geriatr Psychiatry Neurol* 22, no. 3 (Dec. 10, 2008): 188-95.

Melamed M. L., E. D. Michos, W. Post, et al. 25-hydroxyvitamin d levels and the risk of mortality in the general population. *Arch Intern Med* 168, no. 15 (Aug. 11, 2008): 1629-37.

Okinawa Centenarian Study data presented at the American Geriatrics Society annual meeting, 2001. Cited by H. McCord and G. McVeigh, "NutritionNews: 'Magic' Appetite Shutoff from the Orient," *Prevention*, January 2002, pages 52-3.

Paschka, A. G., R. Butler, and C. Y. Young. Induction of apoptosis in prostate cancer cell lines by the green tea component EGCG. *Cancer Letters* 130, no. 1-2 (Aug 14, 1998): 1-7.

Pereira, A. C., D. E. Huddleston, A. M. Brickman, et al. An in vivo correlate of exercise-induced neurogenesis in the adult dentate gyrus. *Proc Natl Acad Sci USA* 104, no. 13 (March 27, 2007): 5638–5643.

Reinberg, Steven. "Many Americans Fall Short on Their Vitamin D," GoodGuide. com, March 24, 2009.

Rozen, T. D., M. L. Oshinsky, C. A. Gebeline, et al. Open label trial of coenzyme Q10 as a migraine preventive. *Cephalalgia* 22 (2002): 137-41.

Sears, Barry. *Omega Rx Zone: The Miracle of the New High-Dose Fish Oil*. New York: HarperCollins, 2005.

Shrubsole, M. J, W. Lu, Z. Chen, et al. Drinking green tea modestly reduces breast cancer risk. *J Nutr* 139, no. 2 (Feb 2009): 310-316.

Simopoulos, Artemis and Jo Robinson. *The Omega Diet: The Lifesaving Nutritional Program Based on the Diet of the Island of Crete*. New York: Harper Paperbacks, 1999.

Snowdon, David. *Aging with Grace: What the Nun Study Teaches Us About Leading Longer, Healthier, and More Meaningful Lives*. New York: Bantam Books, 2001.

Stoll, Andrew. *The Omega-3 Connection*. New York: Simon & Schuster, 2001.

Strandhagen, E., P-O Hansson, I. Bosaeus, et al. High fruit intake may reduce mortality among middle-aged and elderly men. *Eur J Clin Nutrition* 54 (2000): 337-341.

Templeton, David. "Penn State Study: Selenium Slows AIDS Progression," Pittsburg Post Gazette, December 1, 2008.

Tribole, Evelyn. *The Ultimate Omega-3 Diet*. New York: McGraw-Hill, 2007.

Varga, Z. Omega-3 Polyunsaturated fatty acids in the prevention of atherosclerosis. *Orv Hetil* 149, no. 14 (Apr. 6, 2008): 627-37.

Villegas, R., Y. T. Gao, G. Yang, et al. Legume and soy food intake and the incidence of type 2 diabetes in the Shanghai Women's Health Study. *Am J Clin Nutr* 87, no. 1 (January 2008): 162-167.

Acknowledgments

As every author on the planet knows, a book is a collaborative effort. This one might have my name on it but it wouldn't have been possible if a veritable army of very, very smart people had not been willing to take time out of their busy days to answer my questions and generously share their significant intellectual firepower.

To wit: Daniel Amen, M.D.; Suzanne Bennett, D.C.; Ann Knight, D.C.; Mark Houston, M.D.; Dave Leonardi, M.D.; Barry Sears, Ph.D.; and Beth Traylor, M.D. Special thanks are due to Larry McCleary, M.D., who generously read and critiqued the chapter on the brain; Keith McCormick, D.C., who did the same for the section on osteoporosis; and Dan Buettner, whose outstanding work, *The Blue Zones*, inspired much of section III on emotional intelligence. A special thanks goes to Sue Copp, M.S., whose help, always generously available for the asking, is so greatly appreciated.

And then there's that amazing team at Fair Winds Press, my much appreciated publisher, that somehow miraculously transforms my plain old boring Word docs into gorgeous books like this one. This book went through two revisions with two different teams. To all the wonderful people from both Team One and Team Two: a huge hug of appreciation for Ken Fund, Will Kiester, Jill Alexander, Tiffany Hill, Karen Levy, Jenna Patton, and Jess Haberman.

And, of course, my indefatigable and super-talented editors, Cara Connors on the first edition and Meredith Quinn on the second.

A great agent does a lot more than just broker a deal. She nurtures, she cajoles, she suggests book ideas and then helps flesh them out, she "pre-edits," she wrangles, she plays good cop (or bad cop), she's fiercely protective, and she's ultimately the best friend an author can have in the world of publishing. My agent, Coleen O'Shea, of the Allen O'Shea Literary Agency, does all that and more. She is, quite simply, the most perfect agent on the planet. Thank you.

But wait, there's more.

My writing hero, William Goldman, who could no more write a boring word than Aaron Copland could write a bad piece of music or Miles Davis could take a bad solo. The late Ed McBain (Evan Hunter) has been a source of infinite delight to me for decades. (Short, pithy, engaging sentences work in detective novels as well as in nutrition textbooks.) And then, of course, there's the greatest science writer in America, Robert Sapolsky, who proves that humor, style, accessibility, and scholarship can coexist in the same package. I may not always achieve that goal, but the fact that Sapolsky does it every single time he sets pen to paper gives me faith that it is in fact attainable on the Planet Earth.

Professor Ernest van den Haag of the New School for Social Research was instrumental in teaching me how to think, always a good thing if you're planning on writing, teaching, and speaking. I never thanked him, but I'm doing it now.

Allen Stone; Laura Nyro; Miles Davis; Earth, Wind & Fire—the movie's not the same without the soundtrack.

Werner Erhard, wherever you are, my greatest wish is for you to know how much you mean to me and how deeply and profoundly you have altered my life.

Thanks to Howard, Robin, Fred, Gary, and Artie for staying on the air on September 11, 2001. I will never forget that as long as I live.

My family: my dear brother Jeffrey Bowden, my sister-in-law Nancy Fiedler, and my niece and nephew Cadence Bowden and Pace Bowden. I love you all. Even you, Pace.

And then, finally, my "chosen" family, who have sustained and nourished me, some of them for more than thirty years: Anja Christy, without whom I would have not written this book, Peter Breger, Scott Ellis, Christopher Crabb, Susan Wood, Christopher Duncan, Sky London, Doug Monas, Liz Neporent, Lauree Dash, Oliver Beaucamp, Jeannette Lee Bessinger, Kevin Hogan, Billy Stritch. I love you all, and you are with me even if we don't talk for years. (I'm talking to *you*, Scott Ellis).

To paraphrase Peggy Noonan, "Without them, there is no him."

And, finally, Michelle.

You've changed my life in ways I never even knew were possible.

Thank you.

—Jonny

About the Authors

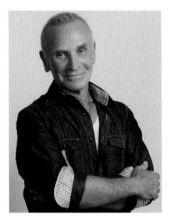

Jonny Bowden, Ph.D., C.N.S., also known as "The Nutrition Myth Buster"™ is a nationally known board-certified nutritionist and expert on diet and weight loss. His no-nonsense, myth-busting approach has made him a popular guest on television, where he has been interviewed over 100 times (including appearances on the *Dr. Oz Show*, Fox News, CNN, MSNBC, ABC, NBC, and CBS. Dr. Jonny has written (or has been quoted in) articles in *The New York Times*, *Forbes*, *The Daily Beast*, *The Huffington Post*, *Vanity Fair Online*, *Men's Heath*, *O* (The Oprah Magazine), *People*, *Prevention*, and dozens of other print and online publications.

Dr. Jonny is the best-selling author of 15 books, including *The 150 Healthiest Foods on Earth*, *Living Low Carb* (now in it's fourth edition), and the controversial number-one Amazon best-seller, *The Great Cholesterol Myth* (co-authored with cardiologist Stephen Sinatra, M.D.). A popular speaker, Dr. Jonny has spoken at academic and consumer events ranging from the American Academy of Anti-Aging Medicine to Beijing University in China, to the WOW Summit—A National Conference on Parenting. In 2012, Dr. Bowden was elected to honorary membership in the DeTao Masters Academy, an international group of 125 thought leaders headquartered in Shanghai.

Dr. Jonny is a columnist for *Clean Eating Magazine*, *Better Nutrition*, *Amazing Wellness*, and *Whole Foods Magazine* and has served on the scientific advisory board for multiple companies in the natural products industry. He is also a consultant for Cenegenics Medical Institute.

In September 2017, Fair Winds Press published the updated and revised 10th anniversary edition of Dr. Jonny's classic best-seller *The 150 Healthiest Foods on Earth*, which has sold over half a million copies and has been translated into four languages.

www.jonnybowden.com
Twitter: @jonnybowden
Facebook: @Dr.JonnyBowdenPhDCNS

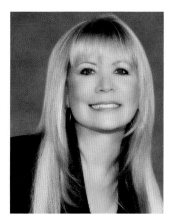

Beth Traylor, M.D. is a Fellow of the American Academy of Family Physicians and a Diplomate of the American Board of Family Medicine. She earned her certification in age management medicine in 2002 and has practiced with the internationally renowned Cenegenics Elite Health Group as a senior partner since that time.

Dr. Traylor has served as the president of the Board of the Cenegenics Education and Research Foundation, whose mission is to train doctors from across the globe on how to apply the science of age management medicine and support research in the field.

Index

S

Salmon. *See* Wild salmon

Salovey, Peter, 213–214

Sanson, Gillian, 133

Sapolsky, Robert, 160, 163–164

Sarcopenia, 131, 139

Sardines, 33, 52, 98, 117, 134, 200, 233, 239

Sardinia, 219

Sassone-Corsi, Paolo, 205

Saturated fats, 33, 34, 98, 119, 167

Saturday Evening Review, 162

Sauerkraut, 78, 238

Savasana, 110

School Sisters of Notre Dame, 237

Schwartz, Barry, 217

Scopolamine, 124

Sears, Barry, 45, 46, 48

Seasonal affective disorder (SAD), 240

Sea vegetables, 200

The Second Brain (Gershon), 77

Sedentary behavior, 88

Selenium, 39, 87, 170, 173, 194, 196, 235–236

Self-awareness, 224

Serotonin, 77, 160, 241

Servan-Schreiber, David, 163

7 x 3 Matrix of Health Aging, 229, 231–243

Sex hormones, 182–190

Sexual function and satisfaction, DHEA and, 202, 203

Shames, Richard, 193

Shape Up (Bowden), 224

Sharma, Hari, 29

Shiitake mushrooms, 103, 172

Shomon, Mary, 197

Short-term memory problems, 111

Shoulder exercises, 143

Silent (chronic) inflammation, 46

Sills, Steven, 227

Simopoulos, Artemis P., 48

Sinatra, Stephen, 24, 35, 104

Sinclair, David, 19, 68, 70, 238

SIRT genes, 68, 70, 238

Sirtuin genes, 15, 68, 70

Sitting and sitting breaks, 35, 88, 208

Skin, aging, 42

Sleep
  biological rhythms and, 89
  cortisol and, 35, 90
  energy and, 90
  epidemiological studies on impact of, 17
  heart disease prevention and, 35
  hormones and, 89–90
  impact of inadequate, 90
  in longevity journal, 247
  melatonin and, 204–205
  overview, 89–90
  recommendations, 89, 209
  7 x 3 Matrix of Healthy Aging recommendations, 241–242
  three tips for better, 90

Smith, Glenn, 114

Smoking, 104, 135. *See also* Tobacco

SNACC detox program, 84–85

Snowdon, David, 222, 237

Social connections and relationships. *See also* Emotional intelligence
  absence of choice and, 216–217
  emotional intelligence and, 91, 213
  epidemiological studies on impact of, 17
  examples of societies with longevity and, 217–220
  face-to-face connection, 245
  health/medical outcomes and, 220, 222–223
  heart disease risk prevention and, 36
  Ikarian culture, 217–218
  importance of, 21, 74, 91
  in Okinawa, Japan, 218–219
  recommendations for, 20
  7 x 3 Matrix of Healthy Aging recommendations, 242–243
  stress and, 63

Social intelligence, 213. *See also* Emotional intelligence

Soda, 136

Sodium, 103, 178

Soy formula, 199

Soy oil, 33

Soy sauce, 78, 199

Soy, thyroid function and, 198–199

SPECT scans, 125

Spices. *See also* specific names of spices
  anti-inflammatory, 51
  antioxidant and anti-inflammatory-rich, 37, 39

Spinach, 51, 103

Squats, 141

Standing squat, 153

Statin drugs, 47

Stenlake, Richard, 138

Steroid hormones, 183, 201

Steroids, 29, 30, 164

Strawberries, 30, 37

Strength training, 140–144, 208, 240

Stress, 61–65
  autoimmune disease and, 195
  brain health and, 63, 90, 111
  deep breathing and, 64
  immunity and, 163–165
  impact of, 90–91
  longevity journal on reducing, 247
  overview, 61–63
  sympathetic nervous system, 64

Stress hormones, 200–203

Stretching exercises, 144–155

Strokes, 81, 167, 187

Sugar. *See also* Glycation
  eliminating from your diet, 179
  gut health and, 78
  increase in consumption of, 85–86
  sugar-insulin connection, 113, 115, 116

Suicide, 241

Sulfides/thiols, 38

Sulforaphane, 38, 86, 208

Sulfuraphane, 99

SunFiber, 79, 80, 81

Sun phobia, 128

Sunshine, 208, 240–241

Superoxide dismutase (SOD), 36

Supplements
  antioxidents, 27
  for bone health, 135–136
  for brain health, 121–129
  carnosine, 59
  fiber, 79, 80, 81
  fish oil, 35, 45, 52
  for heart disease (B vitamins), 102
  heart disease prevention and, 36
  for heart protection, 102, 103–105

Best-selling books by acclaimed nutritionist Jonny Bowden, Ph.D., C.N.S.

SELF CARE

The Most Effective Ways on Earth to
Boost Your Energy
*The Surprising, Unbiased Truth about Using Nutrition,
Exercise, Supplements, Stress Relief, and Personal Empowerment
to Stay Energized All Day*
978-1-59233-468-1

The Great Cholesterol Myth
*Why Lowering Your Cholesterol Won't Prevent Heart Disease—
and the Statin-Free Plan That Will
*Now Includes 100 Recipes for Preventing and Reversing
Heart Disease*
978-1-59233-712-5

The Most Effective Natural Cures on Earth
*The Surprising, Unbiased Truth about What Treatments
Work and Why*
978-1-59233-291-5

FOOD FACTS

The 150 Healthiest Foods on Earth, revised edition
*The Surprising, Unbiased Truth about What You Should
Eat and Why*
978-1-59233-764-4

The Healthiest Meals on Earth
*The Surprising, Unbiased Truth about What Meals to Eat
and Why*
978-1-59233-470-4

RECIPES

150 Healthiest 15-Minute Recipes on Earth
*The Surprising, Unbiased Truth about How to Make the Most
Deliciously Nutritious Meals at Home in Just Minutes a Day*
978-1-59233-442-1

150 Healthiest Slow Cooker Recipes on Earth
*The Surprising, Unbiased Truth about How to Make Nutritious
and Delicious Meals That Are Ready When You Are*
978-1-59233-494-0

150 Healthiest Comfort Foods on Earth
*The Surprising, Unbiased Truth about How to Make Over
Your Diet and Lose Weight While Still Enjoying the Foods
You Love and Crave*
978-1-59233-482-7